Volume 7 in the Series

Major Problems in Neurology

JOHN N. WALTON, T.D., M.D., D.Sc., F.R.C.P.
Consulting Editor

OTHER MONOGRAPHS IN THE SERIES

PUBLISHED

Barnett, Foster and Hudgson: **Syringomyelia,** *1973*
Dubowitz and Brooke: **Muscle Biopsy: A Modern Approach,** *1973*
Pallis and Lewis: **The Neurology of Gastrointestinal Disease,** *1974*
Hutchinson and Acheson: **Strokes,** *1975*
Gubbay: **The Clumsy Child,** *1975*
Hankinson and Banna: **Pituitary and Parapituitary Tumours,** *1976*

FORTHCOMING

Behan and Currie: **Neuroimmunology**
Cartlidge and Shaw: **Head Injury**
Newsom Davis and Cameron: **The Neurology of Breathing and its Disorders**

Neurology of Pregnancy

JAMES O. DONALDSON, M.D.
Assistant Professor of Neurology and Medicine
The University of Connecticut
School of Medicine

1978

W. B. Saunders Company Philadelphia • London • Toronto

W. B. Saunders Company: West Washington Square
Philadelphia, PA 19105

1 St. Anne's Road
Eastbourne, East Sussex BN21 3UN, England

833 Oxford Street
Toronto, Ontario, M8Z 5T9, Canada

Library of Congress Cataloging in Publication Data

Donaldson, James O

Neurology of pregnancy.

(Major problems in neurology; v. 7)

1. Pregnancy, Complications of. 2. Nervous system—Diseases. I. Title. II. Series. [DNLM: 1. Nervous system diseases—In pregnancy. 2. Pregnancy complications. W1 MA492U v. 7 / WQ240 D676n]

RG580.N47D66 618.3 76-58600

ISBN 0-7216-3139-8

Neurology of Pregnancy ISBN 0-7216-3139-8

Last digit is the print number: 9 8 7 6 5 4 3 2 1

To my teachers,
who so generously shared their knowledge,
experience, judgment, and enthusiasm

Editor's Foreword

It is a pleasure to welcome to the series of volumes on Major Problems in Neurology this contribution by Dr. James O. Donaldson on *Neurology of Pregnancy*. Of the previous volumes published, some have been written wholly by authors working in the United Kingdom or Australia, but others have been the product of fruitful trans-Atlantic collaboration. This is the first such volume to have been conceived and produced wholly in the United States of America, a development which as editor of the series I am glad to see and which I am sure will be commended by our readers. I hope that this important monograph will be the first of many from American authors.

When I learned that Dr. Donaldson was planning to write it, I felt sure that it would fulfill admirably the major objective of these monographs—namely, that of bringing to the attention of an experienced and sophisticated clientele of readers some important problems and developing areas in neurologic medicine not specifically dealt with in major current texts. As Dr. Donaldson's teacher and mentor, my good friend Dr. Arthur Asbury, has said in his Foreword, descriptions of the many neurologic disorders that may complicate pregnancy are scattered widely throughout the neurologic and obstetric literature. In this comprehensive and scholarly monograph I believe that Dr. Donaldson has done a signal service to neurologists and obstetricians and to the medical profession in general by reviewing fully those disorders of the central and peripheral nervous system that are known to occur in the pregnant woman. I have found this book clearly written yet succinct, detailed and thorough yet critical and perceptive. It is a volume both to be read and to be used as an invaluable reference source. Dr. Donaldson has done Philadelphia proud, and I am sure that this important monograph will be widely read and consulted.

JOHN N. WALTON

Newcastle upon Tyne, 1977

Foreword

Pregnancy in no way indemnifies women against disorders affecting their nervous systems. It is frequent to encounter neurologic disturbances first appearing during pregnancy, to say nothing of preexisting neurologic diseases that complicate subsequent pregnancy. Despite the commonplace nature of the general problem, the concurrence of neurologic dysfunction and pregnancy creates clinical situations that are difficult and confusing for both the neurologist and the obstetrician. The reasons are easy to determine.

First, the pregnant woman is at risk for a broad range of neurologic conditions. These encompass virtually all clinical neurologic disorders, with the possible exception of aging changes in the nervous system. One need only scan the Table of Contents of this volume to be convinced of the diversity of nervous system disorders occurring during pregnancy.

Second, neurologic disease coinciding with pregnancy often raises special questions. Although many neurologic conditions are banal in nonpregnant individuals, their occurrence in the pregnant woman frequently has unusual implications in terms of both the significance of the disorder and its management. Most neurologists and obstetricians have too little experience with any one neurologic complication of pregnancy to be sure of their ground without referring to the pertinent literature.

Third, and perhaps most important, medical writing on the subject of the neurology of pregnancy, although abundant, is scattered almost to the point of inaccessibility throughout a host of journals and monographs. It requires an assiduous search to track down all that is known about a given neurologic entity in pregnancy.

For all of these reasons, this monograph by Dr. Donaldson will be welcome to neurologists, obstetricians, and many others as well. It is written in a spare, factual manner, and the scholarship is impeccable. The bibliography alone is a worthy contribution. Use of illustrations is generous, and the author's treatment of each subject is appropriately comprehensive.

Finally, it would be remiss not to mention something about the author. Dr. James O. Donaldson, III is a Pennsylvanian by birth and heritage. He attended Haverford College and the University of Pennsylvania School of Medicine, receiving his M.D. degree in 1968. His subsequent training in both internal medicine and neurology was undertaken at the Hospital of the University of Pennsylvania with brief interruptions for service in the Armed Forces and 6 months at the National Hospital, Queen Square, in London. His interest in the present subject goes back to his days as a medical student and was sparked by his wife, who was then a delivery room nurse.

Early in his period of neurologic residency training, Dr. Donaldson first broached the idea for this monograph. Enthusiasm for his endeavor was immediate, both in the Department of Neurology and in the Department of Obstetrics and Gynecology. Over the next 2 years, Dr. Donaldson worked diligently to complete his project and has produced what will be a most useful addition to our working libraries.

ARTHUR K. ASBURY

Philadelphia, Pennsylvania, 1977

Preface

Neurology of Pregnancy covers neurologic conditions that are directly related to pregnancy or the puerperium or, alternatively, neurologic conditions whose course or management is altered by the coexistence of pregnancy. The neurologic complications of the Pill and disorders also associated with menarche, menstruation, and menopause are reviewed. In this process, by viewing pregnancy and menstruation as experimental evidence given us by nature, lessons can be learned concerning the pathogenesis of disease. The focus is upon the woman, with secondary emphasis upon her child. This monograph is intended to complement existing texts of perinatology, pediatric neurology, and medical and surgical problems during pregnancy. These books should be consulted for information on the effects of maternal drug and alcohol addiction, the effects of a long list of infections and toxins, and the prenatal diagnosis of inborn errors of metabolism and neural tube defects.

This book is written for obstetricians and neurologists. Clinical descriptions of even rare neurologic conditions are meant to be complete enough to permit recognition of the syndrome by an obstetrician and to guide his further evaluations and treatment in a logical manner. In addition, I have pointed out the obstetric and fetal factors that must temper a neurologist's advice.

This monograph allows facile access to the collective experiences of many physicians represented by an extensive literature, which is, however, scattered over 150 years through at least 235 journals and 40 books. Bibliographies include material cited in the text plus representative papers from a variety of journals to aid physicians who wish to read further but may be limited by the size of the medical library available to them. I am indebted to the diligent staff of the library of the University of Pennsylvania School of Medicine, who never failed to locate somewhere the requested material, no matter how old or obscure the source.

I have followed Edwin R. Bickerstaff's lead by referring to "oral contraceptives" or "anovulatory hormones" as "the Pill." At first "the

Pill" may sound colloquial, but it is a terse term with an unmistakable definition in this context. Within a decade, "the Pill" has come to mean the same thing around the world in any language. In our pill-conscious societies, this is a telling statement of the impact and importance of the Pill.

I expect the chapter on eclampsia to be controversial. The pathogenesis of the cerebral manifestations of eclampsia is based upon some old but also some relatively new knowledge. In addition to adequately explaining the pathology, it also shows the importance of antihypertensive therapy in the treatment of eclampsia. This will be less controversial than my castigation of magnesium sulfate as an anticonvulsant. I have found this to provoke strong emotions among many obstetricians who have used magnesium sulfate for the duration of their professional lives. I trust that the information presented will not be rejected out of hand.

I am indebted to many people for assistance during the production of this book: to George A. McCarty, with whom I first explored the need for and the contents of this book over many cups of coffee in an Army clinic in Heilbronn, Germany, and who later so carefully reviewed the text; to Arthur K. Asbury for his enthusiastic advice and support throughout; to my colleagues who allowed me to increase my clinical experience by sharing their patients with me; to John N. Walton for his careful critique and suggestions; to John J. Hanley and his staff at the W. B. Saunders Company for their editorial expertise; and, of course, to my family, who wondered when I would quit typing. Special appreciation is extended to the authors and publishers who have allowed me to reproduce their graphs, drawings, and photographs. This collection of illustrations is itself a unique contribution to and a vital part of this monograph. Among these contributors, I especially thank Professor H. L. Sheehan, who generously supplied eleven illustrations.

JAMES O. DONALDSON

West Hartford, Connecticut, 1977

Contents

Chapter One
NEUROANATOMY OF FEMALE REPRODUCTIVE ORGANS 1

Chapter Two
NEUROPATHY 23

Chapter Three
MUSCLE DISEASE 56

Chapter Four
MOVEMENT DISORDERS 74

Chapter Five
INFECTIONS 88

Chapter Six
MULTIPLE SCLEROSIS 111

Chapter Seven
CEREBROVASCULAR DISEASE 115

Chapter Eight
TUMORS 157

Chapter Nine
HEADACHE 182

Chapter Ten
EPILEPSY 190

Chapter Eleven
ECLAMPSIA AND OTHER CAUSES OF PERIPARTUM CONVULSIONS 211

Chapter Twelve
PERIPARTUM PSYCHIATRIC DISEASE 251

INDEX 263

CHAPTER ONE

Neuroanatomy of Female Reproductive Organs

The innervation of the female reproductive organs has long been of interest. The basis of our scientific knowledge is the meticulous anatomic studies made by Lee (1846), Frankenhauser (1867), and Langley and Anderson (1896) in the nineteenth century. Subsequent experiments utilizing surgery, local anesthetics, electric stimulation, pharmacology, and histochemistry have supplied more information. In many cases our concepts of human anatomy have been extrapolated from investigations in other mammals; these may not be valid for humans since these animals have an estrous cycle or extra lumbar vertebrae. Other evidence cannot be ethically tested in humans. Even so, an acceptable scheme of human innervation has emerged which explains many clinical observations.

I shall not deal with the function of the autonomic nervous system within the sexual organs. These functions and their modifications by hormones during the various stages of a woman's life, pregnancy, and labor are the subject of several hypotheses and an extensive literature. That subject is best reviewed by an obstetrician. This chapter will be confined to visceral pain, extrinsic neuronal pathways, and lesions thereof.

VISCERAL PAIN

Visceral pain is a vague, ill-defined, dull, deep ache evoked by an organ which is distended, ischemic, or inflamed. Often visceral pain is referred to a cutaneous sensory field within the same somatotome.

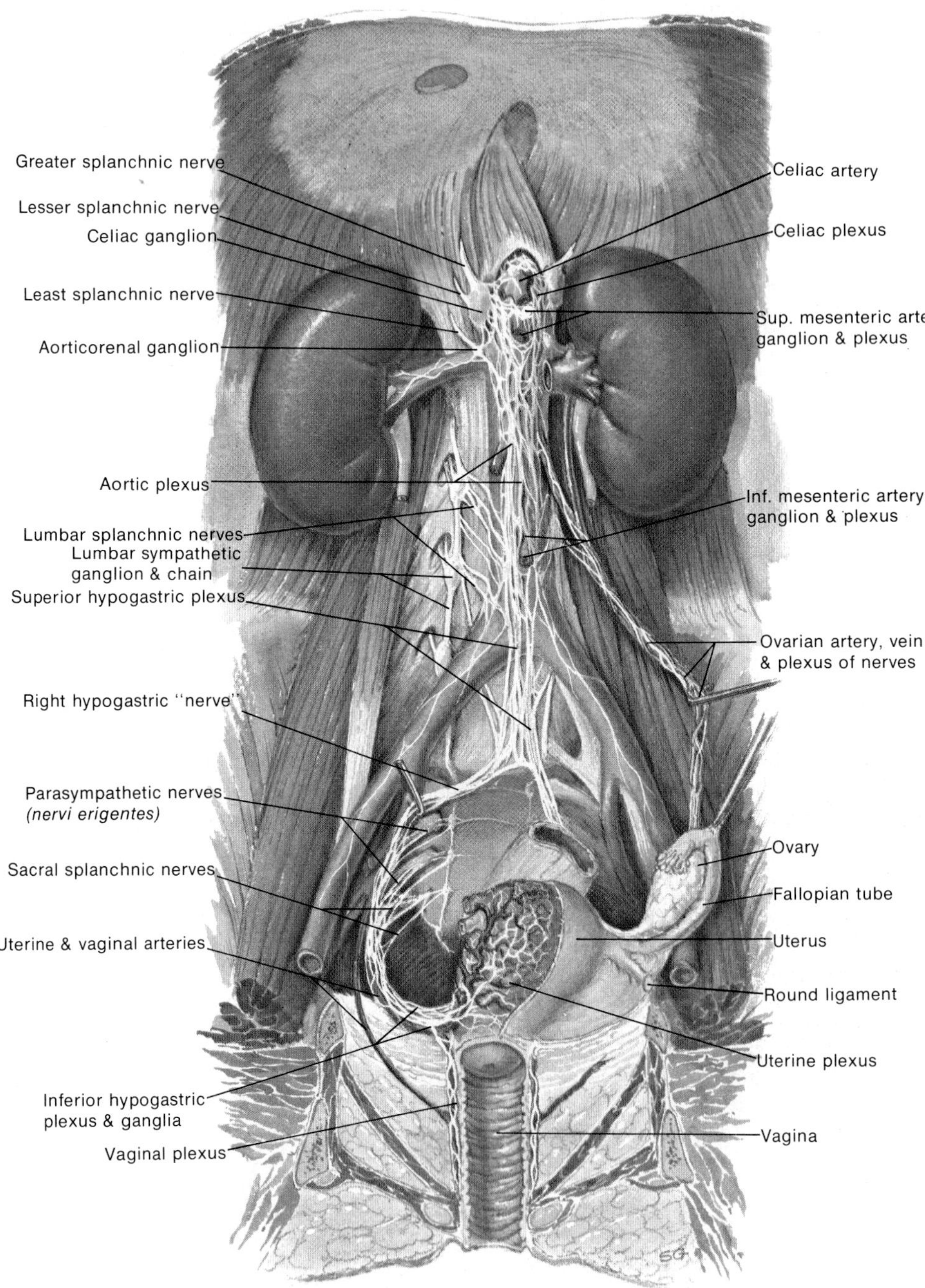

Figure 1.1 Nerve supply of uterus. From Bonica, J. J. (1960) *What's New*, **217**, 16. Plates courtesy Abbott Laboratories.

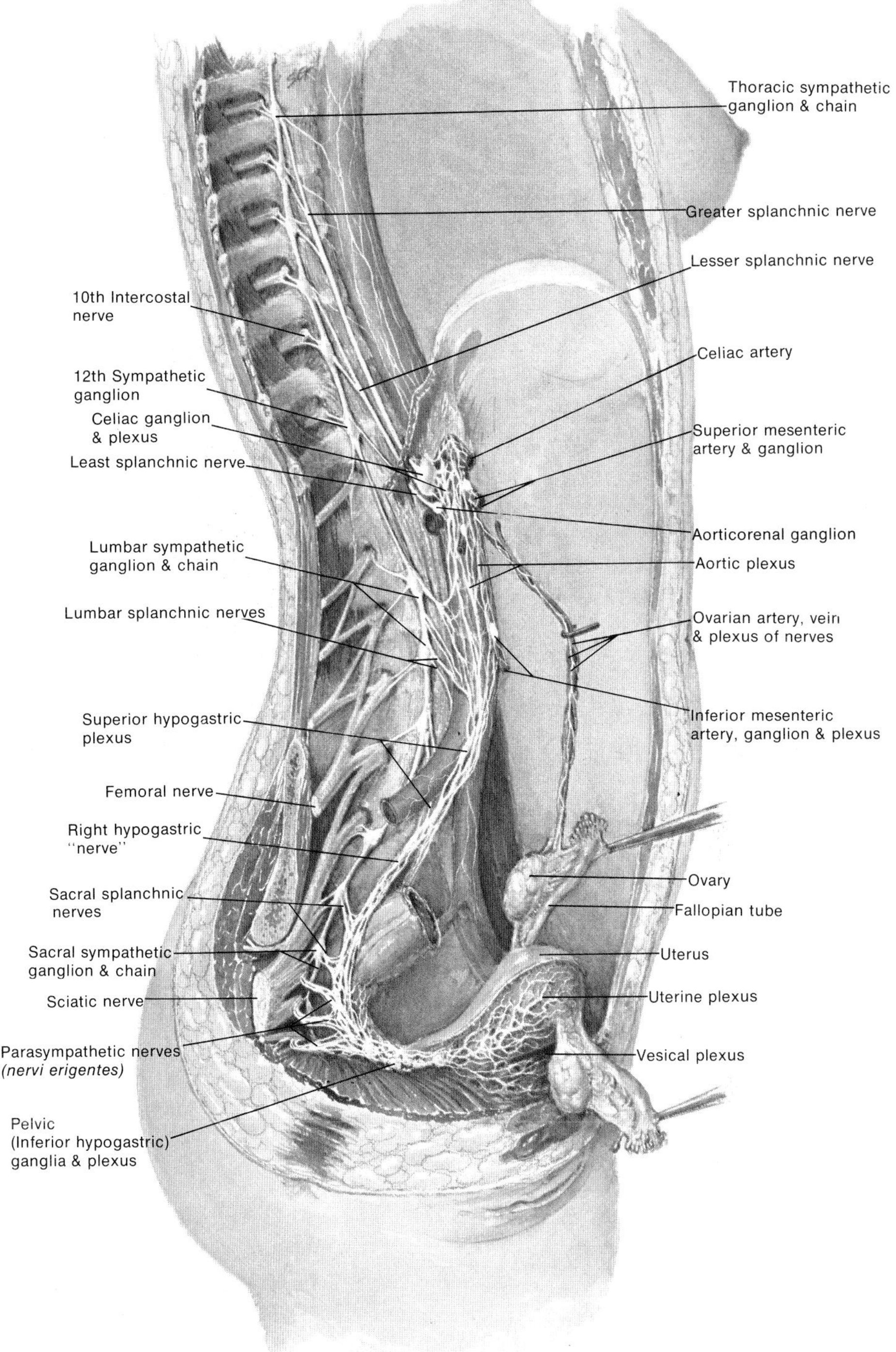

Figure 1.2. Nerve supply of uterus. From Bonica, J. J. (1960) An atlas of mechanisms and pathways of pain in labor. *What's New,* **217,** 16. Plates courtesy Abbott Laboratories.

Hyperesthesia may be demonstrated in this zone, but visceral pain need not be abolished by infiltration of local anesthetics into this area.

A distinction between peritoneal pain and pain arising solely from the uterus or ovary may be neither possible nor clinically helpful. The viscera are insensitive to ordinary stimuli, and the uterus may be incised without pain. A sound may be passed without discomfort. The cervix is insensitive to touch, the grasp or forceps, and biopsy. Distension is the most common cause of pain. Uterine pain is caused by distension, strong myometrial contractions, curettage, and sometimes inflammation. Cervical distension causes pain (Paul et al., 1956).

The association between myometrial contractions and labor pains is so strong that the terms are synonymous in common usage. Presumably, the stronger the contraction, the more intense the pain. This is usually but not always true when intrauterine pressures in humans have been measured during menstruation and parturition.

Dysmenorrhea

Moir (1934) observed regular menstrual contractions that developed intrauterine pressures of up to 100 mm Hg which went unnoticed by the patient. At 120 mm Hg, the level at which arterial pulsations were abolished, the patients had a sensation of heaviness and discomfort but not pain. In women with dysmenorrhea, Moir recorded pressures exceeding 150 mm Hg. He implicated ischemia as one cause of dysmenorrhea.

Woodbury et al. (1947) confirmed these studies. In fact, one of his patients generated an intrauterine pressure of 340 mm Hg. In most subjects, the tension between contractions subsided to 5 to 15 mm Hg. Some patients with dysmenorrhea had inadequate relaxation as judged by high pressures (40 to 70 mm Hg) between contractions. The contractions of these patients were irregularly spaced and of unequal strength. This implied uncoordinated spread of contractions.

Unilateral dysmenorrhea has been described in cases of hematometra in the rudimentary horn of a double uterus (Claye, 1945; Resnick, 1946).

Labor Pain

Hendricks (1962) recorded human uterine activity throughout labor and delivery. During contractions the intrauterine pressure could rise to 100 mm Hg but would always drop below diastolic blood pressure before the next contraction. Postpartum intrauterine tension climbed to 250 to 300 mm Hg. However, postpartum pains are not usually described as being as intense as labor pains. Suckling and intravenous oxytocin promptly increased tension.

Skin Hyperesthesia

Uterine visceral pain and skin hypersensitivity to touch and pin pricks have been associated with labor (Head, 1893), acute salpingitis (Labate, 1937), and uterotubal insufflation (Rubin and Davids, 1942). Head found labor pains to be associated with skin tenderness over T_{11}, T_{12}, and L_1 abdominal dermatomes (Fig. 1.3). During after-pains skin hypersensitivity included these areas plus the S_3 area of the buttock.

Hyperpathia to touch and pin prick associated with acute salpingitis occurs in vertical bands near the midline and below the umbilicus. Another area of sensitivity on the inner upper thigh occurs less frequently. In an individual case, skin hypersensitivity is not helpful in distinguishing salpingitis from other tubal pathology such as an ectopic pregnancy (Labate, 1937).

Visceral pain can increase skeletal muscle tone. Cleland (1933) demonstrated that the abdominal muscles of dogs and cats contracted when the pressure within a uterus distended by a balloon exceeded 100

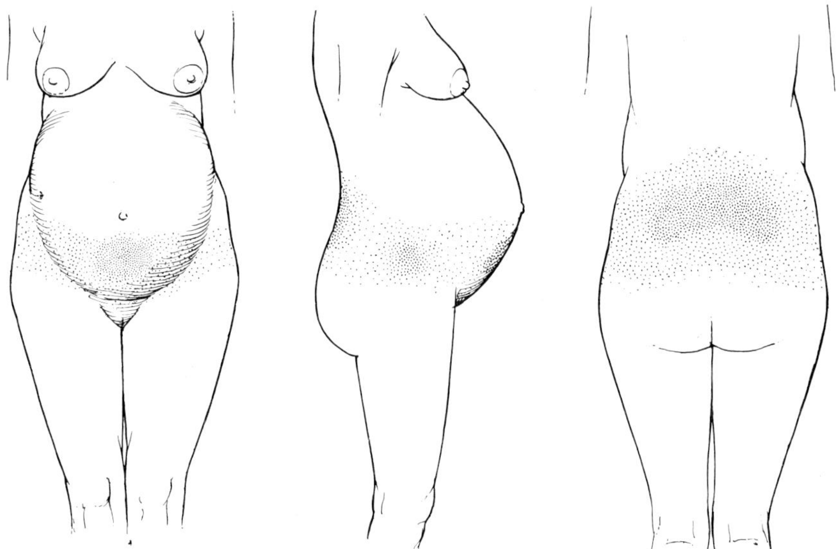

Figure 1.3. Areas of referred pain during first stage labor. Density of stippling indicates intensity of pain. From Bonica, J. J. (1967) *Principles and Practices of Obstetric Analgesia and Anesthesia.* Philadelphia: F. A. Davis Company.

mm Hg. Intestinal stimulation caused the same reaction. No doubt a similar mechanism operates in humans.

ORGAN INNERVATION

The best approach to the study of the innervation of the female reproductive organs is to divide the system into three parts: (1) the ovary and adjacent oviduct, (2) the uterus, most of the oviduct, and cervix, and (3) the vagina and perineum (Figs. 1.1, 1.2, and 1.4). These structures all have sympathetic, parasympathetic, and visceral sensory nerves, but the origins and pathways of the nerves are different. The perineum also has somatic nerves.

Ovary, Ampullary Oviduct, and Fimbria

Frankenhauser (1867) traced the ovarian nerves from their entry into the ovary at its hilus. As the ovarian plexus, most of the fibers follow the ovarian artery proximally to its origin from the aorta. The course of the ovarian nerves is lost in the preaortic and renal plexuses. In the cat the sympathetic nerves, accompanied by the visceral sensory nerves, can be traced from the preaortic plexus through the fourth lumbar sympathetic ganglion and up the sympathetic chain (Labate, 1937).

Sympathetic fibers can arise from any of the levels supplying splanchnic sympathetic outflow from T_{5-6} to L_2. As a rule, most of the sympathetic supply of an organ is derived from the same levels as the visceral sensation (Brodal, 1969). In the ovary T_{10} and T_{11} supply the visceral sensation.

In the baboon the parasympathetic innervation is vagal via the abdominal and ovarian plexuses (LePere et al., 1966). In addition, the ovary may receive a few sacral parasympathetics via the inferior hypogastric plexus.

Uterus, Cervix, and Proximal Oviduct

The uterus is innervated by autonomic and visceral sensory nerves. Many nerves follow the blood vessels, presumably to regulate their caliber. Many other nerves pervade the myometrium. Neuronal cell bodies do not exist within the uterus – only myelinated and unmyelinated nerve processes. Free nerve endings have been described by all investigators. Some have seen encapsulated receptors in the uterine wall. Freeman's careful work (1946) found Pacinian corpuscles only in the periuterine adventitia. A high nerve density in the cervix and lower uterus can be demonstrated by anatomic dissection (Krantz, 1959), and by histochemical staining for both adrenergic (Owman et al., 1967) and cholinergic endings (Coupland, 1962). The secretory cells of the cervix and the myometrium are richly supplied. Few endings exist within the endometrium.

Nerves from Frankenhauser's pelvic plexus enter the uterus at its isthmus on both sides. Frankenhauser's plexuses are extensive reticula of axons and ganglia measuring 2 cm $\times$ 3 cm $\times$ 1 mm which lie in the broad ligaments on each side of the uterus. Each pelvic plexus is composed of contributions from the sacral plexus and the inferior hypogastric plexus. The sacral plexus supplies preganglionic parasympathetic nerves from the sacral cord levels S_2 to S_4. These nerves synapse in a large ganglion, the cervical ganglion, on either side of the cervix. These cells send postganglionic parasympathetic axons to the cervix and uterus.

The visceral sensory and sympathetic nerves are routed through the inferior hypogastric plexus. This plexus can be traced back to the preaortic mesh of nerves. The superior hypogastric plexus appears to be a continuation of the intermesenteric plexuses below the inferior mesenteric artery. As it extends from the body of the fourth lumbar vertebra to the middle of the first sacral segment, the superior hypogastric plexus incorporates more rami from the sympathetic chain. Over the sacrum the superior hypogastric plexus divides into the left and right middle hypogastric plexuses, each of which follows its respective hypogastric (internal iliac) artery. After branches to the ureters have been given off, the middle hypogastric plexus becomes a mass of sympathetic ganglia and nerves called the inferior hypogastric plexus. Many of these nerves find their way to Frankenhauser's pelvic plexus.

The sympathetic fibers arise from the splanchnic set of roots (T_{5-6} to L_2), the bulk of which is contributed by T_{11}, T_{12}, and L_1. The sensory fibers enter the spinal cord in the dorsal roots of T_{11}, T_{12}, and L_1 with some individual variation.

There is no definite evidence that the cervix has sacral visceral sensory afferent nerves. The notion is based upon Head's observation that after-pains were associated with referred pain in the S_3 distribution (Head, 1893). Considering the vagaries of a sensory examination in a cooperative patient resting comfortably, I find these observations of interest, but they are certainly not hard evidence of sacral sensory afferents to the cervix. Indeed, perineal trauma could easily explain the sacral tenderness. However, as outlined by Cleland (1933), the 1922 edition of *Cunningham's Textbook of Anatomy* cited Head's observations as clinical evidence of sacral sensory innervation of the uterus. Kuntz referred to *Cunningham's* in his standard reference book, *The Autonomic Nervous System*. This statement was kept in all four editions which appeared from 1929 to 1953. Of course, many other authors in turn cited Kuntz.

Vagina and Perineum

The upper vagina is almost insensitive. Pain and sensitivity to touch are absent when the organ is formally tested (Klink, 1953). Vaginal pain is not appreciated unless the vaginal adventitia is involved or the introitus is affected. For instance, vaginal moniliasis is not painful until the vulvar infection is perceived. The distribution of nerve endings within the vagina and the external genitalia supports this observation (Krantz, 1958) (Table 1.1). The labia and mons veneris have specialized free endings called Merkel discs. These receptors occur in human lips and external genitalia but are scarce on hairy skin (Brodal, 1969). In contrast to most mechanoreceptors, Merkel discs slowly adapt to continued stimulation with discharges persisting for 5 minutes (Iggo, 1962).

The introitus is innervated by the pudendal nerves (Fig. 1.4). The pudendal nerve is a somatic nerve derived from the S_2 to S_4 roots; it supplies sensory fibers to the perineum and motor fibers to the muscles of the pelvic floor. No nerves to the uterus are contained in the pudendal nerve. Thus, a pudendal nerve block will not relieve labor pains or interrupt the course of labor, but it will relax the pelvis and allow an episiotomy to be performed without pain (Klink, 1953).

CLINICAL APPLICATIONS

As a general rule, chronic lesions that interrupt the uterine innervation will have little if any effect upon the ability of the uterus to expel the fetus. Acute interruption of the autonomic nerves by various types of anesthetics will temporarily slow or stop contractions unless the active stage of labor is well under way.

Paracervical Blocks

Infiltration of local anesthetic into each lateral fornix of the vagina blocks neuronal conduction through Frankenhauser's pelvic plexuses and the paracervical ganglia (Fig. 1.5). Thus, all sensory and autonomic innervation to the uterus and cervix is interrupted. Labor may be

Table 1.1. Quantitative distribution of free nerve endings in selected regions of the female genitalia

	Touch			Pressure	Pain	Other types	
	Meissner corpuscles	Merkel tactile discs	Peritrichial endings	Pacinian corpuscles	Free nerve endings	Ruffini corpuscles	Dogiel-Krause corpuscles
Mons veneris	++++	++++	++++	+++	+++	++++	++
Labia majora	+++	++++	+++	+++	+++	+++	++
Clitoris	+	+	0	++++	+++	+++	+++
Labia minora	++	++	0	++	++	++	+++
Hymeneal ring	0	+	0	0	+++	0	0
Vagina	0	0	0	0	+ Occasionally	0	0

From Krantz, K. E. (1959) Innervation of the human uterus. *Annals of the New York Academy of Science*, **75**, 770–784.

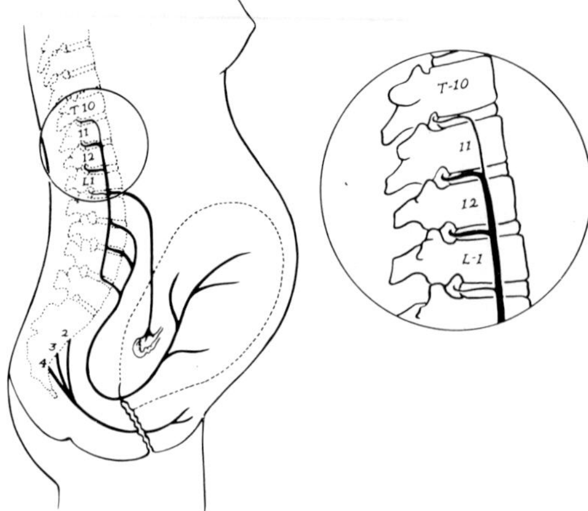

Figure 1.4. Diagram of the sensory (pain) innervation to the ovary, uterus, and perineum. See text for details. From Bonica, J. J. (1975) *Clinical Obstetrics and Gynecology*, **2,** 511.

inhibited unless the cervix is actively dilating. The paracervical nerves have been sectioned for the relief of dysmenorrhea (Doyle and DesRosiers, 1963).

Presacral Neurectomy (Section of the Superior Hypogastric Plexus)

Sensory nerves from both sides of the uterus combine in the superior hypogastric plexus. Cotte (1925) realized that this site was surgically accessible and that interruption of these nerves could offer relief from primary dysmenorrhea. This operation was acceptable until hormonal therapy replaced it.

Presacral neurectomy relieved low abdominal cramps, but some women who had had the operation continued to complain of backaches. Labor in these patients was short and painless until the fetal head dis-

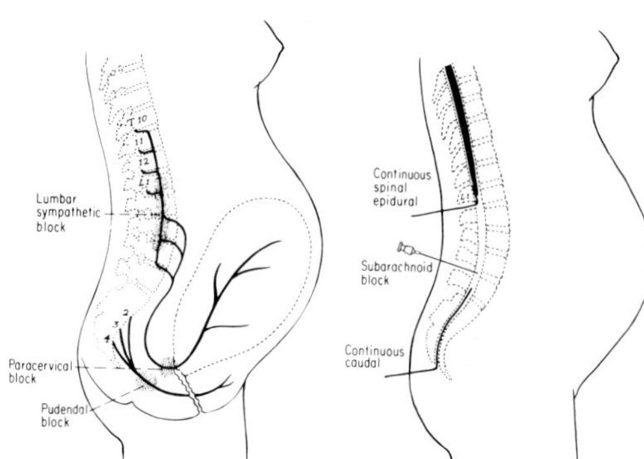

Figure 1.5. Regional anesthetic techniques employed during parturition. From Bonica, J. J. (1975) *Clinical Obstetrics and Gynecology*, **2,** 512.

tended the perineum. Meigs (1939) observed that although subsequent curettage was always painless, cervical dilatation caused backache in two patients in a large series. He offered this observation as further evidence for the presence of sacral sensory nerves in the uterus. Probably the operation had been incomplete.

Infiltration of both second lumbar sympathetic ganglia, through which the sensory and sympathetic nerves pass, will similarly cause uterine analgesia (Bonica, 1968). Block of the T_{11}, T_{12}, and L_1 dorsal roots by direct paravertebral injection of local anesthetic accomplishes the same result (Cleland, 1933) (Fig. 1.5).

Epidural Anesthesia

Epidural and caudal anesthesia must reach the T_{11}–T_{12} level to abolish labor pain (Edwards, 1942) (Fig. 1.5). Segmental epidural anesthesia in the low thoracic or high lumbar region is also effective (Bromage, 1961). The umbilicus serves as a convenient T_{10} landmark.

Tabes Dorsalis

A completely painless childbirth without autonomic dysfunction occurs in one rare condition—tabes dorsalis. The lesion in tabes is a fibrosis of multiple dorsal roots proximal to a healthy dorsal root ganglion. Reports on tabes coexisting with pregnancy are few. Most of them are found in the French literature before 1920 (Gaussel-Ziegelmann, 1910). One remarkable case from the Boston City Hospital (Williams, 1931) was described as follows:

> Mrs. N. L., 29 years old, had been married 6 years. After having had three miscarriages at 5 to 6 months, she had given birth to a full-term baby, which died at the age of 9 months from unmistakable congenital syphilis. The mother and father were then examined. Positive Wassermann reactions were obtained from both. After both parents had been subjected to prolonged antiluetic treatment, and repeated Wassermann tests on both had proven negative, they were advised that it would be safe to again try to produce offspring.
>
> In December 1919, the patient presented herself in the third month of pregnancy. Signs of tertiary lues were then present—an ataxic gait, a coarse jerky tremor of outstretched hands, absent knee and ankle reflexes. diminished pain in both legs, unequal pupils with sluggish light reflexes but normal accommodation. . . .The patient went through her pregnancy without complications other than extreme weakness and difficulty in walking. The delivery at term was practically painless, no anesthetic required. The baby showed a negative Wassermann reaction and has been well since birth.
>
> The patient again became pregnant in 1922 and went through a pregnancy uneventful except for weakness, difficulty in walking, and slight incontinence of

urine. On November 25, being close to term, she was awakened from sleep early in the morning by rupture of the membranes. Thinking that she had voided urine involuntarily and feeling a slight pressure on the rectum, she went to the toilet, and delivered herself, without pain, of a well-formed full-term baby. The mother did not realize what had happened for several minutes, and the baby was drowned in the hopper before its birth was discovered. Although no autopsy was permitted, the child was well formed and not macerated. There could be no doubt that it had been born alive.

During a subsequent pregnancy she suffered from lightning pains and severe gastric crises, for which she was hospitalized but found not to be in labor.

As this case demonstrates, tabetic crises can mimic labor, but labor itself is painless.

Spinal Cord Transections

The possibility of marriage and motherhood for paraplegics has gained importance as more young survivors of spinal cord transections wish to live as full a life as possible. Guttmann's experience is that paraplegics and even quadriplegics can be successful mothers (Guttmann, 1973). Performance of sexual intercourse is not a problem for a paraplegic woman, although orgasm is absent if both spinothalamic tracts are severed (Guttmann, 1973). Fertility is unaffected, although amenorrhea for 2 or 3 months after spinal cord trauma is not unusual.

For our purposes pregnant patients should be classified into three groups: (1) those with lesions below T_{11}, T_{12}, or L_1 (the uterine sensory afferents), (2) those with midthoracic lesions—T_{5-6} to T_{10}, and (3) those with cervical and high thoracic lesions—above T_{5-6}.

All groups should have sacral anesthesia during labor. Patients with cauda equina lesions have relaxed perineal muscles, and those with lesions above T_{11} have painless labor, although they may be able to gauge the time of uterine contractions from other cues. Spasticity—flexor spasms and spontaneous clonus—will be aggravated by labor pains. If the cord level of the lesion is above the splanchnic outflow (i.e., above T_{5-6}), autonomic hyperreflexia exists in addition to somatic hyperreflexia.

Autonomic Stress Syndrome

The autonomic stress syndrome, as delineated by Guttmann and Whitteridge (1947), is the result of overstimulation of the splanchnic nerves, which are uninhibited by higher centers. Stimulation may be caused by bladder distension, rectal digital examination, genital stimulation, or immersion of a foot into ice water (Bors, 1952). Labor is now another recognized stimulus (Guttmann and Frenkel, 1965; Rossier et al., 1969). The diagnosis in pregnant paraplegics may be missed and the patient treated for pre-eclampsia (Oppenhimer, 1971).

The autonomic stress syndrome consists of throbbing headache, facial flushing, dilated pupils, nasal congestion, marked sweating, and severe paroxysmal hypertension. Reflex bradycardia is seen if baroreceptors and the vagus nerves are intact. Premature ventricular beats, ventricular bigeminy, AV nodal block, and prominent U waves have been observed during uterine contractions. Electrocardiographic monitoring is warranted.

The comparison of this syndrome with pheochromocytoma is a good one. The symptoms are caused by a sudden release of catecholamines (Garnier and Gertsch, 1964). Paroxysms associated with hypertension are directly correlated with serum dopamine-β-hydroxylase and urinary normetanephrine excretion (Naftchi et al, 1974). Hexamethonium, an autonomic ganglionic blocking agent, prevents occurrence of the symptoms (Kurnick, 1956). Presumably a beta-receptor blocking agent such as propranolol would also be effective and have fewer side effects.

Obstetric Management of Paraplegics

In the obstetric management of pregnant paraplegic women the physician must be careful to anticipate and avoid complications. Urinary tract infections, which are a potential problem in any pregnancy and in any paraplegic, must be a constant concern (Bradley et al., 1957). Occlusion of an ileal bladder during pregnancy has been reported (Daw, 1973). Constipation will be aggravated. Anemia must be avoided since it lowers tissue resistance to pressure sores (Guttmann, 1973).

Women with lesions above the level of T_{11} are prone to premature labor. Weekly examinations throughout the third trimester, especially with multigravidas, are warranted to detect early cervical dilatation and effacement. Hospitalization before delivery can be justified.

Delivery via the vagina is preferred unless there is an obstetric indication for cesarean section. A bony deformity of the spine or pelvis may compromise the pelvic outlet. Robertson and Guttmann (1963) repair the episiotomy with nonabsorbable sutures (silk or nylon). Catgut sutures are poorly absorbed by paraplegics. Buried sutures often cause sterile abscesses.

Breast feeding has been successful for paraplegics and quadriplegics. The "let-down" phenomenon is normal (Robertson, 1972).

The risk of fetal abnormality, stillbirth, or abortion appears to be increased for pregnant women who become paraplegics but not for paraplegics who become pregnant, although case reports are too sporadic for statistical analysis. Likely hazards are direct trauma and irradiation (Göller and Paeslack, 1970; Robertson, 1972). The extent of the mother's injury must be determined with all necessary radiographs. Since shielding is impossible with spinal radiographs and myelograms, fetal exposure and its consequent risk are unavoidable.

NEUROENDOCRINE CONTROL OF LACTATION

Regular, periodic nursing is usually the stimulus necessary for release of oxytocin and prolactin, which maintain lactation. The afferent limb of the reflex is a polysynaptic tactile sensory pathway from the teat to the hypothalamus. The efferent limb is hormonal. In the milk-ejection (let-down) reflex, there is a 40- to 50-second latent period from the initiation of suckling to the ejection of milk by the oxytocin-induced contraction of the breast's myoepithelial cells.

Milk-Ejection Reflex

The milk-ejection reflex is initiated by stimulation of sensory receptors in the nipple, one of the most highly innervated areas of skin (Cathgart and Gairns, 1948). These impulses reach the spinal cord along the fourth, fifth, and sixth thoracic dorsal roots. Denervation of the nipples (Grosvenor and Findlay, 1968) or section of the dorsal roots (Popovici, 1963) prevents the reflex. Sympathectomy has no effect in the rat (Bacq, 1932).

It is doubtful but has not been proved that the nerves mediating the milk-ejection reflex ever cross the midline. There may be differences among species. In the spinal cord of rats, the fibers ascend adjacent to the ipsilateral spinothalamic tract, at least to the neck (Eayrs and Baddeley, 1956). In the midbrain of the guinea pig, the afferent fibers can again be identified adjacent to the spinothalamic tract. Rostrally the fibers pass medioventrally with respect to the medial geniculate body (Tindal et al., 1967).

In the diencephalon of the guinea pig, the pathway divides into a dorsal path, which enters the hypothalamus close to the third ventrical, and a ventral path, which extends into the subthalamus before entering the lateral hypothalamus (Tindal et al., 1967). In the goat, when one hypothalamic paraventricular nucleus was destroyed, a milk-ejection reflex occurred only in response to stimulation of the contralateral nipple (Popovici, 1963). In rats, the firing rate of paraventricular neurons accelerated 20- to 40-fold during suckling (Wakerley and Lincoln, 1973). The course of the path is lost within the hypothalamus but terminates with the release of oxytocin.

Prolactin is promptly released in response to suckling, but the afferent pathway has not been studied. Presumably it shares the afferent limb of the milk-ejection reflex. The quality of the stimulus is important. Hand milking of cows causes the release of more prolactin than does machine milking (Johke, 1969).

Lesions of the Afferent Pathway

High bilateral spinal cord lesions interrupting the spinothalamic tracts resulted in the cessation of lactation in rabbits (Mena and Beyer, 1963). Rabbits with chronic cord transections produced milk but at a subnormal rate (Beyer and Mena, 1970). In human quadriplegics lactation is said to be normal (Guttmann, 1974). Central conditioned reflexes—visual or auditory—can induce oxytocin release (Grosvenor and Mena, 1967). In the rabbit temporal lobe lesions can induce milk secretion (Mena and Beyer, 1968).

It is interesting that lactation can occur in the presence of syringomyelia (Roussy, 1932; Relkin, 1967). A syrinx typically destroys the nerves destined for the contralateral spinothalamic tract as they cross the midline near the central canal.

Nonpuerperal Galactorrhea

The most common cause of nonpuerperal lactation is drugs which interfere with CNS synaptic transmission by dopamine. The list includes phenothiazines, reserpine, alpha-methyldopa, and the tricyclic antide-

Table 1.2. Galactorrhea induced by persistent stimulation of peripheral nerves

Stimulant (References)
Nonpuerperal suckling (Knott, 1907; Slome, 1956)
Skin lesions
Chest burns (Dowling, 1961)
Dermatitis (McDonald, 1966)
Herpes zoster (Grimm, 1955; Cronin, 1949)
Tabes dorsalis (André-Thomas, 1932; Grimm, 1955)
Breast diseases
Cysts, abscesses (Grimm, 1955)
Chest surgery
Radical mastectomy (Aufses, 1955)
Augmentation mammaplasty (Hartley, 1971)
Thoracoplasty (Salkin, 1949; Grossman, 1950)
Pneumonectomy (Salkin, 1949; Berger, 1966; Crist, 1971)
Median sternotomy with aortic valve surgery (Berger, 1966)

pressants. The exact site (or sites) of action is unproven. More serious causes are tumors of the pineal gland, hypothalamus, and pituitary gland. Less common are cases of the Chiari-Frommel syndrome, testicular choriocarcinoma, and encephalitis.

Rare but interesting cases of nonpuerperal lactation result from peripheral stimulation of the afferent limb of the reflex arcs. (Table 1.2). The amount of milk can be sufficient to nourish an infant. Premenopausal Zulu grandmothers lactated when they used their breasts as nature's pacifier (Slome, 1956). Other cases are recorded back to antiquity.

Lactation attributed to tabes dorsalis presumably is caused by persistent dorsal root irritation during progressive fibrosis. I would not expect a completed lesion to induce lactation.

Lactation provoked by stimulation of the chest can be successfully treated by infiltration of the dorsal roots by local anesthetics.

Diabetes Insipidus

The polyuria and polydipsia of diabetes insipidus result from inadequate production of antidiuretic hormone (ADH, vasopressin). Trauma, surgery, pinealomas (among other tumors), cysts, and granulomas are just a few of the many possible causes. Experimental hypothalamic lesions in animals cause both diabetes insipidus and symptoms referrable to inadequate oxytocin production—uterine atony and failure of milk ejection (Fisher et al., 1938). Similar symptoms are possible when a woman with diabetes insipidus becomes pregnant.

Vasopressin and oxytocin are believed to be fragments of a large precursor protein. Most vasopressin is synthesized by the supraoptic nucleus, and most oxytocin is produced by the hypothalamic paraventricular nucleus (Hays, 1976). Different stimuli release each hormone. Antidiuretic hormone is released by hypertonicity, volume depletion, nicotine, cholinergic drugs, and meperidine. Oxytocin is released not by these stimuli but by suckling (Hays, 1976; Gaitan et al., 1964).

In most cases diabetes insipidus does not affect fertility, gestation, parturition, or lactation; however, exceptions can be found in each instance. Anovulation results if both lobes of the pituitary are affected (Gordon and Bradford, 1970). Dystocia can occur but responds to intravenous oxytocin (Marañón, 1947). Some women never lactate. Others have found that lactation abruptly ceases after several weeks of an adequate milk supply (Hendricks, 1954). Vasopressin replacement therapy has not induced labor or abortion.

Pregnancy has a variable effect upon diabetes insipidus. Since placental oxytocinase can inactivate both vasopressin and oxytocin, the dosage of vasopressin should rise in the second and third trimesters.

This response has been observed but so has every other possibility (Blotner and Kunkel, 1942). The completeness of the lesion no doubt varies from patient to patient. Pregnancy may in some way stimulate the functioning remnant (Pico and Greenblatt, 1969). If diabetes insipidus appears during pregnancy and disappears afterward, I would suspect an active lesion—perhaps a tumor or a cyst.

Suckling may dramatically reduce flow of urine in some patients (Chou et al., 1969).

REFERENCES

Visceral Pain

Claye, A. M. (1945) Unilateral dysmenorrhoea. *British Medical Journal,* **2**, 438.

Cleland, J. G. P. (1933) Paravertebral anaesthesia in obstetrics. Experimental and clinical basis. *Surgery, Gynecology, Obstetrics,* **57**, 51–62.

Head, H. (1893) On disturbances of sensation with especial reference to the pain of visceral disease. *Brain,* **16,** 1–133.

Hendricks, C. H., Eskes, T. K. A. B., and Saameli, K. (1962) Uterine contractility at delivery and in the puerperium. *American Journal of Obstetrics and Gynecology,* **83,** 890–906.

Labate, J. S. (1937) Skin hyperesthesia in acute salpingitis. *Surgery, Gynecology, Obstetrics,* **65**, 321–330.

Lackner, J. E., Krohn, L., and Soskin, S. (1937) The etiology and treatment of primary dysmenorrhea. *American Journal of Obstetrics and Gynecology,* **34**, 248–266.

Moir, C. (1934) Recording the contractions of the human pregnant and non-pregnant uterus. *Transactions of the Edinburgh Obstetrical Society,* **54,** 93–120.

Paul, W. M., Glickman, B. I., Cushner, I. M., and Reynolds, S. R. M. (1956) Cervical tone and pain thresholds. Study in the nongravid human uterus. *Obstetrics and Gynecology,* **7**, 510–517.

Resnick, L. (1946) Unilateral dysmenorrhoea associated with uterine malformation, *South African Medical Journal,* **20**, 370–373.

Routledge, J. H., and Elliott, J. (1962) Pain studies in pelvic viscera. *American Journal of Obstetrics and Gynecology,* **83**, 701–709.

Rubin, I. C., and Davids, A. M. (1942) Study of cutaneous hyperalgesia and the viscerosensory reflex of uterus and tubes by means of uterotubal insufflation. *Journal of Mt. Sinai Hospital,* **9,** 761–766.

Theobald, G. W. (1936) Referred pain and in particular that associated with dysmenorrhoea and labour. *British Medical Journal,* **2,** 1307, 1308.

Theobald, G. W. (1946) Some gynaecological aspects of referred pain, *Journal of Obstetrics and Gynaecology of the British Empire,* **53**, 309–327.

Woodbury, R. A., Torpin, R., Child, G. P. et al. (1947) Myometrial physiology and its relation to pelvic pain. *Journal of the American Medical Association,* **134**, 1081–1085.

Ovarian Innervation

Bors, E. (1950) Perception of gonadal pain in paraplegic patients, *Archives of Neurology and Psychiatry,* **63**, 713–718.

Labate, J. S., and Reynolds, S. R. M. (1937) Sensory pathways of the ovarian plexus, *American Journal of Obstetrics and Gynecology,* **34**, 1–11.

LePere, R. H., Benoit, P. E., Hardy, R. C. et al. (1966) The origin and function of the ovarian nerve supply in the baboon. *Fertility and Sterility,* **17**, 68–75.

Neilson, D., Jones, G. S., Woodruff, J. D. et al. (1970) The innervation of the ovary. *Obstetric and Gynecologic Survey,* **25**, 889–904.

Innervation of the Uterus and Cervix

Alvarez, H., Blanco, Y. S., Panizza, V. G. et al. (1965) Effects of the electrical stimulation of the presacral nerve on contractility of the human pregnant uterus. *American Journal of Obstetrics and Gynecology,* **93**, 131–135.

Beck, T. S. (1846) On the nerves of the uterus. *Philosophical Transactions of the Royal Society* (London), **136**, 213–235.

Corey, E. L., McGaughey, H. S., and Thornton, W. N. (1957) Electromyography of the human uterus. *American Journal of Obstetrics and Gynecology,* **74**, 473–483.

Coupland, R. E. (1962) Histochemical observations on the distribution of cholinesterase in human muscle. *Journal of Obstetrics and Gynaecology of the British Commonwealth,* **69**, 1041–1043.

Davis, A. A. (1933) The innervation of the uterus. *Journal of Obstetrics and Gynaecology of the British Empire,* **40**, 481–497.

Frankenhäuser, F. (1867) *Die Nerven der Gebärmutter und ihre Endigungen in den glatten Muskelfasern; Ein Beitrag zur Anatomie und Gynäkologie.* Jena: Fr. Manke.

Freeman, A. (1946) The distribution of the nerves to the adult human uterus. *American Journal of Clinical Pathology,* **16**, 117–123.

Hirsch, E. F., and Martin, M. E. (1943) The distribution of nerves in the adult human myometrium. *Surgery, Gynecology, Obstetrics,* **76**, 697–702.

Kaminester, S., and Reynolds, S. R. M. (1935) Motility in the transplanted, denervated uterus. *American Journal of Obstetrics and Gynecology,* **30**, 395–402.

Krantz, K. E. (1959) Innervation of the human uterus. *Annals of the New York Academy of Science,* **75**, 770–784.

Langley, J. N. and Anderson, K. H. (1896) The innervation of the pelvic and adjoining viscera, Part VI. Anatomical observations. *Journal of Physiology* (London), **20**, 372.

Lee, R. (1846) On the nervous ganglia of the uterus. *Philosophical Transactions of the Royal Society* (London), **2**, 211.

Nakanishi, H., McLean, J., Wood, C. et al. (1969) The role of sympathetic nerves in control of the nonpregnant and pregnant human uterus. *Journal of Reproductive Medicine,* **2**, 20–33.

Ownan, C. H., Rosengren, E., and Sjöberg, N. O. (1967) Adrenergic innervation of the human female reproductive organs: A histochemical and chemical investigation. *Obstetrics and Gynecology,* **30**, 763–773.

Pauerstein, C. J., and Zauder, H. L. (1970) Autonomic innervation, sex steroids and uterine contractility. *Obstetric and Gynecologic Survey,* **25**, 617–630.

Reynolds, S. R. M. (1965) *Physiology of the Uterus.* New York: Hafner Publishing Company.

Ryan, M. J., Clark, K. E., and Brody, M. J. (1974) Neurogenic and mechanical control of canine uterine vascular resistance. *American Journal of Physiology,* **227**, 547–555.

Shabanah, E. H., Toth, A., and Maughan, G. B. (1964) The role of the autonomic nervous system in uterine contractility and blood flow. *American Journal of Obstetrics and Gynecology,* **89**, 841–859.

Innervation of the Vulva and Vagina

Brodal, A. (1969) *Neurological Anatomy,* 2nd ed. London: Oxford University Press.

Iggo, A. (1962) An electrophysiological analysis of afferent fibres in primate skin. *Acta* Neurovegetativa, **24,** 225–240.

Klink, E. W. (1953) Perineal nerve block; an anatomic and clinical study in the female. *Obstetrics and Gynecology,* **1**, 137–146.

Krantz, K. E. (1958) Innervation of the human vulva and vagina. *Obstetrics and Gynecology,* **12**, 382–396 (1958).

Dysmenorrhea and Presacral Neurectomy

Blinick, G. (1947) Painless labors following presacral neurectomy. *American Journal of Obstetrics and Gynecology,* **54**, 148–151.

Claye, A. M. (1945) Unilateral dysmenorrhoea. *British Medical Journal,* **2**, 438.

Cotte, G. (1925) La sympathectomie hypogastrique a-t-elle sa place dans la thérapeutique gynécologique? *Presse médicale*, **33**, 98.

Davis, A. (1963) Alcohol injection for relief of dysmenorrhea. *Clinical Obstetrics and Gynecology*, **6**, 754–762.

Davis, A. A. (1934) The presacral nerve: Its anatomy, physiology, pathology, and surgery, *British Medical Journal*, **2**, 1–5.

Doyle, J. B., and DesRosiers, J. J. (1963) Paracervical uterine denervation for relief of pelvic pain. *Clinical Obstetrics and Gynecology*, **6**, 742–753.

Fontaine, R., and Herrmann, L. G. (1932) Clinical and experimental basis for surgery of the pelvic sympathetic nerves in gynecology. *Surgery, Gynecology, Obstetrics*, **54**, 133–163.

Hendricks, C. H., Eskes, T. K. A. B., and Saameli, K. (1962) Uterine contractility at delivery and in the puerperium. *American Journal of Obstetrics and Gynecology*, **83**, 890–906.

Ingersoll, F. M., and Meigs, J. V. (1948) Presacral neurectomy for dysmenorrhea. *New England Journal of Medicine*, **238**, 357–360.

Meigs, J. V. (1939) Excision of the superior hypogastric plexus (presacral nerve), for primary dysmenorrhea. *Surgery, Gynecology and Obstetrics*, **68**, 723–732.

Regional Anesthesia

Bonica, J. J. (1968) Autonomic innervation of the viscera in relation to nerve block. *Anesthesiology*, **29**, 793–813.

Bonica, J. J. (1967) *Principles and Practice of Obstetric Analgesia and Anesthesia*. Philadelphia: F. A. Davis Company.

Bromage, P. R. (1961) Continuous lumbar epidural analgesia for obstetrics. *Canadian Medical Association Journal*, **85**, 1136–1140.

Cleland, J. G. P. (1933) Paravertebral anaesthesia in obstetrics: Experimental and clinical basis. *Surgery Gynecology, Obstetrics*, **57**, 51–62.

Edwards, W. B., and Hingson, R. A. (1942) Continuous caudal anesthesia in obstetrics. *American Journal of Surgery*, **57**, 459–464.

Klink, E. W. (1953) Perineal nerve block. An anatomic and clinical study in the female. *Obstetrics and Gynecology*, **1**, 137–146.

Tabes Dorsalis

Allen, E. M. (1917) Coincident pregnancy and tabes dorsalis. *Journal of the American Medical Association*, **67**, 979, 980.

Gaussel-Ziegelmann (1910) Tabes et puerperalite. *Obstetrique* (Paris), **3**, 540–542.

Williams, J. T. (1931) Pregnancy complicated by tabes. *New England Journal of Medicine*, **204**, 119–122.

Paraplegia

Bors, E., and French, J. D. (1952) Management of paroxysmal hypertension following injuries to cervical and upper thoracic segments of the cord. *Archives of Surgery*, **64**, 803–812.

Bradley, W. S., Walker, W. W., and Searight, M. W. (1957) Pregnancy in paraplegia. A case report with urologic complication. *Obstetrics and Gynecology*, **10**, 573–575.

Daw, E. (1973) Pregnancy problems in a paraplegic patient with an ileal conduit bladder. *Practitioner*, **211**, 781–784.

Deyoe, F. S. (1972) Marriage and family patterns with long-term spinal cord injury. *Paraplegia*, **10**, 219–224.

Elkin, D. C. (1922) Spontaneous labor in a case of decentralized uterus. *Journal of the American Medical Association*, **78**, 27–29.

Garnier, B., and Gertsch, R. (1964) Autonome Hyperreflexie und Katecholaminausscheidune beim Paraplegiker. *Schweizerische Medizinische Wochenschrift*, **94**, 124–130.

Göller, H., and Paeslack, V. (1970) Our experiences about pregnancy and delivery of a paraplegic woman. *Paraplegia*, **8**, 161–166.

Good, F. L. (1924) Pregnancy and labor complicated by diseases and injuries of the spinal cord. *Journal of the American Medical Association*, **83**, 416–418.

Guttmann, L., and Whitteridge, D. (1947) Effects of bladder distension on autonomic mechanisms after spinal cord injuries. *Brain,* **70,** 361–404.

Guttmann, L., and Frankel, H. L. (1965) Cardiac irregularities during labour in paraplegic women. *Paraplegia,* **3,** 144–151.

Guttmann, L. (1973) *Spinal Cord Injuries: Comprehensive Management and Research.* Oxford: Blackwell Scientific Publications.

Hardy, A. G., and Warrell, D. W. (1965) Pregnancy and labour in complete tetraplegia. *Paraplegia,* **3,** 182–188.

Hutchinson, H. T., and Vasicka, A. (1962) Uterine contractility in a paraplegic patient. *Obstetrics and Gynecology,* **20,** 675–678.

Jackson, F. E. (1964) Pregnancy complicated by quadriplegia. *Obstetrics and Gynecology,* **23,** 620, 621.

Kurnick, N. B. (1956) Autonomic hyperreflexia and its control in patients with spinal cord lesions. *Annals of Internal Medicine,* **44,** 678–686.

Naftchi, N. E., Wooten, G. F., Lowman, E. W. et al. (1974) Relationship between serum dopamine-β-hydroxylase activity, catecholamine metabolism, and hemodynamic changes during paroxysmal hypertension in quadriplegia. *Circulation Research,* **45,** 850–861.

Oppenhimer, W. M. (1971) Pregnancy in paraplegic patients: two case reports. *American Journal of Obstetrics and Gynecology.* **110,** 784–786.

Robertson, D. N. S., and Guttmann, L. (1963) The paraplegic patient in pregnancy and labour. *Proceedings of the Royal Society of Medicine,* **56,** 380–383.

Robertson, D. N. S. (1972) Pregnancy and labour in the paraplegic. *Paraplegia,* **10,** 209–212.

Rossier, A. B., Ruffieux, M., and Ziegler, W. H. (1969) Pregnancy and labour in high traumatic spinal cord lesions. *Paraplegia,* **7,** 210–216.

Saunders, D., and Yeo, J. (1968) Pregnancy and quadriplegia—the problem of autonomic dysreflexia. *Australian and New Zealand Journal of Obstetrics and Gynaecology,* **8,** 152–154.

Tarabulcy, E. (1972) Sexual function in the normal and in paraplegia. *Paraplegia,* **10,** 201–208.

Ware, H. H. (1934) Pregnancy after paralysis. A report of three cases. *Journal of the American Medical Association,* **102,** 1833–1835.

Milk-Ejection Reflex

Bacq. Z. M. (1932) The effect of sympathectomy on sexual functions, lactation, and the maternal behavior of the albino rat. *American Journal of Physiology,* **99,** 444–453.

Beyer, C., and Mena, F. (1970) Parturition and lactogenesis in rabbits with high spinal cord transection. *Endocrinology,* **87,** 195–197.

Cathgart, E. P., and Gairns, F. W. (1948) The innervation of the human quiescent nipple, with notes on pigmentation, erection, and hyperneury. *Transactions of the Royal Society of Edinburgh.* **61,** 699–717.

Cowie, A. T., and Tindal, J. S. (1971) *The Physiology of Lactation.* London: Edward Arnold.

Eayrs, J. T., and Baddeley, R. M. (1956) Neural pathways in lactation. *Journal of Anatomy* **90,** 161–171.

Grosvenor, C. E., and Mena, F. (1967) Effect of auditory, olfactory and optic stimuli upon milk ejection and suckling-induced release of prolactin in lactating rats. *Endocrinology,* **80,** 840–846.

Grosvenor, C. E., and Findlay, A. L. R. (1968) Effect of denervation on fluid flow into mammary gland. *American Journal of Physiology,* **214,** 820–824.

Grosvenor, C. E., DeNuccio, D. J., King, S. F. et al. (1972) Central and peripheral neural influences on the oxytocin-induced pressure response of the mammary gland of the anaesthetized rat. *Journal of Endocrinology,* **55,** 299–309.

Johke, T. (1969) Prolactin release in response to milking stimulus in the cow and goat estimated by radioimmunoassay. *Endocrinologica Japonica,* **16,** 179–185.

Mena, F., and Beyer, C. (1963) Effect of high spinal section on established lactation in the rabbit. *American Journal of Physiology,* **205,** 313–316.

Mena, F., and Beyer, C. (1968) Induction of milk secretion in the rabbit by lesions in the temporal lobe. *Endocrinology,* **83,** 618–620.

Popovici, D. G. (1963) Recherches neurophysiologiques sur le réflexe d'évacuation du lait. *Revue Biologie* (Bucarest), **8,** 75–81.

Relkin, R. (1965) Galactorrhea: A review. *New York State Journal of Medicine,* **65,** 2800–2807.

Relkin, R. (1967) Neurologic pathways involved in lactation. *Diseases of the Nervous System,* **28,** 94–97.

Roussy, G., deGery, C., and Mosinger, (1932) A propos d'un cas de syringomyelie avec galactorrhee et ileus postoperatoire. *Revue Neurologique,* **1,** 521–531.

Tindal, J. S., Knaggs, G. S., and Turvey, A. (1967) The afferent path of the milk-ejection reflex in the brain of the guinea-pig. *Journal of Endocrinology,* **38,** 337–349.

Wakerley, J. B., and Lincoln, D. W. (1973) The milk-ejection reflex of the rat: A 20- to 40-fold acceleration in the firing of paraventricular neurones during oxytocin release. *Journal of Endocrinology,* **57,** 477–493.

Nonpuerperal Galactorrhea

André-Thomas, and Kudelski, C. (1932) Galactorhee chez une tabetique. *Revue Neurologique,* **2,** 665–668.

Aufses, A. H. (1955) Abnormal lactation following radical mastectomy. *New York State Journal of Medicine,* **55,** 1914, 1915.

Berger, R. L. Joison, J., and Braverman, L. E. (1966) Lactation after incision on the thoracic cage. *New England Journal of Medicine,* **274,** 1493–1495.

Besser, G. M., and Edwards, C. R. W. (1972) Galactorrhoea. *British Medical Journal,* **2,** 280–282.

Crist, T., Hendricks, C. H., and Brenner, W. E. (1971) Lactation following lobectomy. *American Journal of Obstetrics and Gynecology,* **110,** 738–739.

Cronin, D. L. (1949) Galactorrhea. *Journal of the American Medical Association,* **140,** 1375, 1376.

Dowling, J. T., Richards, J. B., Freinkel, N. et al. (1961) Nonpuerperal galactorrhea. *Archives of Internal Medicine,* **107,** 885–893.

Foss, G. L., and Short, D. (1951) Abnormal lactation. *Journal of Obstetrics and Gynaecology of the British Empire,* **58,** 35–46.

Grimm, E. G. (1955) Non-puerperal galactorrhea with case reports. *Quarterly Bulletin of Northwestern University Medical School* **29,** 350–354.

Grossman, S., Buchberg, A. S., Brecher, E. et al. (1950) Idiopathic lactation following thoracoplasty. *Journal of Clinical Endocrinology,* **10,** 729–734.

Hartley, J. H., and Schatten, W. E. (1971) Postoperative complication of lactation after augmentation mammaplasty. *Plastic and Reconstructive Surgery,* **47,** 150–153.

Knott, J. (1907) Abnormal lactation: in the virgin; in the old woman; in the male; in the newborn of either sex ("witches' milk"). *American Medicine,* **2,** 373–378.

McDonald, C. J., and Lerner, A. B. (1966) Atopic dermatitis and persistent lactation. Archives of Dermatology, **93,** 174–176.

Mead, M. (1963) *Sex and Temperament in Three Primitive Societies.* New York: William Morrow & Company, p. 193.

Salkin, D., and Davis, E. W. (1949) Lactation following thoracoplasty and pneumonectomy. *Journal of Thoracic Surgery,* **18,** 580–590.

Slome, C. (1956) Nonpuerperal lactation in grandmothers. *Journal Pediatrics,* **49,** 550–552.

Somlyo, A. P., and Waye, J. D. (1960) Abnormal lactation. *Journal of Mt. Sinai Hospital,* **27,** 5–9.

White, A. E. (1960) Nonpuerperal lactation: A review with case reports. *Annals of Internal Medicine,* **52,** 1264–1272.

Diabetes Insipidus

Blotner, H., and Kunkel, P. (1942) Diabetes insipidus and pregnancy. *New England Journal of Medicine,* **227,** 287–292.

Chau, S. S., Fitzpatrick, R. J., and Jamieson, B. (1969) Diabetes insipidus and parturition. *Journal of Obstetrics and Gynaecology of the British Commonwealth,* **76,** 444–450.

Fisher, C., Magoun, H. W., and Ranson, S. W. (1938) Dystocia in diabetes insipidus: The relation of pituitary oxytocin to parturition. *American Journal of Obstetrics and Gynecology,* **36,** 1–9.

Gaitan, E., Cobo, E., and Mizrachi, M. (1964) Evidence for the differential secretion of oxytocin and vasopressin in man. *Journal of Clinical Investigation,* **43,** 2310–2322.

Gordon, G., and Bradford, W. P. (1970) Pregnancy in a patient with diabetes insipidus following induction of ovulation by clomiphene. *Journal of Obstetrics and Gynaecology of the British Commonwealth,* **77,** 467–469.

Hays, R. M. (1976) Antidiuretic hormone. *New England Journal of Medicine,* **295,** 659–665.

Hendricks, C. H. (1954) The neurohypophysis in pregnancy. *Obstetric and Gynecologic Survey,* **9,** 323–341.

Maronon, G. (1947) Diabetes insipidus and uterine atony. *British Medical Journal,* **2,** 769–771.

Pico, I., and Greenblatt, R. B. (1969) Endocrinopathies and fertility: IV. Diabetes insipidus and pregnancy. *Fertility and Sterility,* **20,** 384–392.

CHAPTER TWO

Neuropathy

CATAMENIAL SCIATICA (ENDOMETRIOSIS)

Catamenial sciatica occurs in menstruating women of childbearing age. Pain commences 2 or 3 days before menstruation begins and continues from 2 days to 3 weeks after the cessation of flow. The pain-free intermenstrual interval progressively shortens as the condition becomes chronic. Numbness, weakness, loss of ankle jerks, and neurogenic bladder have all been observed. The repeated association with menstruation and the absence of some of the characteristics of the pain accompanying a herniated intervertebral disk distinguish this syndrome. Although the pain is intense and radiates down the leg beyond the knee, it either is constant or is aggravated by all movements. Pain is not necessarily relieved by bed rest, and it need not be aggravated by standing or coughing. Myelograms are commonly normal.

Endometriosis is the cause of this rare syndrome. Ectopic endometriosis is rare, but catamenial hemoptysis from pleural and lung involvement is a recognized syndrome (Lattes et al., 1956). Repeated catamenial subarachnoid hemorrhages have been caused by endometriosis of the cauda equina (Lombardo et al., 1968). In 1947 Dagnelie found that he could palpate nodules along the sciatic nerve during a pelvic examination of a woman with catamenial sciatica. Her pain was relieved by testosterone and exacerbated by estrogens. Since then a half dozen tissue-proven cases have been reported; the site of implantation ranges from the cauda equina to an isolated root and from the lumbosacral plexus to the sciatic nerve (Fig. 2.1).

The diagnosis is difficult. One woman saw 17 specialists before one decided that her family physician's initial impression was reasonable and confirmed it at surgery (Zangger and Heppner, 1962). Contrary to my

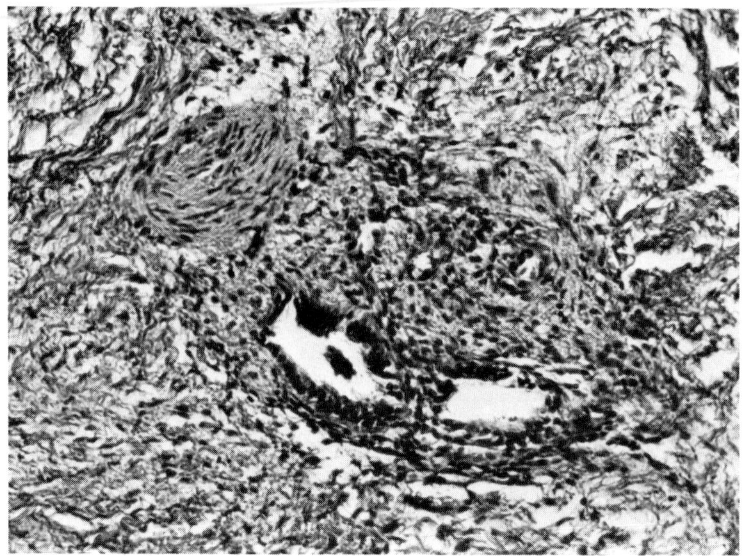

Figure 2.1. Biopsy specimen from right sciatic nerve showing endometrial glands and stroma associated with a nerve bundle (hematoxylin and eosin, × 200). From Head, H. B., Welch, J. S., Mussey, E. et al. (1962) Cyclic sciatica: Report of case with introduction of a new surgical sign. *Journal of the American Medical Association,* **180,** 523. Photomicrograph courtesy H. B. Head and the Publications Department, Mayo Foundation. Copyright 1962, American Medical Association.

expectation, the neural implants may be the only area involved. The woman need not have widespread disease.

Treatment with progesterone preparations or by castration, either surgically or by irradiation, has relieved pain and diminished weakness.

MONONEUROPATHIES DURING PREGNANCY

Bell's Palsy

Bell's palsy is idiopathic facial paralysis of acute onset due to compression of the facial nerve along its course within the temporal bone. Since the lower motor neuron is affected, both the forehead and lower face are involved. Brain stem lesions rarely cause isolated seventh cranial nerve signs.

Clinical Presentation

Onset is sudden. A young adult awakens one morning to find one side of his face paralyzed. He cannot wrinkle his brow, raise his eyebrow, completely close his eye, purse his lips, whistle, or smile. Food accumulates between teeth and cheek. He may bite his tongue, which is still painful since the trigeminal nerve contains the pain fibers from the tongue. Chewing is otherwise normal. Appreciation of taste on the anterior two-thirds of the tongue is lost if the lesion is proximal to the branching of the chorda tympani. If the nerve to the stapedius is involved, loud noises are intensified (hyperacusis). Simultaneous bilateral facial palsy is rare.

Pain is not a prominent symptom, although an ill-defined postauricular ache may be present. The presence of significant pain raises the possibility of otitis media, skull fracture, or a herpes zoster infection of the geniculate ganglion (the Ramsay Hunt syndrome).

Etiology

Epidemics of Bell's palsy suggest a viral agent. Herpes simplex has been implicated (McCormick, 1972). The association of diabetes mellitus and Bell's palsy suggests that some cases are ischemic diabetic mononeuropathies (Korczyn, 1971a). Hilsinger et al. (1975) found an association with the preluteal stage of the menstrual cycle and proved a relationship to pregnancy which was first noted by Bell (1830) (Fig. 2.2). Interstitial edema may be a factor, but no consistent relationship to toxemia has been established.

Bell's Palsy and Pregnancy

The most complete and reliable statistics on Bell's palsy come from the Facial Paralysis Clinic of the Kaiser Permanente Medical Center in California directed by Kedar Adour. Over a 3-year period the incidence of idiopathic facial paralysis in women of all ages and in those of child-bearing age was 17 per 100,000 per year. The frequency of Bell's palsy during pregnancy and the first two postpartum weeks was 57 per 100,000 per exposure year. Seventy-six per cent of these cases occurred in the third trimester and the first two puerperal weeks—an incidence of 118 per 100,000 per exposure year. Neither parity nor toxemia appeared to be a determining factor in this study (Hilsinger et al., 1975). Toxemia was found in about half the patients in two other series (Pope, 1969; Robinson, 1972).

Bell's palsy does not affect the course of pregnancy.

Prognosis and Treatment

The prognosis for recovery of a satisfactory facial expression and function is good if the initial paralysis is partial and fair if it is complete

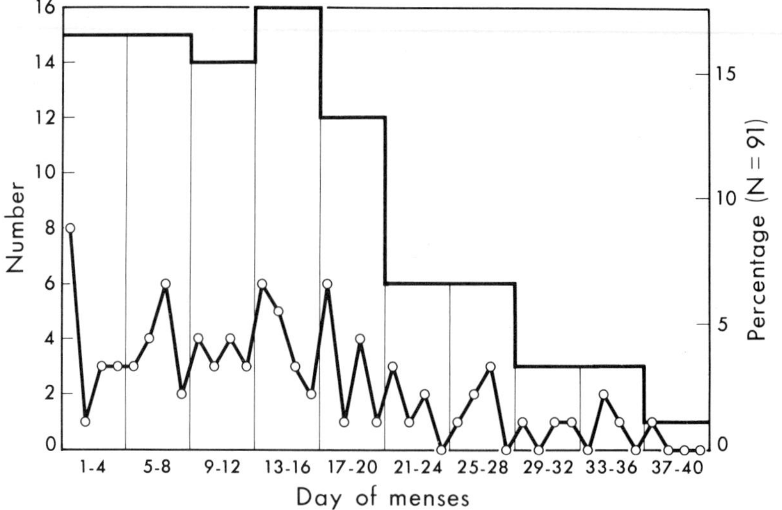

Figure 2.2. Onset of Bell's palsy in 91 women by number of days after onset of menses. From Hilsinger, R. L., Adour, K. K., and Doty, H. E. (1975) Idiopathic facial paralysis, pregnancy, and the menstrual cycle. *Annals of Otology, Rhinology and Laryngology.* Courtesy of R. L. Hilsinger, Jr.

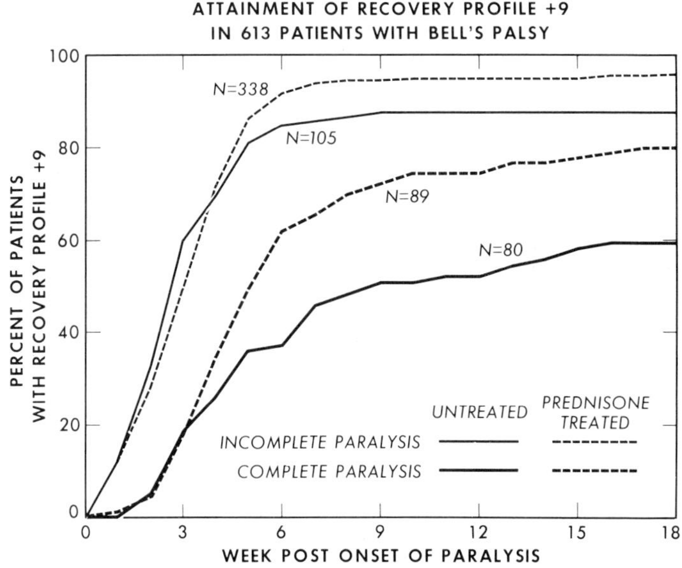

Figure 2.3. Attainment of satisfactory recovery (Adour's recovery profile ≥ + 9) in 613 patients with Bell's palsy according to initial completeness of paralysis and type of treatment. From Adour, K. K. (1975) The bell tolls for decompression? *New England Journal of Medicine,* **292,** 749. Courtesy of K. K. Adour.

(Adour, 1975) (Fig. 2.3). Loss of taste indicates a less favorable prognosis (Diamant et al., 1972). Bell's palsy that appears in the week before delivery can clear spontaneously in the early puerperium (Korczyn, 1971b).

A 10-day course of prednisone 40 to 60 mg per day increases the chances of recovery of function if it can be instituted within a week after onset of paralysis (Thomas, 1955; Taverner, 1966; Adour et al., 1972). Hilsinger et al. (1975) found similar results in pregnant women without apparent ill-effects to either the mother or the infant.

Surgical decompression of the facial nerve is not beneficial (Adour, 1975).

Carpal Tunnel Syndrome

The median nerve is highly vulnerable to compression within the carpal tunnel formed at the wrist by the flexor retinaculum. Any arthritic condition or tenosynovitis can compromise the space available for the nerve. Systemic diseases involving thickening of tissue (e.g., acromegaly, hypothyroidism, amyloidosis) are other possible causes. A transient carpal tunnel syndrome occurs during pregnancy.

Typically, a pregnant or menopausal woman awakens in the early morning hours with painful, burning tingling in one or both hands, usually the dominant hand. A deep aching may be felt along the inner aspect of the forearm. Subjectively the fingers feel useless and are often described as wooden. Pain is relieved by lifting the arm above the head or, for some, by dangling it over the edge of the bed. If this brings no relief, the patient will arise and walk about shaking and rubbing the hand.

In 1880 Putnam described this syndrome under the title of acroparesthesica. Since then there has been confusion about the relationship of median nerve compression to distal paresthesias in all fingers (Benson and Inman, 1956). About one-fifth of pregnant women complain of some pain in the hand (Nicholas et al., 1971), but few have the true carpal tunnel syndrome. Over half of the patients who complain of the characteristic set of symptoms when first seen will state that the tingling occurred in all fingers of the hand, including the little finger. In those instances the examiner must query the patient carefully about the severity of pain in each finger. Since the patient is not seen during the time of distress, a precise history may be difficult to elicit. It is useful to have the patient make notes during an attack. This is important since the diagnosis is mainly a historical one. If the little finger is involved, an additional lesion or another ailment (often postural obstruction of venous return) must be sought.

Upon examination there is little to be found. Occasionally percussion at the wrist over the median nerve elicits Tinel's sign. Transient ischemia produced by a blood pressure cuff may induce the paresthesias. Pin prick is blunted in the cutaneous distribution of the median nerve. Weakness and wasting of abductor pollicus brevis and opponens pollicus is unusual. In long-standing cases, motor nerve conduction across the wrist is slowed. Measurement of the median nerve's sensory action potential is the most sensitive test.

Treatment

Since pregnant women can expect their symptoms to regress after delivery, treatment need not be drastic. The first line of therapy consists of nocturnal splinting of the wrist. A lightweight plastic splint should be applied to the dorsum of the wrist, which should be in a neutral or slightly flexed position (Wilkinson, 1960). Extension of the wrist or the use of a volar splint may actually increase compression and produce more symptoms. The patient should not lie upon the affected arm.

Diuretics for pregnant women and estrogens for menopausal women have been used with variable, usually negligible, success. Those women who become symptomatic shortly after starting to take the Pill often find relief from diuretics for the month or two that paresthesias may last (Sabour, 1970).

The most effective second stage treatment is local injection of steroids into the carpal tunnel (Foster, 1960). Within 2 days approximately 80 per cent find relief which lasts 1 or 2 weeks. A month of weekly injections may give longer relief. Recurrence of signs merits surgery.

Division of the transcarpal ligaments produces immediate and permanent relief (Kremer et al., 1953). It is uncommon for a pregnant woman to require surgery (Tobin, 1967). True hypesthesia and motor involvement indicate surgery as first treatment and suggest a cause other than pregnancy.

Meralgia Paresthetica

Meralgia paresthetica is a minor but bothersome disorder of pregnancy. In 1895 Roth described painful paresthesia in the area innervated by the lateral femoral cutaneous nerve; he named it by combining *meros* and *algos,* the Greek nouns for thigh and pain. Typically, numbness, tingling, and stinging pain occur in the middle third of the lateral thigh. Symptoms are exaggerated by extending the hip when standing and relieved by sitting down. Men often complain that the slapping of coins and keys in their pockets against the leg accentuates the pain. Mild sensory loss to light touch and pin prick may be mapped out in the central area of hyperesthesia (Jones, 1974).

In pregnant women the symptoms of meralgia paresthetica usually begin about the thirtieth week of gestation (Rhodes, 1957). Age and parity are irrelevant. There is no predilection for either side, and the condition may be bilateral (Rhodes, 1957). It may recur with subsequent pregnancies (Price, 1909). In all patients, pregnant or nonpregnant, obesity or a recent rapid weight gain is common (Ecker and Woltman, 1938).

Since the lateral cutaneous nerve of the thigh is a purely sensory nerve, entrapment anywhere along its route will provoke similar symptoms (Fig. 2.4). The nerve is derived from the second and third lumbar roots. It runs interior to the iliacus muscle to exit from the pelvis under the inguinal ligament adjacent to the anterior superior iliac process. Thereafter it pierces the fascia lata and terminates in skin. In most cases the nerve is injured as it passes beneath the inguinal ligament (Keegan and Holyoke, 1962). Obesity and the exaggerated lumbar lordosis of pregnancy tend to stretch the nerve and make it more vulnerable to

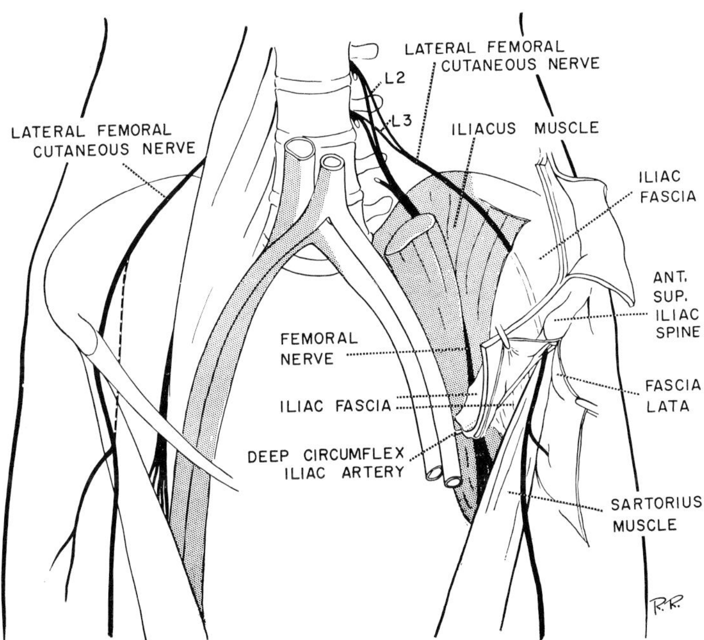

Figure 2.4. Course of the lateral cutaneous nerve of the thigh. From Keegan, J. J., and Holyoke, E. A. (1962) Meralgia paresthetica: An anatomical and surgical study. *Journal of Neurosurgery,* **19,** 342.

trauma (Pearson, 1957). In one patient the nerve was probably compressed within the pelvis as the pain of meralgia paresthetica coincided with the development of an intrapartum lumbosacral plexus palsy (Ecker and Woltman, 1938).

Since resolution of symptoms can be expected within 3 months after delivery, treatment consists of explaining the symptoms to the patient and reassuring her of their transient course in pregnant women; excessive weight gain should also be curbed. Temporary relief may be afforded by infiltrating local anesthetics into the nerve as it passes the inguinal ligament. If symptoms persist, the nerve must be transposed to decompress it (Keegan and Holyoke, 1962).

Recurrent Brachial Plexus Neuropathy

Recurrent brachial plexus neuropathy (neuralgic amyotrophy) has been reported in six families. In the women it is commonly associated with menarche, pregnancy, or the early puerperium. Brachial neutritis presents with severe and persistent pain and simultaneous (or shortly subsequent) rapid onset of weakness in the arm and shoulder. For the majority, pain diminishes as weakness increases. Fasciculations and wasting of the shoulder girdle ensue. The pathogenesis is unknown, but some cases are temporally related to an immunization; however, weakness need not be in the injected arm. It may be bilateral. Laboratory studies are not helpful. Improvement begins in 4 to 8 weeks with full functional recovery for 60 per cent within 1 year and for almost all within 3 years (Tsairis et al., 1972).

Familial mononeuritis multiplex with a brachial predilection is transmitted as an autosomal dominant trait (Taylor, 1960). Its appearance and course are similar to those of brachial neuritis, but it differs in that some patients will also have involvement of the lower cranial nerves and the lumbosacral plexus. The sexes are equally affected. Sixty-five per cent of the women developed one or more attacks during pregnancy or immediately postpartum (Geiger et al., 1974).

POLYNEUROPATHY DURING PREGNANCY

Guillain-Barré Syndrome

Guillain-Barré syndrome is an idiopathic polyneuritis of rapid onset in which weakness is more prominent than sensory loss. The syndrome can be labeled postinfectious polyneuritis if it occurs 1 to 3 weeks after infectious mononucleosis, mumps, measles, varicella, viral hepatitis, mycoplasmin infections, or immunizations. The pathology is a patchy infiltration of inflammatory cells with segmental demyelination throughout the peripheral nervous system (Asbury et al., 1969). The differential diagnosis must include diphtheria, botulism, porphyria, and poisoning with lead, arsenic, or triethyl cresyl phosphate.

Weakness develops over 1 to 3 weeks. Proximal muscles usually lose power before distal ones. Weakness may be symmetrical in distribution but not in degree. Areflexia is the rule. Involvement of respiratory and bulbar muscles may necessitate tracheostomy and assisted ventilation.

Sensory symptoms of pain, numbness, and paresthesia are more prominent than the minimal fading "glove and stocking" hypesthesia often found. In some cases loss of sensation is more predominant than loss of strength. Loss of a sense of joint position in hands and legs may long delay rehabilitation.

Manifestations of autonomic dysfunction include profuse sweating, periods of hypotension or hypertension, and cardiac arrhythmias. Since nasotracheal aspiration may provoke arrhythmias, the patient's pulse or electrocardiogram should be monitored by the nurse at bedside for several minutes after the procedure. Papilledema is found in 5 per cent of cases. Bladder function is not impaired, although the patient may have difficulty in voiding in bed.

The classic laboratory finding is an elevated CSF protein level with a CSF leukocyte count of below 10 cells per cu mm. A normal initial concentration of CSF protein indicates that the spinal roots are unaffected at that time and does not exclude the diagnosis. Repeated CSF examinations are indicated. Routine electrodiagnostic studies early in the course of the disease may be normal because most of the patches of demyelination have occurred proximally in the plexuses, not distally in the limbs where nerve conduction velocities are measured (Eisen and Humphreys, 1974). Serial routine determinations of nerve conduction velocity or special techniques to measure proximal neural conduction may be needed to detect the very slow conduction velocity expected in this disease.

Treatment consists of prevention of complications. This requires consistent, constant care by physicians, nurses, and physical therapists. Pulmonary infections are a constant concern. Bladder catheterization is to be avoided. Even if she is not bedridden, the chances of a pregnant woman developing thrombophlebitis and pulmonary embolism are increased. Cases of definite response to steroids are few and may be lost in large statistical studies. In most cases the hazards of steroids outweigh the low chance of benefit in a disease with a self-remitting course.

Improvement can be expected to begin within 3 or 4 weeks. Complete recovery may take months.

Effect of Pregnancy upon Guillain-Barré Syndrome

Guillain-Barré syndrome occurs in both sexes and in all age groups, although it is less common in the very young and the elderly. The simultaneous occurrence of Guillain-Barré syndrome and pregnancy is probably coincidental. Among 30 women of childbearing age within a 15-year series of 127 cases in Denmark, two women (6.6 per cent) were pregnant (Ravn, 1967). This is approximately the percentage of Danish women of childbearing age expected to be pregnant at any one time. About 30 cases of Guillain-Barré syndrome in pregnant women have been reported. The disease may begin at any time during gestation. Stabilization of the course and initiation of recovery proceed as usual regardless of the pregnancy.

Effect of Guillain-Barré Syndrome upon Pregnancy

A review of reported cases shows that pregnancy, delivery, and the fetus are unaffected by the disease. There does not appear to be any increase in the incidence of spontaneous abortion. Premature birth may be associated with severe cases in the third trimester. Labor and delivery are normal. Uterine contractions are unaffected. Forceps were used in one-half of the deliveries. In all cases the infant was normal. In one French series of eight cases high-dose steroids were used, and no harm to the infants was noted (Notter and Gaja, 1970).

Constant reassurances of eventual recovery and a normal child are of prime importance. Pregnant patients with Guillain-Barré syndrome are apprehensive enough without additional concerns about the pregnancy.

Recurrent Idiopathic Polyneuropathy

Recurrent polyneuropathy clinically similar to but distinct from the idiopathic Guillain-Barré syndrome has been observed in two women with each of their two or three pregnancies, and in one woman who was taking the Pill. The course differs from the Guillain-Barré syndrome in two ways. First, weakness—which seems to begin earlier during gestation with successive pregnancies—slowly progresses to quadriplegia over a period of many weeks. Second, remission of symptoms begins only after delivery. Perception of vibration and joint position is seriously impaired. Recovery to a functional state is slow (e.g., 4 to 10 months) and may not be complete. Infants are normal.

Besides the clinical differences, the antinerve antibodies frequently found in Guillain-Barré syndrome were absent in the one patient tested (Novak and Johnson, 1973). Cerebrospinal fluid is always acellular. The protein concentration in CSF is either normal or slightly elevated. Nerve conduction velocities are slow, and distal latencies are prolonged.

Gestational Distal Polyneuropathy

Gestational distal polyneuropathy is a symmetrical neuropathy caused by distal degeneration or diminution of axons with the longest axons being affected first. A similar neuropathy in alcoholics is more familiar. Fortunately, in countries where an adequate diet, antepartum supplemental vitamins, and effective antiemetics are commonplace, the condition is rare (Chaturachinda and McGregor, 1968). Indeed, it is rare enough that there have been no thorough studies with modern techniques. The condition still develops wherever malnutrition exists.

Gestational distal polyneuropathy presents in two ways: (1) a mild neuropathy which has an acute onset coinciding with the development of the Wernicke–Korsakoff syndrome, and (2) an insidiously progressive, subacute neuropathy which may include encephalopathy as a late manifestation.

Mild Neuropathy with Encephalopathy

It is appropriate that Sergei Korsakoff himself called attention to this association. In 1892 Korsakoff and Serbski published a report on an autopsy of a 27 year old woman in the fourth month of pregnancy. She had continued severe vomiting and became weak, confused, and confabulated but retained knee jerks until her death from parametritis and an iliac fossa abscess. Henderson (1914) noted the frequent association with hyperemesis gravidarum. He did not overlook Korsakoff's observation that polyneuritic symptoms need not always be present with psychosis. Berkwitz and Lufkin (1932) firmly defined the syndrome during pregnancy. Autopsies showed petechial hemorrhages in the mamillary bodies and brain stem—changes characteristic of Wernicke's encephalopathy (Fig. 2.5). Age and parity are irrelevant. Ordinary morning sickness appeared in the first 2 months of pregnancy but became intractable. Curiously, in many cases vomiting abruptly ceased when neurologic symptoms appeared in the third or fourth month of gestation.

Symptoms of paresthesias, dull aching numbness, and dysesthesias (i.e., very tender, painful soles of feet and heel cords) accompany a stocking sensory loss of perception of light touch or pain. As myotactic reflexes are lost, weakness develops. The most distal reflex, the ankle jerk, is the first to go. Joint position perception remains relatively intact.

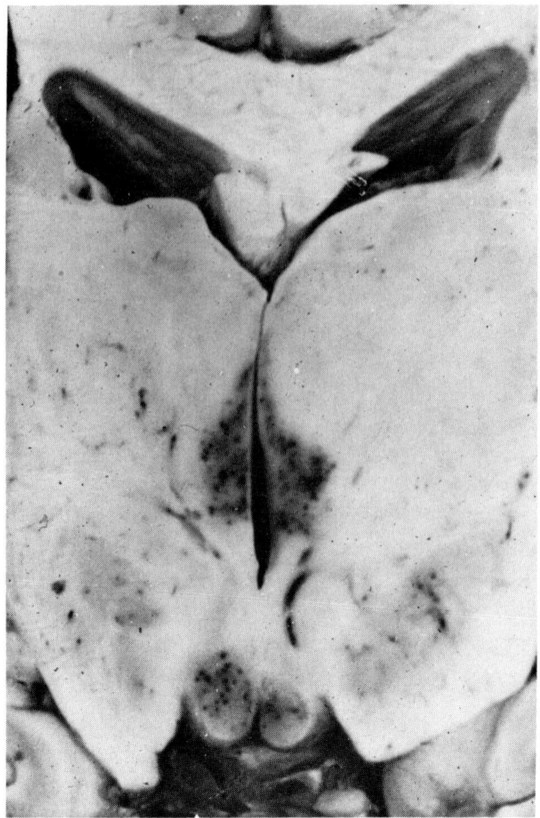

Figure 2.5. Coronal section through the brain of a woman who died of Wernicke's encephalopathy due to hyperemesis gravidarum. Note the petechial hemorrhages in the mammillary bodies and around the third ventricle. From Sheehan, H. L., and Lynch, J. B. (1973) *Pathology of Toxaemia of Pregnancy*. Edinburgh: Churchill Livingstone. Courtesy of Prof. Sheehan.

Almost coinciding with these changes is a global confusion which is more prominent clinically than the mild neuropathy. Sphincter control is disturbed, and tachycardia is found in at least one-half of cases (Berkwitz and Tufkin, 1932). Optic neuritis occurs. The neuropathy and encephalopathy advance together until death from cardiac complications ensues.

Pathogenesis: Although a woman with pernicious vomiting must obviously have a deficiency of several elements, thiamine deficiency must be at least one cause of this syndrome. In the 1930's and 1940's, thiamine deficiency was established as the cause of the Wernicke–Korsakoff syndrome.

The most intriguing chapter of that story began in 1932 on the silver fox ranch of J. S. Chastek in Glencoe, Minnesota. During that winter he fed his 200 foxes whole carp which had been caught in the Great Lakes and quickly frozen. No untoward effects were discovered for 3 to 6 weeks. But then the foxes went off their feed, appeared listless, and staggered with the appearance of weakness. Within a day or two the foxes could not stand, moaned as if in great pain, convulsed, and died. Within 1 month 34 per cent of his foxes died. However, Chastek's financial loss proved to be science's gain.

The cause of Chastek paralysis was a heat labile enzyme capable of inactivating thiamine by cleavage of the molecule (Yudkin, 1949). The condition would not develop if the fish were first cooked. It could be prevented or arrested by large supplements of liver or by parenteral thiamine injections. The pathology was analogous to that of Wernicke's encephalopathy in humans—bilaterally symmetrical hemorrhages in the paraventricular nuclei and in the gray matter of the brain stem (Evans et al., 1942).

Wernicke's encephalopathy is a syndrome with acute onset of nystagmus, extraocular muscle palsies, ataxia, and global confusion. In the United States it is most commonly found in alcoholics but has also been reported in prisoners of war, in patients with pyloric stenosis or chronic digitalis toxicity, and in those undergoing chronic renal dialysis. Thiamine reverses the ophthalmoplegias and the confusion of Wernicke's syndrome (Joliffe et al., 1941), but it does not necessarily improve the residual amnesic psychosis delineated by Korsakoff in his series of papers in the 1890's.

Severe Neuropathy Without Encephalopathy

In other cases severe neuropathy develops without any encephalopathy. From the early stage previously described, the diminished sensibility, weakness, and loss of reflexes proceed proximally in a glove and stocking fashion. Foot drop, wrist drop, and inability to arise from a chair unaided ensue. The patient becomes bedridden and unable to care for herself. Excellent nursing care and physical therapy as well as the use of devices such as foot pushboards and lightweight, cock-up wrist splints are necessary for optimal treatment of these patients.

Boulton described such a case to his colleagues in the Obstetrical Society of London in 1867. A 34 year old multipara developed quadriparesis, sensory loss, anorexia, and weight loss. In her eighth month of pregnancy, a macerated fetus was expelled with subsequent improvement in her strength. To Boulton the remarkable aspect of the case was that although she could answer questions rationally, her memory was completely gone and never did return. Encephalopathy can occur, as it did in this case, but it does so late in the course of the neuropathy and not at its onset. It is related to chronic malnutrition but not necessarily to hyperemesis gravidarum.

The similarities of this syndrome to neuritic beriberi were recognized (Hoffman, 1924; Burgess et al., 1958). Symptomatic beriberi can recur with successive pregnancies. Toxemia of pregnancy with beriberi became an epidemic in Hong Kong in the uncertain years before Japanese occupation in 1942 (King, 1945). Infantile beriberi is recognized (Burgess et al., 1958).

Pathogenesis

The concept of a thiamine-restricted diet causing a thiamine-responsive neuropathy is well founded in the pigeon (Swank, 1940) and to some extent in the rat (Prineas, 1970). With our present knowledge of the pathogenesis of Wernicke's syndrome it is ethically impossible to induce a thiamine deficiency in man. However, two subjects did develop a clinical neuropathy after 10 weeks on a thiamine intake restricted to 0.1 mg per day (Williams et al., 1943). During the next 7 weeks, ankle jerks and then knee jerks were lost as weakness developed. One subject was unable to walk unaided. Apathy, anorexia, emesis, and tachycardia were seen. With thiamine treatment a prompt improvement was noted, but one subject exhibited confusion and weakness 1 month later. Pantothenic acid (Bean et al., 1955) and pyridoxine (Vitler et al., 1953) deficiencies also have induced polyneuropathy in human subjects.

The exact cellular mechanisms are now being elucidated. The conventional wisdom holds that a multifactorial nutritional deficiency compromises the ability of the neuron to synthesize essential substances and to support the flow of metabolites along the axon to distal nerve endings. A supply of energy by oxidative metabolism is crucial to the whole process. Thiamine, as thiamine diphosphate (ThDP), acts as a cofactor for alpha-keto acid decarboxylase and transketolase, which are important in glycolysis and the hexose monophosphate shunt respectively.

However, 5 to 9 per cent of total animal body thiamine exists as a triphosphate (ThTP), which cannot substitute for thiamine diphosphate in the reactions just mentioned. Relatively high levels of thiamine triphosphate and a membrane-bound thiamine triphosphatase (ThTPase) are found in active membranes (Barchi, 1976a). Intriguing research indicates that ThTP and ThTPase are able to regulate the negative charge density on the inner surface of active membranes (Barchi, 1976b). This in turn could influence sodium flux.

While gestational distal polyneuropathy associated with hyperemesis gravidarum is ascribed to acute thiamine deprivation, chronic, more severe neuropathy is at the other end of the spectrum. It is caused by a chronic restriction of thiamine intake and possibly other factors.

Diagnosis and Treatment

Early thiamine deficiency can be documented by measuring erythrocyte transketolase activity (Brin, 1962; Dreyfus, 1962). This has not been done in gestational neuropathy.

Although satisfactory results have been obtained with administration of thiamine alone (Theobald, 1936), it seems prudent to treat these patients with an adequate diet, large doses of parenteral thiamine and other vitamins, and whatever physical therapy is appropriate for the extent of weakness. Strauss and McDonald (1933) had good results with inexpensive liver extract and yeast tablets.

Acute Intermittent Porphyria

Acute intermittent porphyria is an inborn error of heme synthesis which presents in the third and fourth decades with abdominal pain, a variety of mental aberrations, and neuropathy but without the photosensitivity characteristic of other porphyrias. More females than males are symptomatic in a 3:2 ratio, although the disease is transmitted as an autosomal dominant trait. Latent cases with or without porphyrinuria are found.

Clinical Presentation

Almost all patients with acute intermittent porphyria present with abdominal pain (Fig. 2.6). Of those patients, one-half are constipated and one-quarter complain of vomiting. Diarrhea is less common. The deep colicky pain is mainly located in the right iliac fossa and epigastrium, but it can be found in any location and it may be generalized. Pain may last from hours to days. Ileus is evident on an abdominal plain film. Although abdominal tenderness is present, it is much less pronounced than the agony of the patient would suggest. Significant tenderness suggests an acute surgical condition in the abdomen. Ectopic pregnancy has occurred with a porphyric crisis (Friedman and Beard, 1963). Less frequently psychiatric symptoms (e.g., depression) and, rarely, convulsions are the initial manifestations.

Neuropathy is an unusual presentation since it typically follows the abdominal symptoms by 3 days to 4 weeks. The pulse rate, the most sensitive indicator of disease activity, is already elevated before neuropathy is clinically present (Fig. 2.7). Administration of barbiturates doubles the chances that paralysis will develop and is associated with the most severely afflicted patients (Goldberg, 1959) (Fig. 2.10). Psychiatric disturbances are found in about 80 per cent of patients with neuropathy.

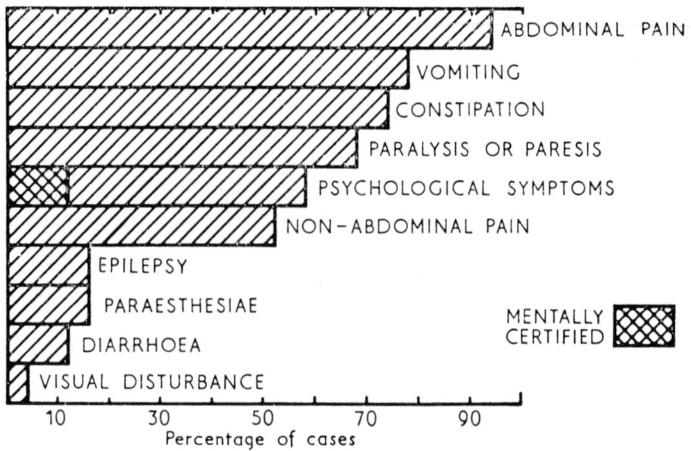

Figure 2.6. Incidence of symptoms in 50 cases of acute intermittent porphyria. From Goldberg, A. (1959) Acute intermittent porphyria: A study of 50 cases. *Quarterly Journal of Medicine*, **28**, 193.

Two clinical features suggestive of porphyric neuropathy may be present: (1) the paradoxical preservation of ankle jerks coexisting with areflexia elsewhere, and (2) a trunk or "bathing suit" distribution of superficial sensory loss (Ridley, 1969). An axonal neuropathy is present (Ridley, 1969; Sweeney et al., 1970).

Autonomic dysfunction is present as dyshydrosis and instability of

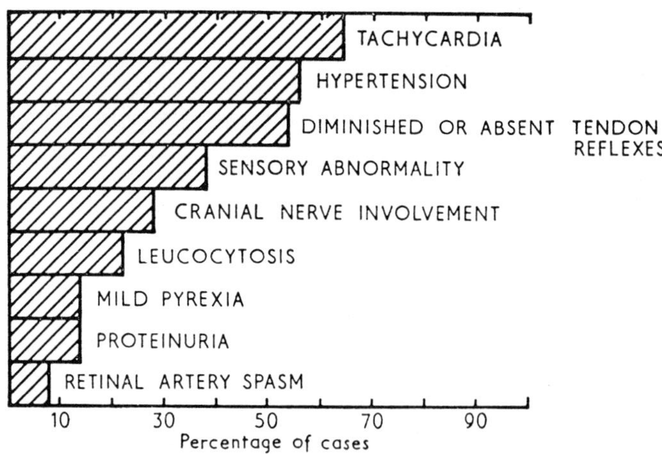

Figure 2.7. Incidence of signs in 50 cases of acute intermittent porphyria. From Goldberg, A. (1959) Acute intermittent porphyria: A study of 50 cases. *Quarterly Journal of Medicine*, **28**, 193.

blood pressure. Hypertension with or without orthostatic hypotension may be the most prominent feature of an attack and is of particular importance in pregnancy. Urinary catecholamines may be elevated (Beattie et al., 1973). Hypertension promptly responds to propranolol.

Seizures are a rare presenting symptom but often occur in the midst of a severe crisis. Hyponatremia secondary to inappropriate secretion of antidiuretic hormone has caused some seizures (Perlroth et al., 1966; Kerr, 1973).

Genetic Defect

The genetic defect is a deficiency of uroporphyrinogen I synthetase (Meyer et al., 1972). The result is insufficient negative feedback control of the rate-limiting step of porphyrin synthesis—the production of δ-aminolevulinic acid synthetase (Fig. 2.8). A 40-fold increase in hepatic mitochondrial δ-aminolevulinic acid synthetase activity has been demonstrated from biopsies of liver specimens taken during fulminant acute intermittent porphyria (Sweeney et al., 1970). The increase in urinary excretion of δ-aminolevulinic acid and porphobilinogen is the hallmark of the laboratory diagnosis of acute intermittent porphyria. Patients may describe burgundy colored urine if porphobilinogen has polymerized while in the bladder. The Watson-Schwartz test will show the characteristic color change.

The factors responsible for the metamorphosis of this condition from latency to acute crisis are poorly understood. Induction of δ-aminolevulinic acid synthetase is at least one effect of an ever-growing

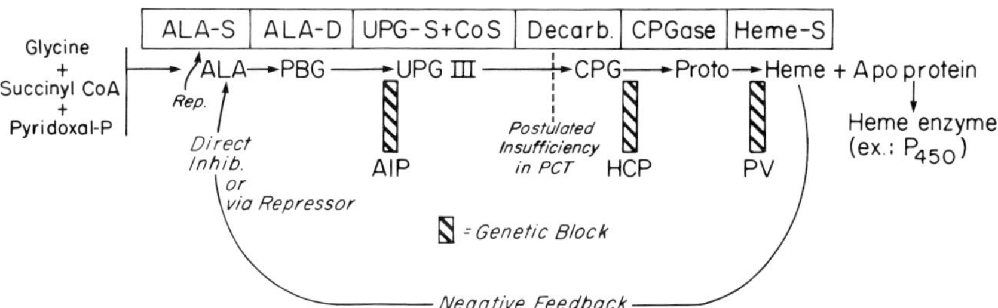

Figure 2.8. Porphyrin biosynthesis and the genetic partial blocks in the hepatic porphyrias. AIP = acute intermittent porphyria; ALA-D = δ-aminolevulinic acid dehydrase; ALA-S = δ-aminolevulinic acid synthetase; CO-S = uroporphyrinogen cosynthetase; CPGase = coproporphyrinogenase; Decarb = decarboxylase; HCP = hepatic coporphyria; Heme-S = heme synthetase (ferrochelatase); PBG = porphobilinogen; PCT = porphyria cutanea tarda; Proto = protoporphyrin; PV = porphyria variegata; Rep = repressor; UPG-S = uroporphyrinogen synthetase. From Watson, C. J. (1975) Hematin and porphyria. *New England Journal of Medicine*, **293**, 605. Courtesy of C. J. Watson.

Table 2.1. Clinical evidence for an interaction between steroid hormones and acute intermittent porphyria (AIP)

AIP becomes manifest after puberty.
Women account for 65 per cent of symptomatic cases.
Average age of onset in women is 25, a decade earlier than in men.
Regular premenstrual attacks occur in some women.
Pregnancy can induce a crisis.
Administration of steroid hormones (e.g., the Pill) may precipitate an attack or induce a remission.

list of substances that are known to provoke porphyric crises. Barbiturates, sulfonamides, griseofulvin, phenytoin, estrogens, progesterone, and oral contraceptives have all been implicated. Also associated are the fasting state, acute febrile illnesses, surgical procedures, and pregnancy. There is no explanation of why these factors may precipitate an attack in some patients but not in others, and why an attack occurs at one time and not at another in some individuals.

An interaction between sex hormones and acute intermittent porphyria is suggested by clinical observation (Table 2.1). Kappas and his colleagues (1974) found that steroids with a 5β configuration stimulated porphyrinogenesis by the liver by inducing formation of δ-aminolevulinic acid synthetase (Fig. 2.9). These investigators postulate that expression of acute intermittent porphyria is related to an increase of steroid hormone production and a shift in the pattern of steroid hormone metabolism from the 5α to the 5β pathway. Both changes occur at puberty.

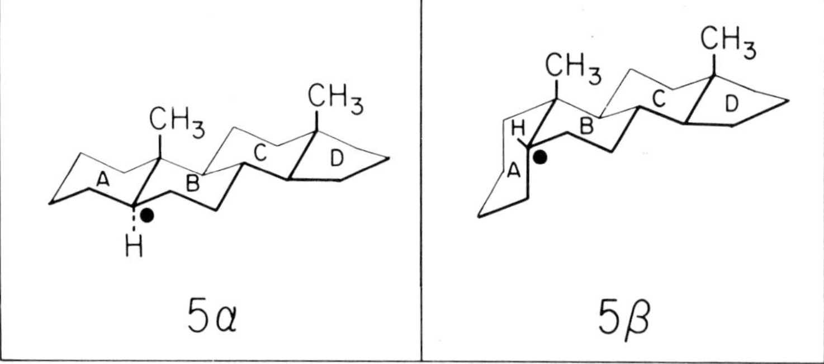

Figure 2.9. Nuclear structures of 5α and 5β steroids. The dot denotes the C5 position at the junction of A and B rings. From Kappas, A., Sassa, S., Granick, S., et al. (1974) Endocrine-gene interaction in the pathogenesis of acute intermittent porphyria. *Research Publications of the Association for Nervous and Mental Diseases,* **53**, 227. Courtesy of A. Kappas.

Effect of Menstruation and the Pill

For one group of women there is a definite relationship between repeated porphyric crises and the menstrual cycle and pregnancy. Relapse occurs most frequently in the premenstrual, luteal stage but has happened about the time of ovulation. For these women long-term combination oral contraceptives have resulted in prolonged remissions (Perlroth et al., 1965; Tschudy et al., 1975). In patients without a definite correlation of all crises with either menstruation or gestation, the Pill may precipitate a crisis. Women who have a blood relative with acute intermittent porphyria should avoid the Pill *(British Medical Journal,* 1972).

In healthy women the Pill causes an increase in daily urinary excretion of δ-aminolevulinic acid (i.e., 2.4 to 4.2 mg.) but no increase in daily porphobilinogen excretion (Koskelo et al., 1966). Excretion of porphyrin precursors is significantly increased in males and females with latent acute intermittent porphyria who were challenged with ethinyl estradiol. One experienced an acute attack. Progesterone can also induce an attack (Levit et al., 1957).

Amenorrhea during severe porphyric crises may occur, as with any severe illness, but it should always raise the question of pregnancy.

Effect of Pregnancy

For most women pregnancy has no ill effect upon acute intermittent porphyria and vice versa. However, over 100 exacerbations during pregnancy have been reported. For some women it is an established pattern.

About 60 per cent of relapses happen in early pregnancy. The majority are transient and do not affect the eventual successful outcome of the pregnancy. Some women habitually abort during these episodes, and remission of symptoms occurs thereafter. A correlation between morning sickness (with its attendant calorie deficit) and porphyric crises has not been attempted.

More serious are the 15 per cent of crises which occur during the second or third trimester. Prominent features are hypertension, hyperemesis, eclampsia, and often pre-existent renal disease. Prematurity and high maternal and fetal mortality rates are also characteristic of these crises.

Postpartum cases account for the remaining 25 per cent. Frequently intrapartum administration of barbiturate has precipitated the attack. Paralysis is common (Fig. 2.10).

The children of porphyric mothers are normal at birth regardless of genotype. In the one infant studied, δ-aminolevulinic acid, porphobilinogen, and coproporphyrins were present in the urine on the day of birth but were absent 6 days later (James and Rudolph, 1961). Amniotic fluid

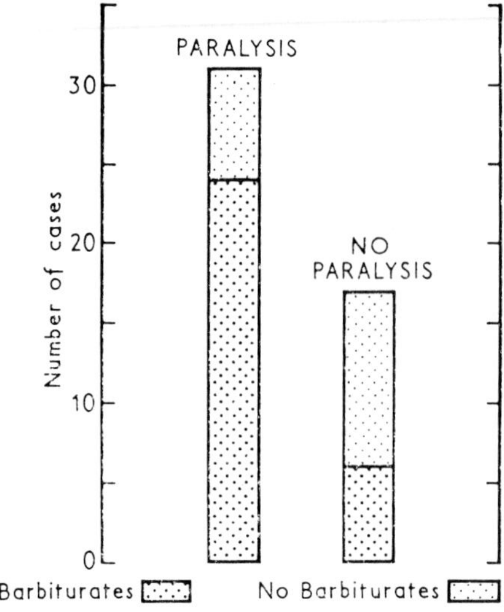

Figure 2.10. The relationship between barbiturate administration and paralysis in 48 patients with acute intermittent porphyria. From Goldberg, A. (1959) Acute intermittent porphyria: A study of 50 cases. *Quarterly Journal of Medicine,* **28,** 190.

contained porphyrins but neither δ-aminolevulinic acid nor porphobilinogen. Breast milk on the seventh postpartum day did not contain porphyrins or their precursors.

The greatest risk to a pregnant woman occurs when the existence of acute intermittent porphyria is unknown. Abdominal pain may prompt an exploratory laparotomy. Barbiturates may be administered, and caloric deficits may be allowed to continue. Consideration of acute intermittent porphyria in the differential diagnosis is the first step toward correct diagnosis. The delay in diagnosis in a group of women studied at the National Institutes of Health ranged from 2 weeks to 20 years (Stein and Tshudy, 1970).

Treatment

Treatment of porphyric crises consists of supportive care, maintenance of caloric needs (Welland, 1964b), and treatment or avoidance of precipitating factors (e.g., barbiturates). Chlorpromazine is the standard treatment for abdominal pain. Propranolol can reverse hypertension and tachycardia (Beattie et al., 1973). Unless propranolol has been given, the pulse rate is the most sensitive indicator of disease activity.

Negative feedback control of delta aminolevulinic acid synthetase by infusion of hematin has dramatically induced remission of central nervous system manifestations (Watson et al., 1973, 1975; Peterson et al., 1976; Watson, 1975).

PERIPARTUM LUMBAR DISC DISEASE

Relaxation of the spinal joints and accentuation of lumbar lordosis predispose pregnant women to low back pain. Mechanical low back pain that may radiate to the thigh is a common complaint during pregnancy. Acute herniation of a lumbar disc during pregnancy is uncommon (King, 1950). A large percentage of women who have back surgery remember that back pain was present years earlier during pregnancy (O'Connell, 1960).

Acute lumbar disc disease causes back pain which radiates down the leg to the foot. It is increased by sitting, standing, and Valsalva's maneuver. Usually only one nerve root is compressed in young patients unless a large protrusion compresses the cauda equina. Neurologic deficits vary according to the root involved.

Unless bowel or bladder sphincter control is lost, the best treatment is prolonged bed rest, local heat and massage, and analgesics. Diazepam, a commonly used sedative and muscle relaxant, should be avoided during pregnancy and lactation (see p. 183). Myelography and surgery can usually be deferred until after childbirth. Laminectomies have been performed during pregnancy without incident (O'Connell, 1960).

MATERNAL OBSTETRIC PALSIES

Compression of a peripheral nerve or nerve trunk can occur during labor and delivery. The injury may be caused by the fetal head, the application of forceps, trauma or hematoma during cesarean section, or improper positioning in leg holders.

Postpartum Foot Drop

The history of postpartum foot drop dates back to 1838 when von Basedow described foot drop after forceps rotation and delivery of a large infant in a deep transverse arrest. That same year Beatty described the second case, retold here.

> Ann Kierman, aged 21, delivered of her first child, November 26th, 1836, after a labour of 7 hours; infant alive. Nothing remarkable occurred during labour, or afterwards, until she complained on the second day, that she could not move her right leg, and that it felt benumbed and dead. On examining the limb, no swelling or pain could be discovered at any part that could indicate the approach of phlegmasia dolens; on the contrary, the sensibility of the limb appeared considerably lessened.
>
> Frictions, with warm turpentine, were ordered to the limb, but without any effect upon the condition of the part. At the end of a fortnight, finding that no improvement had taken place, a course of blisters along the line of the sciatic nerve was commenced, beginning above, and going downwards. This plan, together with attention to her general health, had the effect of gradually restoring the power of the limb. In a month she was able to walk across the ward with the as-

sistance of a stick, but even yet the leg was dragged along with difficulty, and when carried forward, the foot hung loose and vacillating, the toes pointing to the ground. In another month she had regained considerable power over the muscles, her progression was much more firm and steady, and the sensibility of the limb was almost entirely restored. She continued to improve until the month of February, at which time she was walking about nearly well, and preparing to leave the hospital, when puerperal fever made its appearance in our wards.

She died of pericarditis 1 week later.

Romberg (1851) was the first to associate painful spasms of the leg during the labor pains of either natural birth or birth with forceps with the subsequent palsy of the same limb. Hünerman (1892) made the critical observation that maternal palsies had maximum effect on the muscles supplied by the common peroneal (popliteal) nerve and so caused the foot to drop. He correctly ascribed this to the compression of the lumbosacral trunk, composed of fibers from the fourth and fifth lumbar segments, as it crosses the sacral ala that forms the posterior brim of the true pelvis (Fig. 2.11). A shallow concavity of the sacral ala makes the lumbosacral trunk even more vulnerable (Fig. 2.12) (Cole, 1946).

The typical syndrome occurs in a short (5 feet tall) primigravida carrying a relatively large baby (Brown and McDougall, 1957). The average birth weight of the infant is 3750 g or 8¼ pounds. Prolonged labor and midforceps rotation after a transverse arrest are common. The high proportion of midpelvic procedures reflects the fact that the bony

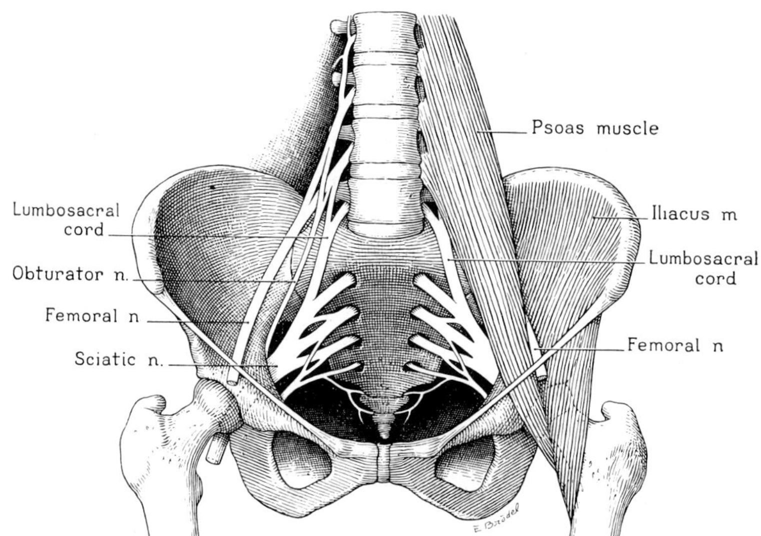

Figure 2.11. The relationship of the lumbosacral cord to the pelvis and the psoas major muscle. From Cole, J. T. (1946) Maternal obstetric paralysis. *American Journal of Obstetrics and Gynecology,* **52,** 374.

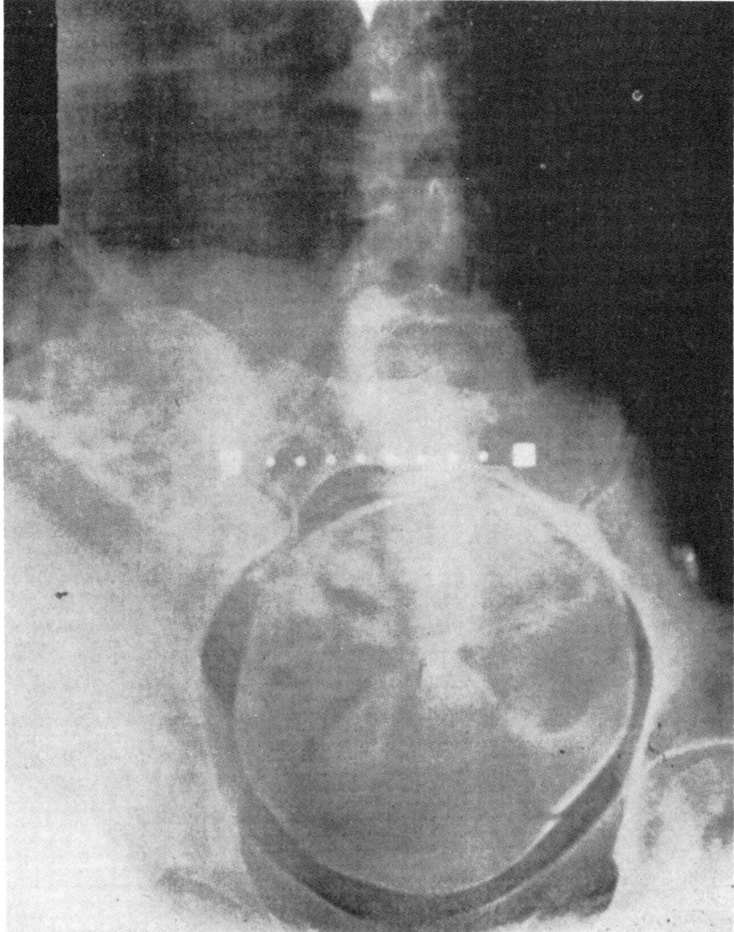

Figure 2.12. Pelvic radiograph of a woman who noted three hours before delivery pain and numbness in her left leg and loss of power in the dorsiflexors of the left ankle. The sacrum is asymmetric. The right sacral ala has a deep anterior concavity. The left sacral ala is shallow. The fetal head lying in the right occipitoanterior presentation impinges upon the left lumbosacral cord. From Cole, J. T. (1946) Maternal obstetric paralysis. *American Journal of Obstetrics and Gynecology,* **52,** 381.

structure of the pelvis interferes with the normal mechanism of rotation and descent during the second stage of labor. Radiographically, a pelvis associated with this complication shows a straight sacrum, a flat wide posterior pelvis, prominent sacroiliac joints, and posterior displacement of the transverse diameter of the inlet (Cole, 1946; Chalmers, 1949). The foot drop, which is almost always unilateral, is on the same side as the infant's brow during descent through the pelvis.

Paralysis is discovered when the woman is allowed out of bed. At first the limp may be attributed to a painful episiotomy. Weakness of ankle dorsiflexion and eversion is easily demonstrated. Numbness, paresthesias, and diminished cutaneous sensation are found along the lateral aspect of the leg and across the dorsum of the foot.

Almost identical symptoms can be produced by compression of the lateral peroneal nerve as it crosses the fibular head. This can be caused by poorly positioned leg holders. In that case the diminished sensibility is limited to the lower lateral aspect of the leg and is not found above the head of the fibula. Electrodiagnostic study will clearly show slow neural conduction across the knee but normal conduction below.

Prognosis

Nerve conduction velocities are helpful in formulating a prognosis after compression of the lumbosacral trunk, even though it is impossible to measure conduction velocity across the injured area. If the injury has been severe enough to damage the axons, the axons distal to the site of injury will conduct artificially stimulated impulses at a normal velocity until 6 days after the insult. Wallerian degeneration then takes place, causing the distal axon to be unexcitable. In this case (i.e., neurotmesis) the prognosis is poor, since the axon must regenerate along the length of the leg, a very slow process that will not always be completed.

If the nerve conduction velocity of the distal peroneal nerve is normal a week after the injury, it can be deduced that the axons are healthy even though compression has disrupted conduction across the injured segment (i.e., neuropraxia). The prognosis in this case is excellent, and full return of function occurs as the myelin sheath is repaired. Recovery can be expected within 3 months and usually sooner.

Treatment

If a foot drop is not treated, the heel cords shorten, resulting in a more severe disability than the foot drop alone. Ambulatory patients need a spring foot-drop splint or a similar device. At night and for bedridden patients, contracture can be prevented by a foot pushboard.

Subsequent Pregnancies

In the management of subsequent pregnancies the physician must attempt to prevent further nerve injury. Although fetal size is difficult to estimate correctly, many women have delivered smaller infants vaginally with problem. If a trial of labor proceeds smoothly, so much the better. Low forceps can be used with caution. However, the use of mid-forceps on a woman with a previous obstetrical lumbosacral trunk palsy invites danger. Cesarean section is prudent if a trial of labor is unsuccessful or if the infant is very large.

Femoral Neuropathy

The femoral (anterior crural) nerve may be injured during a cesarean section, hysterectomy, or other lower abdominal operation. Rarely, femoral neuropathy follows a normal vaginal delivery. The neuropathy is usually unilateral, but it may be bilateral. Indeed, the first report of femoral neuropathy following hysterectomy describes bilateral involvement (Gumpertz, 1896).

The femoral nerve is a large nerve with a root supply from L2, L3, and L4 (Fig. 2.13). Within the abdomen the femoral nerve is cushioned by the iliopsoas muscle, although hemorrhage into the muscle may compress the nerve (Sussens et al., 1968) (Fig. 2.11). The iliopsoas muscle is innervated by a branch just distal to the formation of the femoral nerve. As the femoral nerve exits from the abdomen next to the femoral artery, the nerve is vulnerable to direct trauma. Below the inguinal ligament, the nerve divides into branches that supply the quadriceps and sartorius muscles. Cutaneous branches supply superficial sensation to the anterior thigh and a medial strip that extends from the ankle almost to the groin.

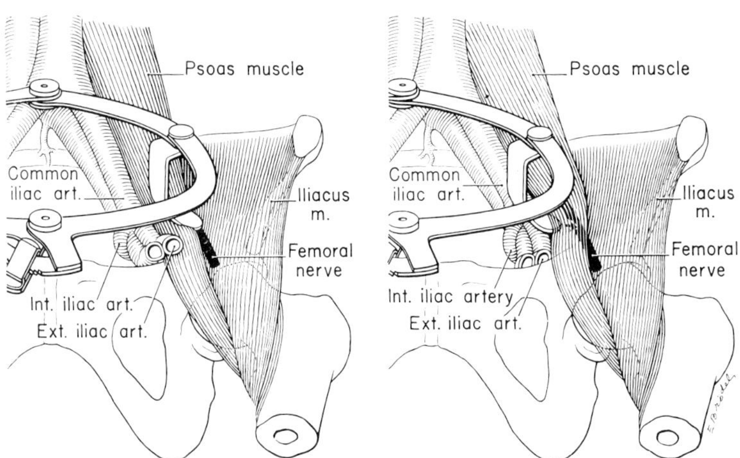

Figure 2.13. Diagrams showing the possible modes of injury to the femoral nerve caused by self-retaining retractors. From Vosburgh, L. F., and Finn, W. F. (1961) Femoral nerve impairment subsequent to hysterectomy. *American Journal of Obstetrics and Gynecology*, **82**, 935.

A typical patient is a thin woman who complains the day following surgery of weakness and numbness of the leg or of paresthesias in the neural distribution just described. Some patients find that they can walk on a level surface but cannot climb steps. The examiner finds severe weakness of the knee extensors (quadriceps femoris) and an absent knee jerk. If the proximal femoral nerve has been damaged, the hip flexors (iliopsoas) will also be weak. Motor involvement is usually more prominent clinically than sensory loss, which varies widely in severity and extent.

Analyses of reported cases found that most cases were managed by the use of self-retaining retractors and a Pfannenstiel incision (McDaniel et al., 1963; Rosenblum, 1966). A thin abdominal wall permits deeper and more lateral insertion of the retractor blades. The pressure exerted by these retractors, positioned against the greater psoas muscle, is at least strong enough to obliterate the femoral pulse (Buchbender and Weiss, 1961). Presumably the nerve is compressed (Fig. 2.13).

The prognosis is almost uniformly excellent, with recovery often beginning 2 or 3 weeks after delivery, although full recovery may take several months.

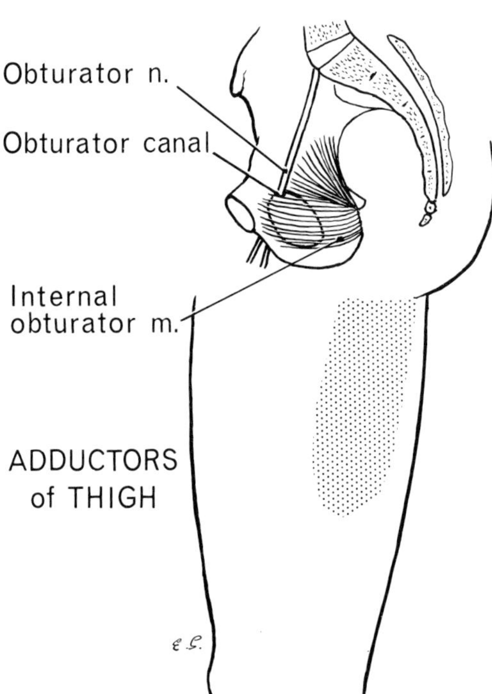

Figure 2.14. Obturator neuropathy is caused by compression along the wall of the pelvis or in the obturator canal. The stippled area shows area of sensory impairment. From Aguayo, A. J. (1975) Neuropathy due to compression and entrapment. In Dyck, P. J., Thomas, P. K., and Lambert, E. H. (eds.): *Peripheral Neuropathy,* Philadelphia: W. B. Saunders Company.

Obturator Neuropathy

Obturator neuropathy is a rare condition caused by a pelvic tumor, hematoma, obturator hernia, or difficult labor. The obturator nerve, composed of fibers from the third and fourth lumbar roots, runs along the pelvic wall underneath the psoas major muscle (Fig. 2.14). It emerges near the pelvic brim where it can be exposed to the fetal head or high forceps. Thereafter the obturator nerve exits through the obturator canal, supplying a cutaneous twig to the upper inner thigh and muscular branches to the large adductors of the thigh, the internal obturator muscle, and the gracilis.

At the time of compression, the woman may complain of a sharp pain in the groin and upper thigh. Later, weakness of hip adduction and rotation will be found, usually accompanied by diminished perception of light touch and pin prick over the upper inner thigh.

REFERENCES

Catamenial Sciatica

Baker, G. S., Parsons, W. R., and Welch, J. S. (1966) Endometriosis within the sheath of the sciatic nerve: Report of two patients with progressive paralysis. *Journal of Neurosurgery,* **25**, 652–655.

Dagnelie, M. J. (1947) Lombo-sciatalgie et endocrinologie: Contribution à l'étude des endométriomes hétérotopiques. *Annales d'Endocrinologie* (Paris), **8**, 26–31.

Denton, R. O., and Sherrill, J. D. (1955) Sciatic syndrome due to endometriosis of sciatic nerve. *Southern Medical Journal,* **48**, 1027–1031.

Granberry, W. M., Henderson, E. D., Miller, R. H. et al. (1959) Endometriosis of the sciatic nerve with evidence of pelvic endometriosis. *Minnesota Medicine,* **42,** 1794–1797.

Guiot, G., Levy, J., Auquier, L., et al. (1965) Sciatique par endométriose (La sciatique cataméniale). *Presse medicale,* **73,** 1397, 1398.

Head, H. B., Welch, J. S., Mussey, E. et al. (1962) Cyclic sciatica: Report of case with introduction of a new surgical sign. *Journal of the American Medical Association,* **180,** 521–524.

Kohorn, E. I. (1963) Neurological complications of endometriosis. *Proceedings of the Royal Society of Medicine,* **56**, 874, 975.

Lattes, R., Shepard, F., Tovell, H. et al. (1956) A clinical and pathologic study of endometriosis of the lung. *Surgery, Gynecology, Obstetrics,* **103**, 552–558.

Lombardo, L., Mateos, J. H., and Barroeta, F. F. (1968) Subarachnoid hemorrhage due to endometriosis of the spinal cord. *Neurology,* **18,** 423–426.

Roth, L. M. (1973) Endometriosis with perineural involvement. *American Journal of Clinical Pathology,* **59**, 807–809.

Zangger, J., and Heppner, F. (1962) Endometriose im Wirbelloch als Ursache einer periodischen Wurzelneuralgia. *Geburtshilfe und Frauenheilkunde,* **22,** 1482–1493.

Bell's Palsy

Adour, K. K. (1975) The bell tolls for decompression? *New England Journal of Medicine,* **292**, 748–750.

Adour, K. K., and Wingerd, J. (1974) Idiopathic facial paralysis (Bell's palsy): Factors affecting severity and outcome in 446 patients. *Neurology,* **24,** 1112–1116.

Adour, K. K., Wingerd, J., and Bell, D. N. (1972) Prednisone treatment for idiopathic facial paralysis (Bell's palsy). *New England Journal of Medicine,* **287,** 1268–1272.

Bell, C. (1830) *The Nervous System of the Human Body*. J. Taylor, Appendix, pp. iv, v. London: Longman, Rees, Orme, Brown, and Green.

Diamant, H., Ekstrand, T., and Wiberg, A. (1972) Prognosis of idiopathic Bell's palsy. *Archives of Otolaryngology,* **95**, 431–433.

Hilsinger, R. L., Adour, K. K., and Doty, H. E. (1975) Idiopathic facial paralysis, pregnancy, and the menstrual cycle. *Annals of Otology, Rhinology and Laryngology,* **84,** 433–442.

Korczyn, A. D. (1971a) Bell's palsy and diabetes mellitus. *Lancet,* **1,** 108–110.

Korcyzn, A. D. (1971b) Bell's palsy and pregnancy. *Acta Neurologica Scandinavica,* **47,** 603–607.

McCormick, D. P. (1972) Herpes simplex virus as a cause of Bell's palsy. *Lancet,* **2,** 937, 938.

Pope, T. H., and Kenan, P. D. (1969) Bell's palsy in pregnancy. *Archives of Otolaryngology* **89**, 830–834.

Robinson, J. R., and Pou, J. W. (1972) Bell's palsy: A predisposition of pregnant women. *Archives of Otolaryngology,* **95**, 125–129.

Thomas, M. H. (1955) Treatment of Bell's palsy with cortisone and other measures. *Neurology,* **5**, 882–886.

Taverner, D., Fearnley, M. E., and Kemble, F. (1966) Prevention of denervation in Bell's palsy. *British Medical Journal,* **1**, 391–393.

Carpal Tunnel Syndrome

Benson, R. C., and Inman, V. T. (1956) Brachialgia statica dysesthetica in pregnancy. *Western Journal of Surgery,* **64**, 115–130.

Foster, J. B. (1960) Hydrocortisone and the carpal tunnel syndrome. *Lancet,* **1**, 454–456.

Hamlin, E., and Lehman, R. A. W. (1967) Carpal tunnel syndrome. *New England Journal of Medicine,* **276**, 849, 850.

Kremer, M., Gilliatt, R. W., Golding, J. S. R. et al. (1953) Acroparaesthesiae in the carpal tunnel syndrome. *Lancet,* **2**, 590–595.

Layton, K. B. (1958) Acroparaesthesia in pregnancy and the carpal tunnel syndrome. *Journal of Obstetrics and Gynaecology of the British Empire,* **65**, 823–825.

Nicholas, G. G., Noone, R. B., and Graham, W. P. (1971) Carpal tunnel syndrome in pregnancy. *Hand,* **3,** 80–83.

Putnam, J. J. (1880) A series of cases of paraesthesia, mainly of the hands, of periodic recurrence, and possibly of vaso-motor origin. *Archives of Medicine,* **4**, 147–162.

Sabour, M. S., and Fadel, H. E. (1970) The carpal tunnel syndrome—a new complication of the "pill." *American Journal of Obstetrics and Gynecology,* **107**, 1265–1267.

Tobin, S. M. (1967) Carpal tunnel syndrome in pregnancy. *American Journal of Obstetrics and Gynecology,* **97**, 493–498.

Wilkerson, M. (1960) The carpal tunnel syndrome in pregnancy. *Lancet,* **1**, 453, 454.

Wood, A. (1961) Paraesthesia of the hand in pregnancy. *British Medical Journal,* **2**, 680–682.

Meralgia Paresthetica

Ecker, A. D., and Woltman, H. W. (1938) Meralgia paresthetica: A report of one hundred and fifty cases. *Journal of the American Medical Association,* **110**, 1650–1652.

Jones, R. K. (1974) Meralgia paresthetica as a cause of leg discomfort. *Canadian Medical Association Journal,* **111**, 541, 542.

Keegan, J. J., and Holyoke, E. A. (1962) Meralgia paresthetica: An anatomical and surgical study. *Journal of Neurosurgery,* **19**, 341–345.

Musser, J. H., and Sailer, J. (1900) Meralgia paresthetica (Roth), with the report of ten cases. *Journal of Nervous Mental Diseases,* **27**, 16–40.

Pearson, M. G. (1957) Meralgia paresthetica: With reference to its occurrence in pregnancy. *Journal of Obstetrics and Gynaecology of the British Empire,* **64**, 427–430.

Peterson, P. H. (1952) Meralgia paresthetica related to pregnancy. *American Journal of Obstetrics and Gynecology,* **64**, 690, 691.

Price, G. E. (1909) Meralgia paresthetica, recurring with repeated pregnancies. *American Medicine,* **4,** 210–212.

Rhodes, P. (1957) Meralgia paresthetica in pregnancy. *Lancet*, **2**, 831.

Roth, V. K. (1895) Meralgia paresthetica. *Meditsinskoye Obozrieniye (Moskow)*, **43**, 678–688.

Recurrent Brachial Plexus Neuropathy

Bradley, W. G., Madrid, R., Thrush, D. C. et al. (1975) Recurrent brachial plexus neuropathy. *Brain*, **98**, 381–398.

Geiger, L. R., Mancall, E. L., Penn, A. S. et al. (1974) Familial neuralgic amyotrophy: Report of three families with review of the literature. *Brain*, **97**, 87–102.

Jacob, J. C., Andermann, F., and Robb, J. P. (1961) Heredofamilial neuritis with brachial predilection. *Neurology*, **11**, 1025–1033.

Taylor, R. A. (1960) Heredofamilial mononeuritis multiplex with brachial predilection. *Brain*, **83**, 113–137.

Tsairis, P., Dyck, P. J., and Mulder, D. W. (1972) Natural history of brachial plexus neuropathy: Report of 99 patients. *Archives of Neurology*, **27**, 109–117.

Ungley, C. C. (1933–34) Recurrent polyneuritis in pregnancy and the puerperium affecting three members of a family. *Journal of Neurology and Psychopathology*, **14**, 15–26.

Guillain-Barré Syndrome

Asbury, A. K., Arnason, B. G., and Adams, R. D. (1969) The inflammatory lesion in idiopathic polyneuritis. *Medicine*, **48**, 173–215.

Betson, J. R., and Golden, M. L. (1960) Guillain-Barré syndrome in pregnancy. *Obstetrics and Gynecology*, **15**, 391–393.

Eisen, A., and Humphreys, P. (1974) The Guillain-Barré syndrome: A clinical and electrodiagnostic study of 25 cases. *Archives of Neurology*, **30**, 438–443.

Elstein, M., Legg, N. J., Murphy, M. et al. (1971) Guillain-Barré syndrome in pregnancy: Respiratory paralysis. *Anaesthesia*, **26**, 216–224.

Kalstone, B. M., and Pearce, F. (1959) Guillain-Barré syndrome in a pregnant woman. *American Practitioner*, **10**, 674–676.

Maisel, J. J., and Woltman, H. W. (1934) Neuronitis of pregnancy without vomiting. *Journal of the American Medical Association*, **103**, 1930, 1931.

Osler, L. D., and Sidell, A. D. (1960) The Guillain-Barré syndrome: The need for exact diagnostic criteria. *New England Journal of Medicine*, **262**, 964–969.

Notter, A., and Gaja, R. (1970) Syndrome de Guillain-Barré et grossesse (À propos de 8 observations). *Lyon Medical*, **223**, 156–162.

Radman, H. M. (1967) Guillain-Barré disease complicating pregnancy. *Maryland Medical Journal*, **16**, 54–56.

Ravn, H. (1967) The Landry-Guillain-Barré syndrome. *Acta Neurologica Scandinavica*, Suppl. 30, **43**, 1–64.

Rudolph, J. H., Norris, F. H., Garvey, P. H. et al. (1965) The Landry-Guillain-Barré syndrome in pregnancy: A review. *Obstetrics and Gynecology*, **26**, 265–271.

Sudo, N., and Weingold, A. B. (1975) Obstetric aspects of the Guillain-Barré syndrome. *Obstetrics and Gynecology*, **45**, 39–43.

Zfass, H. S., Zfass, I. S., Troland, C. E. et al. (1954) Guillain-Barré syndrome: Report of a case in pregnancy and a review of the literature. *Virginia Medical Monthly*, **81**, 72–75.

Recurrent Idiopathic Polyneuropathy

Calderon-Gonzales, R., Gonzales-Cantu, N., and Rizzi-Hernandez, H. (1970) Recurrent polyneuropathy with pregnancy and oral contraceptives. *New England Journal of Medicine*, **282**, 1307, 1308.

Novak, D. J., and Johnson, K. P. (1973) Relapsing idiopathic polyneuritis during pregnancy. *Archives of Neurology*, **28**, 219–223.

Gestational Distal Polyneuropathy

Barchi, R. L. (1976a) Thiamine triphosphatases in the brain. *In* Gubler, C., Fujiwara, M., and Dreyfus, P. (eds.) *Thiamine*. New York: John Wiley & Sons, pp. 195–212.

Barchi, R. L. (1976b) The nonmetabolic role of thiamine in excitable membrane function.

In Gubler, C., Fujiwara, M., and Dreyfus, P. (eds.): *Thiamine*. New York: John Wiley & Sons, pp. 283–305.

Bean, W. B., Hodges, R. E., Daum, K. et al. (1955) Pantothenic acid deficiency induced in human subjects. *Journal of Clinical Investigation,* **34**, 1073–1084.

Berkwitz, N. J., and Lufkin, N. H. (1932) Toxic neuronitis of pregnancy: A clinicopathological report. *Surgery, Gynecology, Obstetrics,* **54**, 743–757.

Boulton, P. (1867) Case of paraplegia occurring during pregnancy. *Transactions of the Obstetrical Society of London,* **9**, 12–15.

Brin, M. (1962) Erythrocyte transketolase in early thiamine deficiency. *Annals of the New York Academy of Science,* **98**, 528–541.

Burgess, R. C., Platt, B. S., Follis, R. H,, Handler, P., and Denny-Brown, D. (1958) Beriberi. *Federation Proceedings,* **17**, 3–56.

Chaturachinda, K., and McGregor, E. M. (1968) Wernicke's encephalopathy and pregnancy. *Journal of Obstetrics and Gynaecology of the British Commonwealth,* **75**, 969–971.

Dreyfus, P. M. (1962) Clinical application of blood transketolase determinations. *New England Journal of Medicine,* **267**, 596–598.

Evans, C. A., Carlson, W. E., Green, R. G. (1942) The pathology of Chastek paralysis in foxes: A counterpart of Wernicke's hemorrhagic polioencephalitis of man. *American Journal of Pathology,* **18**, 79–89.

Henderson, D. K. (1914) Korsakow's psychosis occurring during pregnancy. *Bulletin of the Johns Hopkins Hospital,* **25**, 261–270.

Hoffman, A. J. (1924) Beriberi in Chinese women and its relation to childbearing. *China Medical Journal,* **38**, 987–993.

Ironside, R. (1939) Neuritis complicating pregnancy. *Proceedings of the Royal Society of Medicine,* **32**, 588–595.

Jolliffe, N., Wortis, H., and Fein, H. D. (1941) The Wernicke syndrome. *Archives of Neurology and Psychiatry,* **46**, 569–597.

King, G., and Ride, L. T. (1945) The relation of vitamin B_1 deficiency to the pregnancy toxaemias. *Journal of Obstetrics and Gynaecology of the British Empire,* **52**, 130–147.

Korsakow, S., and Serbski, W. (1892) Ein Fall von polyneuritischer Psychose mit Autopsie. *Archiv für Psychiatrie und Nervenkrankheiten,* **23,** 112–134.

McGoogan, L. S. (1942) Severe polyneuritis due to vitamin B deficiency in pregnancy. *American Journal of Obstetrics and Gynecology,* **43,** 752–762.

Prineas, J. (1970) Peripheral nerve changes in thiamine-deficient rats. *Archives of Neurology,* **23**, 541–548.

Reynolds, E. S. (1897) Peripheral neuritis connected with pregnancy and the puerperal state. *British Medical Journal,* **2**, 1080–1082.

Sheehan, H. L., and Lynch, J. B. (1973) *Pathology of Toxaemia of Pregnancy*. Baltimore: The Williams & Wilkins Company.

Strauss, M. B., and McDonald, W. J. (1933) Polyneuritis of pregnancy: A dietary deficiency disorder. *Journal of the American Medical Association,* **100**, 1320–1323.

Swank, R. L. (1940) Avian thiamine deficiency: A correlation of the pathology and clinical behavior. *Journal of Experimental Medicine,* **71**, 683–702.

Theobald, G. W. (1936) Neuritis in pregnancy successfully treated with vitamin B_1. *Lancet,* **1**, 834–837.

Victor, M., Adams, R. D., and Collins, G. H. (1971) *The Wernicke-Korsakoff Syndrome*. Philadelphia: F. A. Davis Company.

Vitler, R. W., Mueller, J. F., and Glazer, H. S. (1953) The effect of vitamin B_6 deficiency induced by desoxypyridoxine in human beings. *Journal of Laboratory and Clinical Medicine,* **42,** 335–356.

Whitfield, D. W. (1889) Peripheral neuritis due to vomiting of pregnancy. *Lancet,* **1**, 627, 628.

Williams, P. F., Griffith, G. C., and Fralin, F. G. (1940) The relation of vitamin B_1 to the reproductive cycle. *American Journal of Obstetrics and Gynecology,* **40**, 181–193.

Williams, R. D., Mason, H. I., Power, M. H. et al. (1943) Induced thiamine (vitamin B_1) deficiency in man. *Archives of Internal Medicine,* **71**, 38–53.

Yudkin, W. H. (1949) Thiaminase, the Chastek-paralysis factor. *Physiological Reviews,* **29**, 389–402.

Acute Intermittent Porphyria

General References

Goldberg, A. (1959) Acute intermittent porphyria: A study of 50 cases. *Quarterly Journal of Medicine,* **28**, 183–209.

Kappas, A., Sassa, S., Granick, S. et al. (1974) Endocrine-gene interaction in the pathogenesis of acute intermittent porphyria. *Research Publications of the Association for Research in Nervous and Mental Disease,* **53,** 225–237.

Meyer, U. A., Strand, L. J., Doss, M. et al. (1972) Intermittent acute porphyria – Demonstration of genetic defect in porphobilinogen metabolism. *New England Journal of Medicine,* **286**, 1277–1282.

Perlroth, M. G., Tschudy, D. P., Marver, H. S. et al. (1966) Acute intermittent porphyria: New morphologic and biochemical findings. *American Journal of Medicine,* **41**, 149–162.

Ridley, A. (1969) The neuropathy of acute intermittent porphyria. *Quarterly Journal of Medicine,* **38**, 307–333.

Stein, J. A., and Tschudy, D. P. (1970) Acute intermittent porphyria: A clinical and biochemical study of 46 patients. *Medicine,* **49,** 1–16.

Sweeney, V. P., Pathak, M. A., and Asbury, A. K. (1970) Acute intermittent porphyria: Increased ALA-synthetase activity during an acute attack. *Brain,* **93**, 369–380.

Tschudy, D. P., Valsamis, M., and Magnussen, C. R. (1975) Acute intermittent porphyria: Clinical and selected research aspects. *Annals of Internal Medicine,* **83**, 851–864.

Effect of Exogenous Hormones

British Medical Journal (1972) The Pill and porphyria. *British Medical Journal,* **3**, 603, 604.

Koskelo, P., Eisalo, A., and Toivonen, I. (1966) Urinary excretion of porphyrin precursors and coproporphyrin in healthy females on oral contraceptives. *British Medical Journal,* **1**, 652–654.

Levit, E. J., Nodine, J. H., and Perloff, W. H. (1957) Progesterone-induced porphyria: Case report. *American Journal of Medicine,* **22**, 831–833.

Perlroth, M. G., Marver, H. S., and Tschudy, D. P. (1965) Oral contraceptive agents and the management of acute intermittent porphyria. *Journal of the American Medical Association,* **194**, 1037–1042.

Redecker, A. G. (1963) The effect of the administration of oestrogens on acute porphyria. *South African Journal of Laboratory and Clinical Medicine,* **9**, 302, 303.

Remington, C., and DeMatteis, F. (1965) Oral contraceptives and acute intermittent porphyria. *Lancet,* **1**, 270.

Tschudy, D. P., Valsamis, M., and Magnussen, C. R. (1975) Acute intermittent porphyria: Clinical and selected research aspects. *Annals of Internal Medicine,* **83**, 851–864.

Watson, C. J., Runge, W., and Bossenmaier, I. (1962) Increased urinary porphobilinogen and uroporphyrin after administration of stilbestrol in a case of latent porphyria. *Metabolism,* **11**, 1129–1133.

Welland, F. H., Hellman, E. S., Collins, A. et al. (1964a) Factors affecting the excretion of porphyrin precursors by patients with acute intermittent porphyria: II. The effect of ethinyl estradiol. *Metabolism,* **13,** 251–255.

Zimmerman, T. S., McMillin, J. M., and Watson, C. J. (1966) Onset of manifestations of hepatic porphyria in relation to the influence of sex hormones. *Archives of Internal Medicine,* **118**, 229–240.

Effect of Pregnancy

Freedman, A., Yeagley, J. D., and Brooks, J. B. (1952) Acute porphyria with improvement during and following pregnancy. *Annals of Internal Medicine,* **36**, 1111–1120.

Friedman, M., and Beard, R. W. (1963) Acute intermittent porphyria complicated by a secondary abdominal pregnancy. *British Medical Journal,* **2**, 298.

Hughes, R. T. (1957) Acute porphyria in pregnancy. *Lancet,* **1**, 301–303.

Hunter, D. J. S. (1971) Acute intermittent porphyria and pregnancy. *Journal of Obstetrics and Gynaecology of the British Commonwealth,* **78**, 746–750.

James, C. W., Rudolph, S. G., and Abbott, L. D. (1961) Delta-aminolevulinic acid, porphobilinogen, and porphyrin excretion throughout pregnancy in a patient with acute intermittent porphyria with "passive porphyria" in the infant. *Journal of Laboratory and Clinical Medicine,* **58**, 437–444.

Kerr, G. D. (1973) Acute intermittent porphyria and inappropriate secretion of antidiuretic hormone in pregnancy. *Proceedings of the Royal Society of Medicine,* **66**, 763–764.

Neilson, D. R., and Neilson, R. P. (1958) Porphyria complicated by pregnancy. *Western Journal of Surgery,* **66**, 133–149.

Shapiro, H. I., Mazur, J. R., and Emich, J. P. (1969) Acute intermittent porphyria and pregnancy. *Obstetrics and Gynecology,* **34**, 189–193.

Tricomi, V., and Baum, H. (1958) Acute intermittent porphyria and pregnancy: A review. *Obstetric and Gynecologic Survey,* **13**, 307–318.

Tweedy, J. A., and Mattox, J. H. (1965) Acute intermittent porphyria and eclampsia. *Obstetrics and Gynecology,* **25**, 493–494.

TREATMENT

Beattie, A. D., Moore, M. R., Goldberg, A. et al. (1973) Acute intermittent porphyria: Response of tachycardia and hypertension to propranolol. *British Medical Journal,* **3**, 257–260.

Peterson, A., Bossenmaier, I., Cardinal, R. et al. (1976) Hematin treatment of acute porphyria: Early remission of an almost fatal relapse. *Journal of the American Medical Association,* **235**, 520–522.

Watson, C. J., Dhar, J., Bossenmaier, I. et al. (1973) Effect of hematin in acute porphyric relapse. *Annals of Internal Medicine,* **79**, 80–83.

Watson, C. J. (1975) Hematin and porphyria. *New England Journal of Medicine,* **293**, 605, 606.

Welland, F. H., Hellman, E. S., Gaddis, E. M. et al. (1964b) Factors affecting the excretion of porphyrin precursors by patients with acute intermittent porphyria: I. The effect of diet. *Metabolism,* **13**, 232–250.

Postpartum Foot Drop

Adler, E., Jarus, A., and Magora, A. (1956) Rare peripheral nerve complications in obstetrical and gynaecological conditions. *Acta Psychologica et Neurologica Scandinavica,* **31**, 1–7.

von Basedow, K. A. (1838) Über Neuralgia puerperarum cruralis. *Wochenschrift für die gesammte Heilkunde,* **6**, 636–639.

Beatty, T. E. (1838) Paralysis after delivery. *Irish Journal of Medical Science,* **12**, 304–306.

Brown, J. T., and McDougall, A. (1957) Traumatic maternal birth palsy. *Journal of Obstetrics and Gynaecology of the British Empire,* **64**, 431–435.

Burkhart, F. L., and Daly, J. W. (1966) Sciatic and peroneal nerve injury: A complication of vaginal operations. *Obstetrics and Gynecology,* **28**, 99–102.

Chalmers, J. A. (1949) Traumatic neuritis of the puerperium. *Journal of Obstetrics and Gynaecology of the British Empire,* **56**, 205–216.

Cole, J. T. (1946) Maternal obstetric paralysis. *American Journal of Obstetrics and Gynecology,* **52**, 372–386.

Hill, E. C. (1962) Maternal obstetric paralysis. *American Journal of Obstetrics and Gynecology,* **83**, 1452–1460.

Hünerman (1892) Über Nervenlähmung im Gebiete des Nervus ischiadicus infolge von Entbindungen. *Archiv für Gynaekologie,* **42**, 489–512.

Kleinberg, S. (1927) Maternal obstetrical sciatic paralysis. *Surgery, Gynecology, Obstetrics,* **45**, 61–64.

Mills, C. K. (1893) Neuritis and myelitis, and the forms of paralysis and pseudo-paralysis following labor. *Transactions of the College of Physicians,* **15**, 17–50.

Mills, E. M. (1945) Peroneal palsy as a complication of parturition. *Journal of Obstetrics and Gynaecology of the British Empire,* **52**, 278–282.

Romberg, M. H. (1851) *Diseases of the Nervous System,* Vol. 2. Sydenham Society, p. 390.

Tillman, A. J. B. (1935) Traumatic neuritis in the puerperium. *American Journal of Obstetrics and Gynecology,* **29**, 660–666.

Urist, M. R. (1953) Obstetric fracture-dislocation of the pelvis: Report of a case with injury to lumbosacral trunk and first sacral nerve root. *Journal of the American Medical Association,* **152,** 127–129.

Whittaker, W. G. (1958) Injuries to the sacral plexus in obstetrics. *Canadian Medical Association Journal,* **79**, 622–626.

Femoral Neuropathy

Adelman, J. U., Goldberg, G. S., and Puckett, J. D. (1973) Postpartum bilateral femoral neuropathy. *Obstetrics and Gynecology,* **42**, 845–850.

Buchbender, E., and Weiss, R. (1961) Drei Fälle von Femoralisparese nach gynakologischer Bauchoperation. *Nervenarzt,* **32,** 413–415.

Calverley, J. R., and Mulder, D. W. (1960) Femoral neuropathy. *Neurology,* **10,** 963–967.

Cary, N. A. (1925) Complete paralysis of the anterior crural nerve following childbirth. *Journal of Bone and Joint Surgery,* **23,** 451–457.

Gumpertz, K. (1896) Narkosenlähmung des Nervus cruralis. *Deutsche Medizinische Wochenschrift,* **22**, 504, 505.

Hopper, C. L., and Baker, J. B. (1968) Bilateral femoral neuropathy complicating vaginal hysterectomy. *Obstetrics and Gynecology,* **32**, 543–547.

McDaniel, G. C., Kirkley, W. H., and Gilbert, J. C. (1963) Femoral nerve injury associated with the Pfannenstiel incision and abdominal retractors. *American Journal of Obstetrics and Gynecology,* **87**, 381–385.

Rosenblum, J., Scharz, G. A., and Bendler, E. (1966) Femoral neuropathy—A neurological complication of hysterectomy. *Journal of the American Medical Association,* **195**, 410–415.

Susens, G. P., Hendrickson, C. G., Mulder, M. J. et al. (1968) Femoral nerve entrapment secondary to a heparin hematoma. *Annals of Internal Medicine,* **69**, 575–579.

Obturator Neuropathy

Aguayo, A. J. (1975) Neuropathy due to compression and entrapment. In Dyck, P. J., Thomas, P. K., and Lambert, E. H. (eds.): *Peripheral Neuropathy,* Philadelphia: W. B. Saunders Company.

CHAPTER THREE

Muscle Disease

MYASTHENIA GRAVIS

Myasthenia gravis is a disease of the motor end plates of striated muscle and is characterized by fluctuating fatigability of particular muscle groups. Muscles innervated by cranial nerves are more affected than limb muscles. Smooth muscles, myocardium, and myometrium are unaffected.

The concept of myasthenia gravis as an autoimmune disorder, first postulated by John Simpson (1961), has been fruitful. The number of muscle acetylcholine receptors is decreased in these patients (Fambrough et al., 1973). Acetylcholine receptor antibodies have been demonstrated in 70 per cent of patients with myasthenia gravis (Appel et al., 1975). Acetylcholine antibodies were present in an infant with transient neonatal myasthenia gravis and later showed a decay in titer (Keesey et al., 1977). Immunoglobulins from patients can produce weakness and electromyographic evidence of myasthenia (Toyka et al., 1977). Rabbits immunized with acetylcholine receptor protein developed myasthenic symptoms (Patrick and Lindstrom, 1973).

Clinical Presentation

Common manifestations are ptosis, diplopia secondary to external ophthalmoplegia, dysphagia, and dysarthria. Since the facial muscles are weak, an attempt to smile results in the "myasthenic snarl." Speech has a nasal quality, and the patient will tire while reciting. The neck can loll forward and can be lifted from a pillow only with difficulty. Hypoventilation can precede pneumonia and death.

Repetitive action tires the muscles of myasthenic patients abnormally. Rest improves muscle power. The patient may note this while chewing, talking, singing, brushing hair, typing, dancing, or participating in sports. The effect can be demonstrated electromyographically by repetitive stimulation of a motor nerve at the rate of 2 to 5 impulses per second. In a normal subject, the amplitude of the muscle action potential remains unchanged. In a patient with untreated myasthenia gravis, this amplitude decreases by more than 10 per cent by the third response.

In spite of severe weakness, reflexes are characteristically brisk. Repeated striking may diminish the reflex.

Treatment

The introduction of anticholinesterases by Mary Walker (1934) was a great advance. Pyridostigmine, neostigmine, and edrophonium are quarternary ammonium compounds which do not cross the blood-brain barrier as can a tertiary compound such as physostigmine. Placental transfer of quarternary ammonium ions is minimal (Edery et al., 1966).

The administration of edrophonium is used as a diagnostic test or, by some neurologists, as a guide to the adequacy of treatment. Thirty seconds after an intravenous injection of 10 mg of edrophonium, muscle power dramatically returns for 5 minutes.

Pyridostigmine and neostigmine are longer acting therapeutic anticholinesterases. Both are effective 1 to 4 hours after oral administration. Both are available in oral and parenteral preparations (Table 3.1). Pyridostigmine is preferred because it causes a lower degree of muscarinic side effects—sweating, bronchorrhea, diarrhea, and tachycardia. A time-release capsule of pyridostigmine, 180 mg, sustains many patients throughout the night, but it is not sufficient if the patient is awake and active. The dosage and its timing vary with the individual. Oral doses are often given 1 hour before meals.

Anticholinesterases can improve strength only to a certain point. Further increases in dosage will only intensify muscle weakness. Some muscles may be "cholinergic," while others need still more medication.

Table 3.1. Equivalent dosages of anticholinesterase drugs

	Oral	Parenteral
Neostigmine bromide	15 mg	
Neostigmine methylsulfate		0.5 mg IV 1.5 mg IM
Pyridostigmine bromide	60 mg	2.0 mg

The most vital functions—breathing and swallowing—should be at their maximal levels. An excellent measure of vital capacity can be obtained by asking the patient to inhale deeply and then count audibly as high as possible. Once a patient is trained, this number is reliable. If it should drop, a standard measure of vital capacity should be used.

Parenteral injections are used if oral administration is impossible or unwise (i.e., pre- or postoperatively or during labor). During early gestation a morning injection may be needed if emesis gravidarum is significant.

Atropine may be needed to limit bronchorrhea and lessen gastrointestinal hypermotility. It will not prevent fasciculations which accompany "cholinergic" weakness. Steroids in various regimens have prompted remissions in refractory cases (Engle et al., 1974).

Regular rest is important, especially during gestation.

Drug Interactions

Any drug with a curare effect is contraindicated in myasthenia gravis. The list of neuromuscular blocking agents includes diethyl ether, curare, and the aminoglycoside antibiotics—neomycin, streptomycin, kanamycin, and gentamicin. Hypermagnesemia, quinine, quinidine, and large amounts of procaine are contraindicated. The quinine in a gin-and-tonic may be harmful.

Thymectomy

Myasthenia gravis is associated with thymoma and with persistence of the thymus into adult life. Tomograms of the anterior mediastinum may be needed since routine lateral chest radiographs or even cross-table lateral views may not demonstrate thymic enlargement.

Thymectomy early in the course of myasthenia gravis prompts a remission, especially in patients who do not have thymic germinal centers (Genkins et al., 1975). Remission occurs after a delay if germinal centers are present (Perlo et al., 1971).

Epidemiology

Myasthenia gravis is principally a disease of women of childbearing age and older men (Fig. 3.1) Young women with myasthenia gravis often possess the HL-A8 antigen. Since a fluctuating course is typical, any correlation between the course of myasthenia gravis and menstruation is

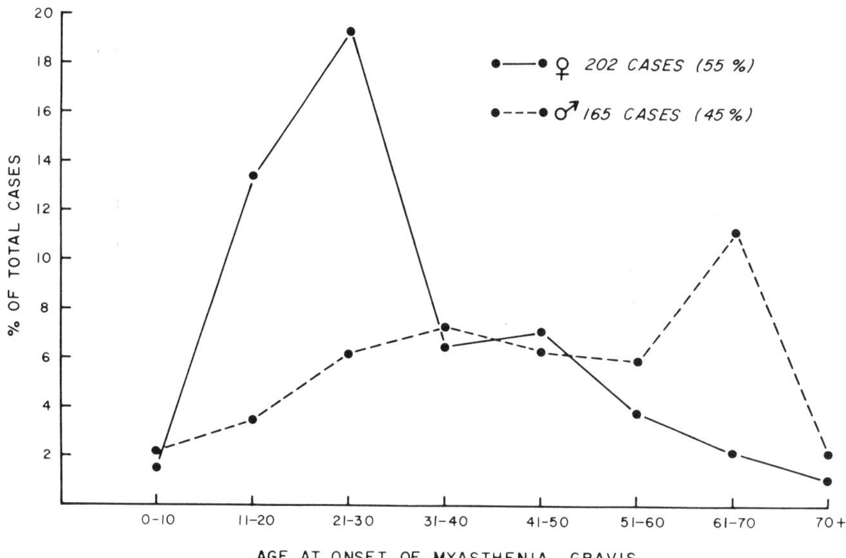

Figure 3.1. Distribution of the age of onset of myasthenia gravis according to sex in 367 patients. From data in Schwab, R. S., and Leland, C. C. (1953) Sex and age in myasthenia gravis as critical factors in incidence and remission. *Journal of the American Medical Association*, **153**, 1270–1273.

difficult to make, Nonetheless, in statistical studies of large groups and in some individual patients, a definite association exists.

Effect of Menstruation upon Myasthenia Gravis

Adolph Strumpell (1896) first noted the exacerbation of myasthenia gravis about the time of menstruation. About 40 per cent of women patients experience worsening of myasthenic symptoms just before menses (Keynes, 1952; Osserman, 1958); in some women the symptoms are very much worse (Adam, 1946). Improvement begins during menstruation, usually the first or second day. After thymectomy this association disappears in 50 per cent of patients (Keynes, 1952).

Before thymectomy, the urinary excretion of pregnanediol of women with myasthenia gravis is at or below the lower limit or normal whether measured in the proliferative or the luteal stage of the menstrual cycle (Schrire, 1959). Within 4 weeks of thymectomy, this measure of progesterone metabolism has doubled or quadrupled. Two years after thymectomy pregnanediol excretion may be ten times the normal rate.

The Pill has not been reported to have an effect upon myasthenia gravis. Estrogen therapy is not beneficial (Vacca and Knight, 1957). Administration of progesterone in oil, 50 mg daily, further weakened one woman, who experienced frequent premenstrual exacerbations (Frenkel and Ehrlich, 1964).

Effect of Pregnancy upon Myasthenia Gravis

Pregnancy has an unpredictable but often profound effect upon myasthenia gravis. This was as true before the advent of anticholinesterases as it was afterward (Viets et al., 1942; Osserman, 1958). Collins (1897) was the first to note the initial symptoms of myasthenia gravis during pregnancy. Another woman had remissions of the disease during her first two pregnancies, but severe exacerbations occurred during the next five (Laurent, 1931)

In a large population of treated myasthenic women, one-third improved during pregnancy, one-third were unaffected, and one-third became worse (Osserman, 1958). The effect of each pregnancy in the same woman can be different, but the pattern is usually set during the first trimester. Abortion does not alter the course of a relapse (Plauche, 1964). Remissions can last for months postpartum.

As first reported by Wharton Sinkler (1899), relapses of varying severity occurred in about 40 per cent of women in the postpartum weeks and months. The diagnosis is not infrequently made in the puerperium. One factor could be the lack of rest until the infant sleeps through the night. For this reason alone, breast feeding is not encouraged in such patients.

Lactation is not a risk provided the mother is well rested. No adverse neonatal effects have been ascribed to lactation. It remains to be determined whether or not anticholinesterases are excreted in human milk. Even if the concentration of pyridostigmine in human milk equals the peak concentration in maternal blood (Cohan et al., 1976), the breast-fed infant would recieve less than 0.01 mg of pyridostigmine daily.

Effect of Pregnancy upon the Thymus

The bulk of the thymus is reduced by estrogen, testosterone, and pregnancy. Involution begins at puberty. In adulthood the thymus is a hardly recognizable remnant which is difficult to distinguish from normal fat in the anterior mediastinum. Myasthenia gravis is associated with thymic hyperplasia and thymoma. The effect of pregnancy upon thymic hyperplasia associated with myasthenia gravis is unknown.

Pregnancy probably affects malignant thymoma adversely (Goldman, 1974). Rarely does malignant thymoma spread beyond the thorax. Four or five patients with malignant thymoma who became pregnant developed extrathoracic metastases. The fifth patient spontaneously aborted in the first trimester. Therapeutic abortion seems indicated if a woman with malignant thymoma becomes pregnant.

Effect of Myasthenia Gravis upon Pregnancy

The effect of myasthenia gravis upon pregnancy is small. Myasthenia gravis does not increase the risk of premature delivery, toxemia, uterine inertia, or postpartum hemorrhage (Osserman, 1958). A myasthenic mother must be sure to rest regularly while pregnant and afterward.

Before a pregnant woman with myasthenia gravis is admitted to the hospital for labor and delivery, the nursing and medical staffs should be well aware of the special problems and limitations imposed by myasthenia gravis (McNall and Jafarnia, 1965; Engel et al., 1974). Myasthenic patients need their medicine at certain times which do not always correspond to the usual floor schedule. Some myasthenic women tire when doing simple tasks, such as brushing their hair, but hesitate to ask for help. Expressed willingness by the staff to do extra things is greatly appreciated by the patient. Injectable anticholinesterase preparations should be readily available.

Obstetric Management

Labor and delivery are normal. Uterine inertia, if it occurs, responds to oxytocin (Osserman, 1965). Low forceps are commonly used to speed delivery. Magnesium sulfate is contraindicated if toxemia develops. Cesarean section is warranted for obstetric reasons only. The fears of physicians who formerly recommended elective cesarean section were not justified (Kennedy and Moersch, 1937).

Anesthesia

Regional anesthesia—paracervical, caudal, epidural, or low spinal—is preferred. Small amounts of procaine have been used without mishap, but large amounts can be toxic since its hydrolysis by plasma cholinesterase has been inhibited (Kalow, 1952). Lidocaine, which, unlike most local anesthetics, is an aminoacyl amide, does not possess this potential for danger (Mathews and Derrick, 1957).

If inhalation anesthetic is to be used, a nitrous oxide–oxygen mixture is acceptable. Ether should be avoided. Narcotics and analgesics should be used carefully with the patient's respiratory function always in mind. Scopolamine is contraindicated.

Equipment for neonatal resuscitation should be at hand for several hours after birth. The infant requires careful observation for at least 72 hours, since infants who develop neonatal myasthenia gravis may be normal at birth.

Counseling

If a woman with stable myasthenia gravis wishes to have a baby, I would advise her to have a thymectomy first. If the condition is still under control 1 year later or in remission, pregnancy can be attempted. This is arbitrary advice. The relapse rate during pregnancy after thymectomy has not been determined. The baby has a one in eight chance of developing transient neonatal myasthenia.

Neonatal Myasthenia Gravis

Neonatal myasthenia gravis is a transient disease that affects offspring of myasthenic mothers (Table 3.2), whereas congenital myasthenia gravis is a persistent disease of infants born to mothers without myasthenia gravis (Levin, 1949). (See Table 3.2). Ptosis and ophthalmoplegia are more typical of congenital myasthenia than of the neonatal variety.

Neonatal myasthenia gravis is presumably caused by placental transfer of maternal antibody (Keesey et al., 1977) (Fig. 3.2). Exchange transfusion for hyperbilirubinemia promptly cured neonatal myasthenia gravis in a 2 day old infant (Dunn, 1976).

Approximately 12 per cent of babies at risk develop neonatal myasthenia gravis (Namba et al., 1970). There is no relationship between neonatal illness and maternal age, the duration or severity of maternal disease, the maternal dose of anticholinesterases (or lack of it), or the presence of antiskeletal muscle antibodies in the mother's serum. Maternal thymectomy does not protect the infant from neonatal myasthenia gravis (Geddes and Kidd, 1951). At least four mothers of affected infants have subsequently delivered normal infants (Namba et al., 1970).

Neonatal myasthenia gravis can appear up to 4 days after birth. However, 80 per cent of neonates become symptomatic within the first day of life. A week-old infant who has not exhibited any signs of myasthenia can be safely discharged from the hospital. The delay in onset has been attributed to the placental transfer of maternal anticholinesterases. Placental transfer of pyridostigmine has been demonstrated in the rat but only to a minor degree (Roberts et al., 1970). Only negligible amounts remained after 24 hours. Metabolites are present in fetal tissue (Roberts et al., 1970). On indirect evidence, Blackhall and his co-

Table 3.2. Clinical features of congenital and neonatal myasthenia gravis

	Congenital	Neonatal
Myasthenic mother	No	Yes
Duration of symptoms	Persistent	Transient
Severity of symptoms	Mild	Mild to severe
Ptosis and ophthalmoplegia	Common	Uncommon

workers implicated these metabolites in the pathogenesis of neonatal myasthenia. However, neonatal myasthenia can develop whether or not the mother has taken anticholinesterases (Namba et al., 1970).

Symptoms of myasthenia in the neonate include feeding problems, "floppiness," a weak Moro reflex, a feeble cry, respiratory distress, and an expressionless facies (Table 3.3). The diagnosis can be confirmed by rapid improvement of sucking, crying, and moving after intramuscular injection of edrophonium chloride, 1.0 mg. Neostigmine methylsulfate, 0.1 mg, has been used, but atropine, 0.06 mg, is needed to prevent muscarinic effects.

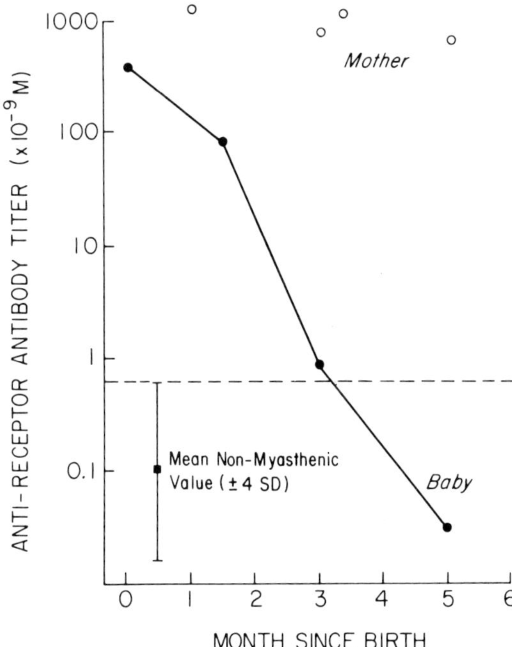

Figure 3.2. Anti-acetylcholine receptor antibody titer in neonatal myasthenia gravis. Anticholinesterase drugs were needed for the first month of life, and strength continued to improve over the next 5 months. Antibody levels do not correlate well with the severity of adult myasthenia gravis. From Keesey, J., Lindstrom, J. et al. (1977) Anti-acetylcholine receptor antibody in neonatal myasthenia gravis. *New England Journal of Medicine*, **296**, 55.

Table 3.3. Common manifestations of neonatal myasthenia gravis in 52 babies (per cent)

Feeding problems	87
Weak sucking and swallowing	71
Tube feeding required	29
Regurgitation	25
Muscle signs	69
Hypotonia (floppy muscles)	48
Weak limb movements	35
Absent moro reflex	19
Absent grasp reflex	12
Respiratory difficulty	65
Feeble cry	60
Cyanosis	27
Mucus in pharynx	23
Expressionless face	37
Open mouth	21
Ptosis and ophthalmoplegia	15

Adapted from Namba et al. (1970) Neonatal myasthenia gravis: Report of two cases and a review of the literature. *Pediatrics,* **45**, 488–504.

Treatment

Careful observation, intensive nursing care, and good general medical care are most important. Endotracheal intubation and assisted ventilation may be necessary until the situation is well under control. Frequent aspiration of secretions will be needed, especially after injections of neostigmine. Feeding by nasogastric tube is preferable to intravenous fluids if normal oral feeding is a problem.

Only 80 per cent of affected infants require anticholinesterase drugs (Namba et al., 1970). Both neostigmine and pyridostigmine have been used, administered intramuscularly, orally, or via nasogastric tube (Table 3.4). Pyridostigmine is preferable since it produces fewer and

Table 3.4. Dosage of anticholinesterase drugs in neonatal myasthenia gravis

	Initial dose		Usual oral maintenance dose (every 4 hr)
	IM	*Oral*	
Pyridostigmine bromide	0.15 mg	4.0 mg	4 to 10 mg
Neostigmine methylsulfate	0.10 mg		
Neostigmine bromide		1.0 mg	1 to 2 mg

From Namba et al. (1970) Neonatal myasthenia gravis: Report of two cases and a review of the literature. *Pediatrics,* **45**, 488–504; and Osserman, K. E. (1965) Myasthenia gravis. In *Medical, Surgical and Gynecological Complications of Pregnancy.* Rovinsky, J. J., and Guttmacher, A. F. (eds.): 2nd ed. Baltimore: The Williams & Wilkins Company.

milder muscarinic side effects (Moore, 1955). Doses are administered 30 to 60 minutes before feeding, depending upon the route of administration. The dose should be large enough to permit adequate swallowing and breathing, but it need not be enough to produce a strong cry and vigorous movements. The dose should be kept low to prevent cholinergic weakness as the disease spontaneously abates in 2 to 4 weeks, if not sooner. As the patient improves, the dose can be reduced or the interval between doses lengthened.

Prognosis

Recovery is complete without any need for continued anticholinesterase drugs. Death occurred in 10 per cent of reported cases, but half of these patients had not received anticholinesterases.

MYOTONIC DYSTROPHY

Myotonic muscular dystrophy is an inherited systemic disease characterized by weakness and wasting of voluntary muscles of the neck, face, and distal limbs primarily. Myotonia can be clinically demonstrated in the thenar muscles and tongue. The typical "dive-bomber" electromyographic pattern is produced by many muscles. Zonular cataracts, cardiac arrhythmias, frontal balding in males, chronic respiratory acidosis, and impaired gut motility have all been reported. Most patients become symptomatic between adolescence and 50 years of age, but the diagnosis may be overlooked for many years. Neonatal myotonia is a severe disease in infants of usually mildly affected mothers.

Evidence is accumulating that the basic defect is an abnormality of membrane chloride permeability (Barchi, 1975). The existence of the T-tubular system in striated muscle provides the conditions which make myotonia possible. Smooth muscle may be involved in the dystrophic process (Harvey et al., 1965) but will not exhibit myotonia since it lacks a T-tubular system. Myotonia can be treated with phenytoin, quinine, or procainamide. The dystrophic process cannot be altered.

Fertility

Testicular atrophy develops in 80 per cent of males with myotonic muscular dystrophy at some stage of their disease. Secondary sexual characteristics may remain normal, although serum testosterone levels are significantly lower (Harper et al., 1972). Serum LH and, especially, FSH levels are significantly higher in severely affected males (Harper et al., 1972). Seminiferous tubules are destroyed, but Leydig cells are morphologically normal until the late stages of disease. Spontaneous abortion has been reported in marriages in which the husband has myotonic dystrophy (Maas, 1937).

Ovarian function in myotonic dystrophy has been relatively poorly investigated. Eighty per cent of women are said to be fertile (Drucker et al., 1961). Spontaneous and habitual abortion is not unusual (Maas, 1937; Holland, 1956; Shore and MacLachlan, 1971). Thomasen (1948) reported that among 33 women with myotonic dystrophy "menstrual irregularities [were] more frequently found in women with severe degrees of muscle dystrophy." Menstrual disorders need not be due to ovarian dysfunction. Hypothalamic dysfunction has been documented in one woman with myotonic dystrophy and amenorrhea (Febres et al., 1975).

Pregnancy and Myotonic Dystrophy

Disability from weakness and myotonia increases or remains constant during pregnancy. Some women show the initial symptoms of myotonia during pregnancy. Impairment of muscular function can increase during any stage of gestation but occurs most commonly during the third trimester. Prolonged bed rest should be avoided since disuse of the muscles will further weaken any patient with muscle disease.

Spontaneous abortion and premature labor are not uncommon. Although the length of labor is normal for most of these women, prolongation of any stage has been attributed to myotonic dystrophy. Uterine inertia has been ascribed to myometrial involvement (Shore and MacLachlan, 1971). Oxytocin stimulates the uterine contractions of women with myotonic dystrophy (Sciarra and Steer, 1961). A prolonged second stage of labor is attributed to an inability to "bear down" forcibly and may result in fetal distress requiring intervention (Davis, 1958; Gardy, 1963; Shore and MacLachlan, 1971). Failure of the emptied uterus to contract promptly has caused profuse postpartum hemorrhage (Hopkins and Wray, 1967; Kuhn et al., 1969).

Anesthesia

A regional anesthetic should be used whenever possible (Hook et al., 1975). Nerve blocks will not prevent myotonia, which is an intrinsic phenomenon of muscle. A myotonic muscle infiltrated with procaine becomes flaccid. Depolarizing "muscle relaxants" cause severe spasms and hyperthermia in myotonic dystrophy. Non-depolarizing agents (e.g., curare) can be used safely. If the patient is taking quinine for myotonia, the dose of curare should be decreased by 50 per cent at least (Hook et al., 1975).

If antepartum hypoventilation and chronic respiratory acidosis exist, thiopental and other respiratory depressants should be avoided (Kaufman, 1959). Electrocardiographic monitoring will alert the staff to any abnormality in cardiac conduction.

Fetal and Neonatal Myotonic Muscular Dystrophy

Infants can develop the dystrophy in utero. Striated muscle from limb muscles, diaphragm, tongue, larynx, and pharynx are severely involved with the pathologic features of immaturity (Sarnat and Silbert, 1976). This can become clinically apparent before delivery as polyhydramnios caused by fetal swallowing dysfunction (Dunn and Dierker, 1973; Sarnat et al., 1976). Arthrogryposis multiplex congenita is another manifestation of intrauterine involvement (Shore, 1975).

Infants with neonatal myotonic dystrophy present as floppy babies with facial diplegia. They may be unable to smile or to suck vigorously. Delay in reaching developmental milestones is common. Neonatal deaths are caused by respiratory distress and feeding problems (Dodge, et al., 1965).

The diagnosis is established by family history. Although these infants have the dystrophy, myotonia is not present either clinically or electromyographically. If a child is suspected of having neonatal myotonic muscular dystrophy, the mother must be examined unless there is a clear family history. Even when her child is severely involved, the mother may have only mild symptoms which have been overlooked.

Counseling

Myotonic dystrophy is inherited through an autosomal dominant gene. The linkage of this gene with a secretor gene allows prenatal diagnosis of myotonic dystrophy in some cases (Renwick et al., 1971; Renwick and Bolling, 1971). Secretor-positive individuals, whether homozygotic (Se/Se) or heterozygotic (Se/se), secrete the substances of the ABH blood group into body fluids, including amniotic fluid. The ideal genetic situation for prenatal diagnosis is depicted in Figure 3.3. If sufficient data can be obtained, predictions can be made in 37.5 per cent of matings (Schrott and Omenn, 1975).

More than 95 per cent of babies with myotonic muscular dystrophy are the offspring of affected mothers (Harper and Dyken, 1972). Neonatal disease can be severe in contrast to mild maternal disease. The reason is unknown.

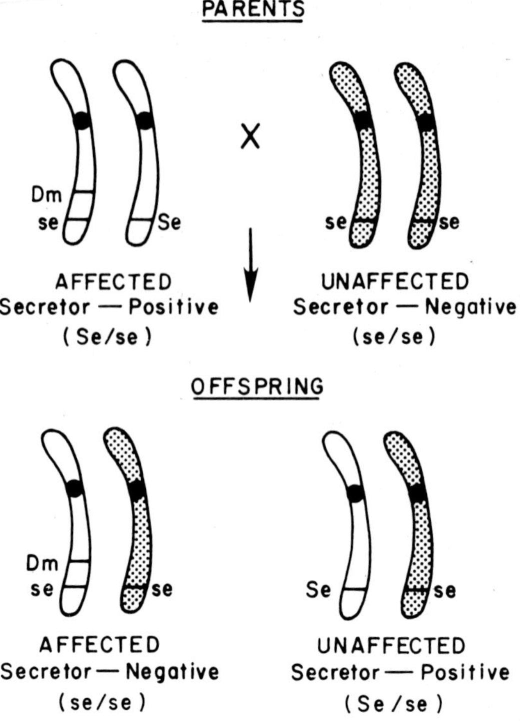

Figure 3.3. The prenatal diagnosis of myotonic muscular dystrophy is possible in this ideal situation because it is not possible to find ABH blood group substances in the amniotic fluid. Adapted from Schrott, H. G., and Omenn, G. S. (1975) Myotonic dystrophy: Opportunities for prenatal prediction. *Neurology*, **25**, 789–791.

MYOTONIA CONGENITA (THOMSEN'S DISEASE)

Thomsen (1876) reported myotonia congenita as a hereditary muscle disorder which afflicted himself and many of his family only after one of his sons was accused of malingering in order to avoid military service (Johnson, 1968). Thomsen's disease is transmitted as an autosomal dominant trait.

Myotonic symptoms become evident from the time the child begins to walk. Myotonia affects limb muscles more than cranial muscles, and proximal muscles more than distal muscles. Muscle strength is normal. Sudden movement, as in arising from a chair, may cause all muscles to become myotonic simultaneously, thus causing a fall. In contrast to myotonic muscular dystrophy, cataracts, mental deterioration, and infertility do not occur. Myotonia congenita is compatible with long life—Thomsen died at the age of 81.

In only two instances has the effect of pregnancy on congenital myotonia been described (Gardiner, 1901; Hakim and Thomlinson, 1969). In both cases myotonia worsened in the second half of gestation and improved after childbirth. No obstetric problems were encountered.

Although symptoms usually do not appear until later in childhood, infants may have difficulty in feeding owing to a stiff tongue. Delay in walking may occur (Walton and Nattrass, 1954).

MYOPHOSPHORYLASE DEFICIENCY

Myophosphorylase deficiency (McArdle's disease) is a rare myopathy characterized by muscle fatigue and painful cramps during exercise. Myoglobinuria and very high serum creatine phosphokinase (CPK) levels can occur during exercise. Smooth muscle and myometrium are not involved. A normal pregnancy, labor, and delivery can be expected (Cochrane and Alderman, 1973).

POLYMYOSITIS

Polymyositis is a subacute inflammatory disease affecting the proximal muscles more than the distal ones. More severely involved muscles are tender. The erythrocyte sedimentation rate (ESR) and CPK level are elevated. Muscle biopsy is diagnostic. The current treatment is prednisone.

Fewer than ten cases of polymyositis in conjunction with pregnancy have been reported. All but two patients (Spellacy, 1964; Tsai and Lindheimer, 1973) had polymyositis before becoming pregnant. The effect of pregnancy upon muscle weakness was variable. Four of nine infants died. The unfavorable course of the disease is probably related to maternal disease underlying polymyositis. In young adults the most common group of associated diseases is the collagen-vascular type of disorder, including systemic lupus erythematosus and scleroderma.

REFERENCES

Myasthenia Gravis

General References

Appel, S. H., Almon, R. R., and Levy, N. (1975) Acetylcholine receptor antibodies in myasthenia gravis. *New England Journal of Medicine,* **293**, 760, 761.

Bender, A. N., Ringel, S. P., Engel, W. K. et al. (1975) Myasthenia gravis: A serum factor blocking acetylcholine receptors of the human neuromuscular junction. *Lancet,* **1**, 607, 609.

Cohan, S. L., Pohlmann, J. L. W., Miksszewski, J. et al. (1976) The pharmacokinetics of pyridostigmine. *Neurology,* **26,** 536–539.

Engel, W. K., Festoff, B. W., Patten, B. M. et al. (1974) Myasthenia gravis. *Annals of Internal Medicine,* **81**, 225–246.

Fambrough, D. M., Drachman, D. B., Satyamurti, S. (1973) Neuromuscular junction in myasthenia gravis: Decreased acetylcholine receptors. *Science,* **182**, 293–295.

Genkins, G., Papatestas, A. E., Horowitz, S. H. et al. (1975) Studies in myasthenia gravis: Early thymectomy. *American Journal of Medicine,* **58,** 517–523.

Kalow, W. (1952) Hydrolysis of local anesthetics by human serum cholinesterase. *Journal of Pharmacology and Experimental Therapeutics,* **104**, 122–134.

Mathews, W. A., and Derrick, W. S. (1957) Anesthesia in the patient with myasthenia gravis. *Anesthesiology,* **18**, 443–453.

Osserman, K. E. (1958) *Myasthenia Gravis.* New York: Grune & Stratton.

Perlo, V. P., Arnason, B., Poskanzer, D. et al. (1971) The role of thymectomy in the treatment of myasthenia gravis. *Annals of the New York Academy of Science,* **183**, 308–315.

Schwab, R. S., and Leland, C. C. (1953) Sex and age in myasthenia gravis as critical factors in incidence and remission. *Journal of the American Medical Association,* **153**, 1270–1273.

Viets, H. R. (1953) A historical review of myasthenia gravis from 1672 to 1900. *Journal of the American Medical Association,* **153**, 1273–1280.

Walker, M. B. (1934) Treatment of myasthenia gravis with physostigmine. *Lancet,* **1**, 1200, 1201.

Pregnancy

Adam, G. S. (1946) Myasthenia gravis and pregnancy. *Journal of Obstetrics and Gynaecology of the British Empire,* **53**, 557–561.

Chambers, D. C., Hall, J. E., and Boyce, J. (1967) Myasthenia gravis and pregnancy. *Obstetrics and Gynecology,* **29**, 597–603.

Collins, J. (1897) Asthenic bulbar paralysis. *Internal Medicine Magazine,* **5**, 203–212.

Fraser, D. (1963) Myasthenia gravis and pregnancy. *Proceedings of the Royal Society of Medicine,* **56,** 379–381.

Fraser, D., and Turner, J. W. H. (1953) Myasthenia gravis and pregnancy. *Lancet,* **2,** 417–419.

Hay, D. M. (1969) Myasthenia gravis and pregnancy. *Journal of Obstetrics and Gynaecology of the British Commonwealth,* **76**, 323–329.

Kennedy, K. S., and Moersch, F. P. (1937) Myasthenia gravis: A clinical review of eighty-seven cases observed between 1915 and the early part of 1932. *Canadian Medical Association Journal,* **37**, 216–223.

Keynes, G. (1952) Obstetrics and gynaecology in relation to thyrotoxicosis and myasthenia gravis. *Journal of Obstetrics and Gynaecology of the British Empire,* **59**, 173–182.

Laurent, I. P. E. (1931) Remissions and relapses associated with pregnancy in myasthenia gravis. *Lancet,* **1**, 753, 754.

McNall, P. G., and Jafarnia, M. R. (1965) Management of myasthenia gravis in the obstetric patient. *American Journal of Obstetrics and Gynecology,* **92**, 518–525.

Osserman, K. E. (1965) Myasthenia gravis. *In* Rovinsky, J. J., and Guttmacher, A. F. (eds.): *Medical, Surgical and Gynecological Complications of Pregnancy,* 2nd ed. Baltimore: The Williams & Wilkins Company, pp. 455–462.

Plauche, W. C. (1964) Myasthenia gravis in pregnancy. *American Journal of Obstetrics and Gynecology,* 404–409.

Schlezinger, N. S. (1955) Pregnancy in myasthenia gravis and neonatal myasthenia gravis. *American Journal of Medicine,* **19**, 718–720.

Sinkler, W. (1899). Asthenic bulbar paralysis. *Journal of Nervous and Mental Disease,* **26,** 536–544.

Strümpell, A. (1896) Über die asthenische Bulbärparalyse (Bulbärparalyse ohne anatomischen Befund; Myasthenia gravis pseudoparalytica). *Deutsche Zeitschrift für Nervenheilkunde,* **8,** 16–40.

Viets, H. R., Schwab, R. S., and Brazier, M. A. B. (1942) The effect of pregnancy on the course of myasthenia gravis. *Journal of the American Medical Association,* **119**, 236–242.

HORMONAL INFLUENCE

Frenkel, M., and Ehrlich, E. N. (1964) The influence of progesterone and mineralocorticoids upon myasthenia gravis. *Annals of Internal Medicine,* **60**, 971–981.

Schrire, I. (1959) Progesterone metabolism in myasthenia gravis. *Quarterly Journal of Medicine,* **28**, 59–75.

Vacca, J. B., and Knight, W. A. (1957) Estrogen therapy in myasthenia gravis: Report of two cases. *Missouri Medicine,* **54**, 337–340.

THYMUS GLAND DURING PREGNANCY

Goldman, K. P. (1974) Malignant thymoma in pregnancy. *British Journal of Diseases of the Chest,* **68**, 279–283.

McLean, J. M., Mosley, J. G., and Gibbs, A. C. C. (1974) Changes in the thymus, spleen and lymph nodes during pregnancy and lactation in the rat. *Journal of Anatomy* **118**, 223–229.

Millar, K. G., Mills, P., and Baines, M. G. (1973) A study of the influence of pregnancy on the thymus gland of the mouse. *American Journal of Obstetrics and Gynecology,* **117**, 913–918.

Persike, E. C. (1940) Involution of thymus during pregnancy in young mice. *Proceedings of the Society for Experimental Biology and Medicine,* **45,** 315–317.

Selye, H. (1941) Effect of dosage on the morphogenetic actions of testosterone. *Proceedings of the Society for Experimental Biology and Medicine,* **46,** 142–146.

CONGENITAL MYASTHENIA GRAVIS

Conomy, J. P., Levinsohn, M., and Fanaroff, A. (1975) Familial myasthenia gravis: A cause of sudden death in young children. *Journal of Pediatrics,* **87**, 428–430.

Herrmann, C. (1971) The familial occurrence of myasthenia gravis. *Annals of the New York Academy of Science,* **183**, 334–350.

Levin, P. M. (1949) Congenital myasthenia in siblings. *Archives of Neurology and Psychiatry,* **62**, 745–758.

Walker, R. P. (1953) Congenital myasthenia gravis. *American Journal of Diseases of Children,* **86,** 198–200.

NEONATAL MYASTHENIA GRAVIS

Dunn, J. M. (1976) Neonatal myasthenia. *American Journal of Obstetrics and Gynecology,* **125**, 265, 266.

Geddes, A. K., and Kidd, H. M. (1951) Myasthenia gravis of the newborn. *Canadian Medical Association Journal,* **64**, 489.

Greer, M., and Schotland, M. (1960) Myasthenia gravis in the newborn. *Pediatrics,* **26**, 101–108.

Keesey, J., Lindstrom, J. et al. (1977) Anti-acetylcholine receptor antibody in neonatal myasthenia gravis. *New England Journal of Medicine,* **296**, 55.

Millichap, J. G., and Dodge, P. R. (1960) Diagnosis and treatment of myasthenia gravis in infancy, childhood, and adolescence. *Neurology,* **10**, 1007–1014.

Moore, H. (1955) Advantages of pyridostigmine bromide (Mestinon) and edrophonium chloride (Tensilon) in the treatment of transitory myasthenia gravis in the neonatal period. *New England Journal of Medicine,* **253**, 1075, 1076.

Namba, T., Brown, S. B., and Grob, D. (1970) Neonatal myasthenia gravis: Report of two cases and a review of the literature. *Pediatrics,* **45**, 488–504.

Stern, G. M., Hall, J. M., and Robinson, D. C. (1964) Neonatal myasthenia gravis. *British Medical Journal,* **2**, 284–286.

Strickroot, F. L., Schaeffer, R. L., and Bergo, H. E. (1942) Myasthenia gravis occurring in an infant born of a myasthenic mother. *Journal of the American Medical Association,* **120,** 1207–1209.

PLACENTAL TRANSFER OF ANTICHOLINESTERASE DRUGS

Blackhall, M. I., Buckley, G. A., Roberts, D. V. et al. (1969) Drug-induced neonatal myasthenia. *Journal of Obstetrics and Gynaecology of the British Commonwealth,* **76**, 157–162.

Edery, H., Porath, G., and Zahavy, J. (1966) Passage of 2-hydroxyiminomethyl-*N*-methyl-pyridium methanesulfonate to the fetus and cerebral spaces. *Toxicology and Applied Pharmacology,* **9**, 341–346.

Roberts, J. B., Thomas, B. H., and Wilson, A. (1970) Placental transfer of pyridostigmine. *British Journal of Pharmacology,* **38,** 202–205.

Myotonic Dystrophy

Barchi, R. L. (1975) Myotonia: An evaluation of the chloride hypothesis. *Archives of Neurology,* **32,** 175–180.

Davis, H. A. (1958) Pregnancy in myotonica dystrophia. *Journal of Obstetrics and Gynaecology of the British Empire,* **65**, 479–480.

Dodge, P. R., Gamstorp, I., Byers, R. K. et al. (1965) Myotonic dystrophy in infancy and childhood. *Pediatrics,* **35**, 3–19.

Drucker, W. D., Rowland, L. P., Sterling, K. et al. (1961) On the function of the endocrine glands in myotonic muscular dystrophy. *American Journal of Medicine,* **31**, 941–950.

Dunn, L. J., and Dierker, L. J. (1973) Recurrent hydramnios in association with myotonia dystrophica. *Obstetrics and Gynecology,* **42**, 104–106.

Febres, F., Scaglia, H., Lisker, R. et al. (1975) Hypothalamic-pituitary-gonadal function in patients with myotonic dystrophy. *Journal of Clinical Endocrinology,* **41**, 833–840.

Gardy, H. H. (1963) Dystrophia myotonica in pregnancy. *Obstetrics and Gynecology,* **21**, 441–445.

Gordon, P., Griggs, R. C., Nissley, S. P. et al. (1969) Studies of plasma insulin in myotonic dystrophy. *Journal of Clinical Endocrinology,* **29**, 684–690.

Harper, P., Penny, R., Foley, T. S. et al. (1972) Gonadal function in males with myotonic dystrophy. *Journal of Clinical Endocrinology,* **35**, 852–856.

Harper, P. S., and Dyken, P. R. (1972) Early-onset dystrophia myotonica: Evidence supporting a maternal environmental factor. *Lancet,* **2**, 53–55.

Harvey, J. C., Sherbourne, D. H., and Siegel, C. I. (1965) Smooth muscle involvement in myotonic dystrophy. *American Journal of Medicine,* **39**, 81–90.

Hook, R., Anderson, E. F., Noto, P. (1975) Anesthetic management of a parturient with myotonia atrophia. *Anesthesiology,* **43**, 689–692.

Hopkins, A., and Wray, S. (1967) The effect of pregnancy on dystrophia myotonica. *Neurology,* **17**, 166–168.

Kaufman, L. (1960) Anaesthesia in dystrophia myotonica: A review of the hazards of anaesthesia. *Proceedings of the Royal Society of Medicine,* **53**, 183–188.

Kuhn, E., Lohe, K., and Runnebaum, B. (1969) Beeinträchtigung des Geburtsverlaufes bei Myotonia dystrophica. *Geburtshilfe und Frauenheilkunde,* **29,** 742–745.

Maas, O. (1937) Observations on dystrophia myotonica. *Brain,* **60,** 498–524.

Renwick, J. H., Bundey, S. E., Ferguson-Smith, M. A. et al. (1971) Confirmation of linkage of the loci for myotonic dystrophy and ABH secretion. *Journal of Medical Genetics,* **8**, 407–416.

Renwick, J. H., and Bolling, D. R. (1971) An analysis procedure illustrated on a triple linkage of use for prenatal diagnosis of myotonic dystrophy. *Journal of Medical Genetics,* **8**, 399–406.

Schrott, H. G., and Omenn, G. S. (1975) Myotonic dystrophy: Opportunities for prenatal prediction. *Neurology,* **25**, 789–791.

Sciarra, J. J., and Steer, C. M. (1961) Uterine contractions during labor in myotonic muscular dystrophy. *American Journal of Obstetrics and Gynecology,* **82**, 612–615.

Shore, R. N., and MacLachlan, T. B. (1971) Pregnancy with myotonic dystrophy: Course, complications and management. *Obstetrics and Gynecology,* **38**, 448–454.

Shore, R. N. (1975) Myotonic dystrophy: Hazards of pregnancy and infancy. *Developmental Medicine and Child Neurology,* **17**, 356–361.

Sarnat, H. B., O'Connor, T., and Byrne, P. A. (1976) Clinical effects of myotonic dystrophy on pregnancy and the neonate. *Archives of Neurology,* **33**, 459–465.

Sarnat, H. B., and Silbert, S. W. (1976) Maturational arrest of fetal muscle in neonatal myotonic dystrophy. *Archives of Neurology,* **33**, 466–474.

Thomasen, E. (1948) *Myotonia: Thomsen's Disease (Myotonia Congenita), Paramyotonia, and Dystrophia Myotonica: A Clinical and Heredobiologic Investigation.* London: M. K. Lewis.

Watters, G. V., and Williams, T. W. (1967) Early onset myotonic dystrophy. *Archives of Neurology,* **17**, 137–152.

Myotonia Congenita

Gardiner, C. F. (1901) A case of myotonia congenita. *Archives of Pediatrics* **18**, 925–928.

Hakim, C. A., and Thomlinson, J. (1969) Myotonia congenita in pregnancy. *Journal of Obstetrics and Gynaecology of the British Commonwealth,* **76**, 561, 562.

Johnson, J. (1968) Thomsen and myotonia congenita. *Medical History,* **12**, 190–194.

Thomsen, J. (1876) Tonische Kraempfe in Willkuerlich beweglichen Musklen in Folge von ererbter psychischer Disposition. *Archiv für Psychiatrie und Nervenkrankheiten,* **6**, 702.

Walton, J. N., and Nattrass, F. J. (1954) On the classification, natural history and treatment of the myopathies. *Brain,* **77,** 169.

Myophosphorylase Deficiency

Cochrane, P., and Alderman, B. (1973) Normal pregnancy and successful delivery in myophosphorylase deficiency (McArdle's disease). *Journal of Neurology, Neurosurgery and Psychiatry,* **36**, 225–227.

Polymyositis

Bohan, A., and Peter, J. B. (1975) Polymyositis and dermatomyositis. *New England Journal of Medicine,* **292**, 344–347, 403–407.

Glickman, F. S. (1958) Dermatomyositis associated with pregnancy. *U.S. Armed Forces Medical Journal,* **9,** 417–425.

Massé, M. R. (1962) Grossesses et dermatomyosite. *Bulletin de la Societe Francaise de Dermatologie et de Syphiligraphie,* **69**, 921–923.

Spellacy, W. N. (1964) Scleroderma and pregnancy. *Obstetrics and Gynecology,* **23**, 297–300.

Tsai, A., Lindheimer, M. D., and Lamberg, S. I. (1973) Dermatomyositis complicating pregnancy. *Obstetrics and Gynecology,* **41**, 570–573.

CHAPTER FOUR

Movement Disorders

CHOREA GRAVIDARUM

Chorea gravidarum is the term given to chorea of any cause occurring during pregnancy. Chorea is characterized by abrupt, brief, nonrhythmical, involuntary movements of any limb and nonpatterned facial grimaces. Emotional stress aggravates the movements. Sleep is peaceful. The chorea may be unilateral—hemichorea—and often is during pregnancy.

Felix Meyer (1907) found the first recorded case in the works of Horstius, published in 1661. He translated the Latin as follows:

> The following case, which occurred to the wife of a schoolmaster in childbirth, is, I think, of a peculiar nature. For more than twelve years since that event, for some reason or other, the whole of her left side is thus affected. When she is awake it is constantly in motion, which she cannot control by will. She is perpetually winking her eyes; her lips are continually opening and shutting; her arm keeps jumping up; her fingers gesticulate; and her foot is never quiet. Yet all this occurs without feeling or pain. But when she is asleep, everything is at rest.

Flagrant chorea is obvious to any observer, but often the patient will attempt to disguise chorea by incorporating it into a mannerism or gesture. Hypotonia of the affected limbs is the rule. Knee jerks are pendular and joints are floppy. Shoulder hypotonia can be demonstrated by having the patient stand and rotating his shoulders back and forth in a quarter circle. Normally the arms dangle at the sides but with hypotonia they flail about. The wrist and fingers assume the shape of a dinner fork with abduction of the thumb (Brain, 1928). Continuous muscular contractions may be impossible to sustain. The extended tongue will dart in and out uncontrollably. Varying hand strength is referred to as "milkmaid's grip."

Incidence

Willson and Preece (1932) found that the overall incidence of chorea gravidarum was about one case per 3000 deliveries. The condition must be much rarer now. Zegart and Schwarz (1968) found that only one case had been encountered in the course of 139,000 deliveries at three major Philadelphia hospitals.

Patient Profile

Most women with chorea gravidarum are young—the average age is 22 (Fig. 4.2) (Willson and Preece, 1932). Almost all reported patients have been Caucasians, but this is a biased sample since the bulk of the old literature is European. Eighty per cent of initial attacks occur during first pregnancies (Fig. 4.3) (Willson and Preece, 1932). One-half start in the first trimester; one-third in the second (Fig. 4.1). Sixty per cent of afflicted women have previously had chorea. A family history of transient chorea is not unusual.

Prognosis

Chorea gravidarum seldom persists indefinitely, unlike the woman described by Horstius. Without treatment the disease abates in 30 per

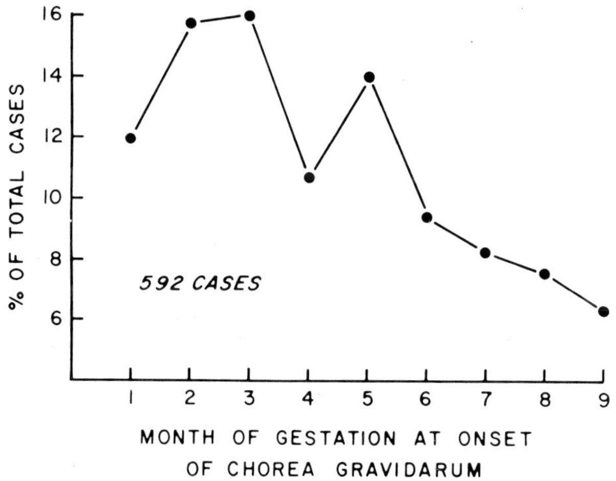

Figure 4.1. The month of gestation at the onset of chorea gravidarum in 592 cases. From data in Willson, P., and Preece, A. A. (1932) Chorea gravidarum. *Archives of Internal Medicine*, **49**, 672.

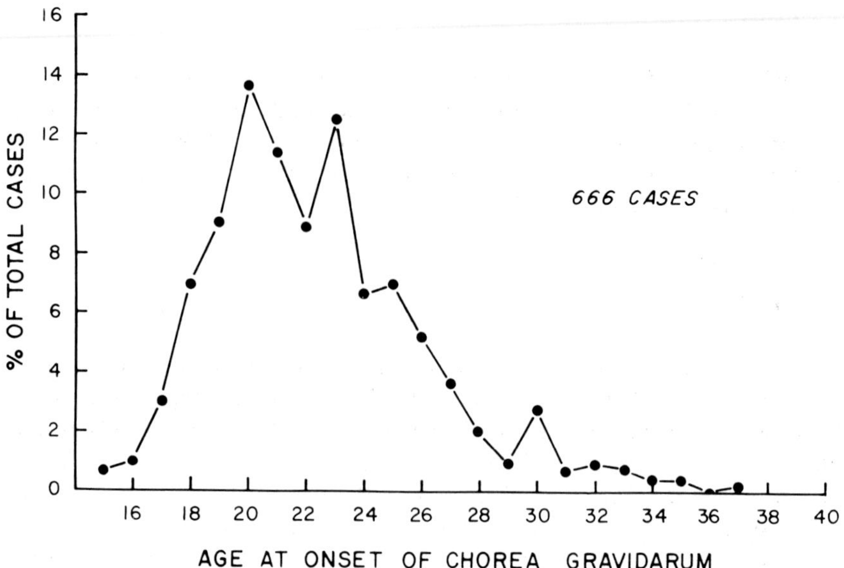

Figure 4.2. Age at onset of chorea gravidarum in 666 cases. Redrawn from Willson, P., and Preece, A. A. (1932) Chorea gravidasum. *Archives of Internal Medicine,* **49,** 522.

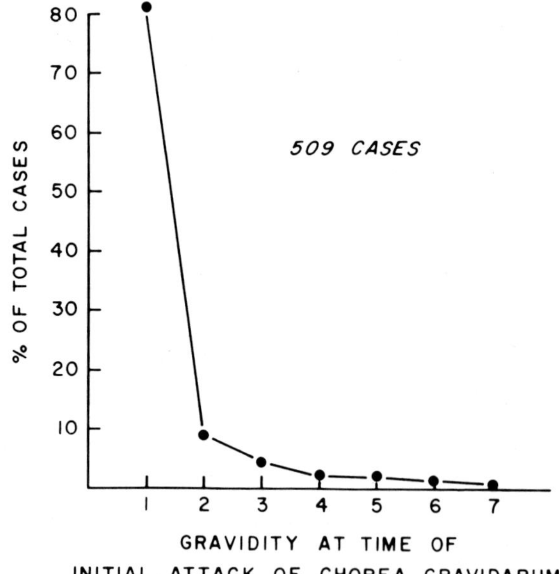

Figure 4.3. Gravidity at time of initial attack of chorea gravidarum in 509 cases. Redrawn from Willson, P., and Preece, A. A. (1932) Chorea gravidarum. *Archives of Internal Medicine,* **49,** 524.

cent of patients before birth. In almost two-thirds, the chorea lasts until the puerperium. Symptoms often dramatically disappear in the days after childbirth.

Mortality is now rare (Lewis and Parsons, 1966). The mortality rate of 12 per cent reported by Willson and Preece (1932) reflected death due to underlying rheumatic heart disease.

Treatment

The traditional treatment has been rest, seclusion, and careful feeding (Wall and Andrews, 1903). Sedation, steroids (Forrest and Hales, 1956), and phenothiazines (Winkelbauer, 1956) have benefited some patients. Haloperidol is an effective treatment for Sydenham's chorea and other involuntary movement disorders (Shenker et al., 1973; Axley, 1972). Chorea gravidarum is not an indication for abortion or premature interruption of pregnancy (Lewis and Parsons, 1966).

Fetal Prognosis

Spontaneous abortion occurs at a normal rate (Zegart and Schwarz, 1968). Infants are healthy. Willson and Preece mentioned two nineteenth century cases of neonatal chorea. One turned out to be a microcephalic child with athetoid cerebral palsy (Barnes, 1869). The other child was said to have transient chorea, but the movements were not described further (Purefoy et al., 1901).

Future Pregnancy

Twenty per cent of women with chorea gravidarum will have recurrent chorea with subsequent pregnancies (Willson and Preece, 1932). Several cases have been described in which attacks occurred in three, four, and even five pregnancies (Fleischman, 1953).

Relationship to Rheumatic Heart Disease

Chorea gravidarum is strongly linked with rheumatic fever. At least 35 per cent of patients have a definite history of acute rheumatic fever and Sydenham's chorea. Four per cent of those with chorea gravidarum had acute rheumatic fever (Willson and Preece, 1932). Women who had normal pregnancies before contracting rheumatic fever have developed chorea during subsequent pregnancies (Black, 1900; Matthews, 1911). Carditis was found in 87 per cent of fatal cases (Willson and Preece, 1932).

Sydenham's chorea may follow the onset of other manifestations of rheumatic fever by up to 7 months (Taranta and Stollermen, 1956). Both are related to group A streptococcal infections. Isolated recurrences of chorea among a group of 60 children with a history of Sydenham's chorea followed an episode of streptococcal pharyngitis by a week, 3 months, or even 6 months (Taranta, 1959). By the time chorea develops, antistreptolysin O titers may have returned to normal. But this does not imply that all cases of chorea gravidarum are related to an immediately preceding streptococcal infection. First, the fact that chorea recurs in several pregnancies in the same woman is statistically against this. Second, Jonas et al. (1972) was able to document that a woman with chorea and a history of acute rheumatic fever had been free of streptococcal infection for 15 months prior to the presentation of chorea in the sixth month of her pregnancy.

Sydenham's chorea is not the only manifestation of "rheumatic brain disease" (Aron et al., 1965). Not infrequently some change in mental status occurs, ranging from emotional lability or hysterical traits to psychotic delusions and hallucinations. Seizures (Warren and Chernyak, 1947) and papilledema (Chun et al., 1961) can occur.

Rheumatic encephalopathy is reflected in the electroencephalogram (EEG) (Usher and Jasper, 1941). Electroencephalographic changes are not limited to patients with clinical manifestation of chorea. Slow waves (3 to 6 Hz) can occur continually or in intermittent rhythmical paroxysms. This activity may be generalized or may occur predominantly over the frontal and central regions. Changes may be unilateral in hemichorea (Buchanan et al., 1942). Improvement in the EEG pattern parallels recovery from rheumatic carditis and chorea, usually within 6 months.

The pathology of rheumatic brain disease is that of a nonspecific arteritis with endothelial swelling, perivascular lymphocytic infiltration, and petechial hemorrhages. Aschoff bodies are not present in the brain (Greenfield and Wolfsohn, 1922; Winkelman and Eckel, 1932). These changes are evident to some degree throughout the cerebrum but are most prominent in the corpus striatum. The same pathologic signs have been reported for chorea gravidarum, but almost all those patients also had cardiac disease (Willson and Preece, 1932). Brain tissue from patients with acute rheumatic fever with or without chorea has not been studied for the presence of antistreptococcal antibodies. Presumably, as the inflammation resolves and the chorea disappears, degenerative changes are left in small arterioles.

The most probable cause of chorea gravidarum is the reactivation by some mechanism of subclinical damage to the basal ganglia resulting from previous rheumatic encephalopathy.

The Pill could activate the same mechanism. At least 15 cases of chorea in association with a course of the Pill have been reported (Fernando, 1966; Lewis and Harrison, 1969; Gamboa et al., 1971; Riddoch et al., 1971; Malcolm, 1971; Buchtal, 1972; Bickerstaff, 1969, 1975). Most are young nulliparae who have taken the Pill less than 4 months. Recovery can occur within 2 days after it is stopped. Six women (40 per cent) previously had Sydenham's chorea and rheumatic fever. Another earlier had had chorea gravidarum (Gamboa et al., 1971). Whether or not subsequent pregnancy will trigger chorea in these women has not been reported.

How hormonal steroids activate chorea is unknown. End arterioles in the basal ganglia are a possible locus of action. An analogy can be drawn to the spider nevi of pregnancy (Bean et al., 1949). Both chorea and cutaneous vascular changes appear in the first and second trimesters; both can dramatically disappear after delivery, and both involve small arteries.

Differential Diagnosis

The differential diagnosis (Table 4.1) is long, but through it runs the thread of small artery disease. Acute rheumatic fever must be ruled out by a careful cardiac examination, electrocardiogram, sedimentation rate, ASO titer, and throat culture. Wilson's disease, although rare, must be excluded as a cause of any movement disorder in adolescents and young adults by determination of serum ceruloplasmin and 24-hour concentration of urinary copper.

The most common cause of a movement disorder is probably a phenothiazine-induced dyskinesia. Prochlorperazine (Compazine) may have been prescribed to control nausea or vomiting. Acute dystonia is unlike true chorea. It can be readily treated by administration of benztropine mesylate. Tardive dyskinesia may be clinically indistinguishable from a chorea.

Systemic lupus erythematosus (SLE), another vascular disease known to cause chorea, is aggravated by pregnancy (Garsenstein et al., 1962). One case of SLE causing chorea gravidarum has been reported (Donaldson and Espiner, 1971).

Huntington's chorea is unusual in the young without a strong family history. Other causes are polycythemia, hyperthyroidism, and idiopathic hypoparathyroidism.

Table 4.1. Differential diagnosis of chorea gravidarum

Condition	Test
Acute rheumatic fever	Cardiac examination Electrocardiogram Sedimentation rate ASO titer Throat culture Electroencephalogram
Wilson's disease	Slit-lamp examination Serum ceruloplasmin Urinary copper (24 hr)
Systemic lupus erythematosus	Sedimentation rate Antinuclear antibody
Phenothiazine reaction	History Therapeutic trial of benztropine (IV)
Polycythemia	Hemoglobin/hematocrit
Hyperthyroidism	Thyroxine (T_4)
Hypoparathyroidism	Skull radiographs Serum calcium, phosphate

WILSON'S DISEASE

Wilson's disease (hepatolenticular degeneration) is an undetermined inborn error of copper metabolism which is transmitted as an autosomal recessive trait. Symptomatic onset usually begins in the second decade of life. The hallmarks of the disease, which may vary clinically from family to family, are cirrhosis of the liver and its sequela, the Kayser-Fleischer ring of copper deposition in Descemet's membrane of the cornea, and central nervous system dysfunction. The latter may appear as an impairment of higher intellectual functions, personality changes, or a movement disorder which can vary from akinesia to a gross flapping tremor. Dysarthria, dysphagia, and a broad silly smile are common. Other abnormalities are a proximal renal tubular acidosis and, more rarely, a hemolytic anemia.

Typical laboratory findings are: (1) a very low serum ceruloplasmin concentration, (2) a normal or low total serum copper level but elevated albumin-bound nonceruloplasmin copper, and (3) increased urinary copper excretion. The diagnosis can be unequivocally determined by a copper assay of liver tissue or by a histologic demonstration of liver copper with a rubeanic acid stain. Routine hematoxylin and eosin staining is not sufficient.

Before Walshe introduced D-penicillamine treatment in 1956, affected women either died, had severe cirrhosis with amenorrhea and infertility, or were seriously handicapped by central nervous system involvement before reaching maturity. Only rare cases of Wilson's disease in pregnant women were reported. Most women had a spontaneous abortion in the third or fourth month of gestation. Only rarely did pregnancy proceed to term delivery (Baldi and Somoza, 1957).

With D-penicillamine, the relentless fatal course of the condition has been checked. Forty-three infants have been born to 28 women with Wilson's disease treated with penicillamine for 1 to 16 years (Scheinberg and Sternlieb, 1975; Walsche, 1977). All infants have been unaffected at birth and have remained asymptomatic for the period observed so far (up to 5 years) (Walsche, 1977).

Most of these mothers took 1 g of D-penicillamine daily. All patients on maintenance doses of penicillamine should have monthly platelet and leukocyte counts and a urinalysis for protein and blood. Vitamin B_6, 50 or 100 mg daily, is recommended to correct the antipyridoxine effect of D-penicillamine (Jaffe et al., 1964). If a cesarean section is planned, Scheinberg and Sternlieb (1975) recommend a reduction in the daily dose of D-penicillamine to 0.25 g daily for the 6 weeks prior to delivery. Wound healing is impaired by D-penicillamine (Geever et al., 1967). Complete withdrawal of D-penicillamine should be avoided.

Penicillamine may be a hazard to the fetus. Besides forming an inert complex with copper excreted by the kidney, penicillamine binds cysteine and is used to treat cystinuria. The urine of an infant of a cystinuric mother who had received 1 g D-penicillamine daily during her pregnancy did contain penicillamine-cysteine complexes (Crawhall et al., 1967). Another infant, born of a woman taking 2 g D-penicillamine throughout her pregnancy, had a congenital connective tissue defect consisting of lax skin, hyperflexibility of joints, fragile veins, and impaired wound healing (Mjølnerød et al., 1971).

The one child born of a woman taking the new drug triethylene tetramine was healthy at birth (Walsche, 1977).

Fetal Copper Metabolism

Ceruloplasmin, an alpha-2–globulin which binds eight copper atoms per molecule, normally accounts for at least 95 per cent of total serum copper. This large protein does not cross the placenta. Serum copper and ceruloplasmin concentrations are normally several times higher in maternal blood than in cord blood (Scheinberg et al., 1954; Sherwin et al., 1960). If the mother has Wilson's disease, ceruloplasmin levels are normal in cord blood and actually higher than maternal levels (Sherwin et al., 1960). Copper loosely bound to albumin equilibrates between maternal and fetal circulations (Scheinberg et al., 1954). Nonceruloplasmin copper is elevated in Wilson's disease.

An improvement in neurologic manifestations has been noted during pregnancy (Sherwin et al., 1960). This improvement could be due to a decrease in maternal total body copper stores caused by the need to supply fetal needs. However, in absolute terms, the body of a newborn infant contains little copper—about 12 mg (Scheinberg and Sternlieb, 1975). In one case studied, breast milk contained normal amounts of copper (Dreifuss, 1966).

Estrogen Effects upon Copper Metabolism

In normal subjects the effect of estrogen administration and pregnancy upon copper metabolism is to at least double the serum ceruloplasmin and thus serum copper levels (Johnson et al., 1959; Markowitz et al., 1955 Dokumov, 1968). The Pill accomplishes the same result (Schenker et al., 1972). In fact, the green plasma of some women who either are taking the Pill or are pregnant has been attributed to this increased ceruloplasmin concentration (Tovey, 1968).

With Wilson's disease there is no consistent change, if any, in any aspect of copper metabolism with either pregnancy or estrogen administration (German and Bearn, 1961; Russ et al., 1957). Any chemical change persists only for the duration of the period of estrogen excess. There is no clinical benefit from estrogen therapy (German and Bearn, 1961).

ENCEPHALITIS LETHARGICA

Epidemics of encephalitis lethargica swept the world from 1916 to 1926. The responsible virus is not known to exist any longer, but its legacy of postencephalitic Parkinsonism remains. This review of the disease in approximately 200 pregnant women is included for its historical interest. Frederick Roques made this aspect of encephalitis lethargica the subject of his doctoral thesis, to which little can be added (Roques, 1928a).

Baron Constantin von Economo delineated the clinical and pathological features of the disease, which he observed in Vienna during the winter of 1916–1917. He did not confuse encephalitis lethargica, as he called it, with the influenza pandemic of the same era (von Economo, 1917). In the acute stage, perivascular round cell cuffing and neuronal degeneration was found in the gray matter of the midbrain, substantia nigra, pons, and, less frequently, in the medulla, cerebral cortex, and spinal cord. The chronic stage is characterized by diffuse neuronal degeneration, especially of the substantia nigra if Parkinson's syndrome has developed.

Epidemics usually flourished during the winter. Young adults were disproportionately afflicted, but no age group was spared. Symptoms varied in presentation, duration, and severity within an outbreak as well as among epidemics. The three most constant features were generalized headache, a disturbance in sleep, and diplopia. Often these symptoms followed up to a week of nonspecific nausea, catarrh, fever, or myalgia.

As the name encephalitis lethargica implies, an overpowering urge to sleep was the most common symptom. But this was not the only irregularity of the normal diurnal rhythm. Some patients were asleep by day, awake at night. A few experienced insomnia for days. Von Economo was so intrigued by this aspect of his disease that he studied the physiologic process of sleep during the last decade of his life.

A wide variety of visual symptoms reflected the prevalence of midbrain involvement. The most common complaint was diplopia due to ophthalmoplegia, failure of conjugate gaze, or nystagmus. Blurred vision resulted from paresis of accommodation. Mild ptosis was frequent. The most dramatic visual disturbance—painful oculogyric crises—usually occurred in the chronic phase. Papilledema and optic atrophy were rare.

Extrapyramidal movement disorders were more typical of the chronic stage than the acute encephalitis lethargica. In early epidemics, chorea during the acute stage was common, whereas it was a rare chronic manifestation. Chorea gravidarum was the initial diagnosis in some cases (Roques, 1928a). Parkinson's syndrome could develop immediately following the acute stage, but more often there was a symptom-free interval of months or years.

Brain stem disease was also manifest by hiccups, irregular respiratory patterns, painful abdominal myoclonus, and cranial nerve paresis. In severe cases convulsions denoted involvement of the cerebral cortex.

Treatment consisted of symptomatic, supportive care. The mortality rate varied among different series, but overall it was 40 per cent.

Influence of Pregnancy upon Acute Encephalitis Lethargica

Pregnancy had little if any effect upon encephalitis lethargica (Roques, 1928a). A predictable percentage, approximately 2.5 per cent of large series consisted of pregnant women. Roques found the prevalence of various signs and symptoms to be almost identical between pregnant and nonpregnant groups with the exception of headache, which was a less frequent complaint among pregnant women. Mortality was equal. As an immediate sequela postencephalitic Parkinsonism was two to three times more frequent (75 per cent) among the 20 pregnant women affected in the Sheffield epidemic of 1924. No long-term follow-up study considering pregnancy as a factor was done. Whether or not the incidence of postencephalitic Parkinson's syndrome a decade later differed was never studied.

Influence of Encephalitis Lethargica upon Pregnancy

Spontaneous abortion during early pregnancy would not be unexpected in any serious maternal disease. Such was the case with encephalitis lethargica. Otherwise, if the expectant mother survived, the pregnancy was unaffected.

Pregnancy and Postencephalitic Parkinsonism

An inability to shift weight easily from one foot to another is a problem for anyone with Parkinson's syndrome. The postural changes and extra weight of pregnancy can only increase this difficulty. It can be imagined how a pregnant woman with Parkinson's syndrome would shuffle along. Thus, it is to be expected that Roques (1928a) found cases in which pregnancy aggravated Parkinsonism; this occured during each of one woman's three pregnancies. It is debatable whether or not pregnancy causes any central effect, hormonal or otherwise, as can be postulated in cases of chorea gravidarum. Postencephalitic Parkinsonism does not alter the course of pregnancy (Critchley, 1928; Kanter and Klawans, 1939).

Influence of Encephalitis Lethargica upon the Fetus

The greatest risk to the fetus is maternal death. Almost all infants of affected mothers who survived were described as healthy at birth. No long-term follow-up study was done. In only rare instances were autopsies performed on fetuses or stillborn infants. Marinesco (1921) found perivascular cuffing in the brain of a fetus whose mother had contracted acute encephalitis during the fifth month of her pregnancy and died 3 weeks later. Santi (1920) also found typical changes in a neonate. Thus, while transplacental infection was possible, its frequency was undetermined.

REFERENCES

Chorea Gravidarum

Barnes, R. (1869) On chorea in pregnancy. *Transactions of the Obstetrical Society, London,* **10**, 147–196.

Bean, W. B., Cogswell, R., Dexter, M. et al. (1949) Vascular changes of the skin in pregnancy. *Surgery, Gynecology and Obstetrics,* **88**, 739–752.

Beresford, O. D., and Graham, A. M. (1950) Chorea gravidarum. *Journal of Obstetrics and Gynaecology of the British Empire,* **57**, 616–625.

Black, M. (1900) Two cases of chorea in pregnancy. *Glasgow Medical Journal,* **54**, 441–444.

Donaldson, I. M., and Espiner, E. A. (1971) Disseminated lupus erythematosus presenting as chorea gravidarum. *Archives of Neurology,* **25**, 240–244.

Fleischman, M. J. (1953) A case report of chorea gravidarum complicating five pregnancies. *American Journal of Obstetrics and Gynecology,* **66**, 1328–1330.

Garenstein, M., Pollak, V. E., and Kark, R. M. (1962) Systemic lupus erythematosus and pregnancy. *New England Journal of Medicine,* **267**, 165–167.

Jonas, S., Spagnuolo, M., and Kloth, H. H. (1972) Chorea gravidarum and streptococcal infection. *Obstetrics and Gynecology,* **39**, 77–79.

Lewis, B. V., and Parsons, M. (1966) Chorea gravidarum. *Lancet,* **1**, 284–286.

Matthews, A. A. (1911) Chorea complicating pregnancy. *Northwest Medicine,* **15**, 372.

McElin, T. W., Lovelady, S. B., and Woltman, H. W. (1948) Chorea gravidarum. *American Journal of Obstetrics and Gynecology,* **55**, 992–1006.

Meyer, F. (1907) Chorea gravidarum. *Intercolonial Medical Journal,* **12**, 79–95.

Purefoy, R. D., Lloyd, H. C., and Carton, P. C. (1901) Clinical report of the Rotunda Lying-In Hospital. *Dublin Journal of Medical Science,* **3**, 185–193.

Wall, C., and Andrews, H. R. (1903) On chorea in pregnancy. *Journal of Obstetrics and Gynaecology of the British Empire,* **3**, 540–547.

Willson, P., and Preece, A. A. (1932) Chorea gravidarum. *Archives of Internal Medicine,* **49**, 471–533, 671–697.

Zegart, K. N., and Schwarz, R. H. (1968) Chorea gravidarum. *Obstetrics and Gynecology,* **32**, 24–27.

Chorea and the Pill

Bickerstaff, E. R. (1969) Involuntary movements and the Pill. *British Medical Journal,* **4**, 556, 557.

Bickerstaff, E. R. (1975) *Neurological Complications of Oral Contraceptives.* Oxford: Clarendon Press.

Buchtal, A. (1972) Chorea minor unter Anwendung von Ovulationshemmern. *Nervenarzt,* **43**, 541, 542.

Fernando, S. J. M. (1966) An attack of chorea complicating oral contraceptive therapy. *Practitioner,* **197**, 210, 211.

Gamboa, E. T., Isaacs, G., and Harter, D. H. (1971) Chorea associated with oral contraceptive therapy. *Archives of Neurology,* **25**, 112–114.

Lewis, P. D., and Harrison, M. J. G. (1969) Involuntary movements in patients taking oral contraceptives. *British Medical Journal,* **4**, 404, 405.

Malcolm, A. D. (1971) Chorea and oral contraceptives. *British Medical Journal,* **4**, 491.

Riddoch, D., Jefferson, M., and Bickerstaff, E. R. (1971) Chorea and oral contraceptives. *British Medical Journal,* **4**, 217, 218.

Sydenham's Chorea

Aron, A. M., Freeman, J. M., and Carter, S. (1965) The natural history of Sydenham's chorea. *American Journal of Medicine,* **38**, 83–95.

Buchanan, D. N., Walker, A. E., and Case, T. J. (1942) The pathogenesis of chorea. *Journal of Pediatrics,* **20**, 555–575.

Chun, R. W. M., Smith, N. J., and Forster, F. M. (1961) Papilledema in Sydenham's chorea. *American Journal of Diseases of Children,* **101**, 641–644.

Greenfield, J. G., and Wolfsohn, J. M. (1922) The pathology of Sydenham's chorea. *Lancet,* **2**, 603–606.

Taranta, A. (1959) Relation of isolated recurrences of Sydenham's chorea to preceding streptococcal infections. *New England Journal of Medicine,* **260**, 1204–1210.

Taranta, A., and Stollerman, G. H. (1956) The relationship of Sydenham's chorea to infection with Group A Streptococci. *American Journal of Medicine,* **20**, 170–175.

Usher, S. J., and Jasper, H. H. (1941) The etiology of Sydenham's chorea: electroencephalographic studies. *Canadian Medical Association Journal,* **44**, 365–371.

Warren, H. A., and Chornyak, J. (1947) Cerebral manifestations of acute rheumatic fever. *Archives of Internal Medicine,* **79**, 589–601.

Winkelman, N. W., and Eckel, J. L. (1932) The brain in acute rheumatic fever. *Archives of Neurology and Psychiatry,* **28**, 844–870.

TREATMENT

Axley, J. (1972) Rheumatic chorea controlled with haloperidol. *Journal of Pediatrics,* **81**, 1216, 1217.

Forrest, A. D., and Hales, I. B. (1956) Severe chorea gravidarum treated with corticotrophin. *Lancet,* **2**, 874, 875.

Shenker, D. M., Grossman, H. J., and Klawans, H. L. (1973) Treatment of Sydenham's chorea with haloperidol. *Developmental Medicine and Child Neurology,* **15**, 19–24.

Winkelbauer, R. G., and Kimsey, L. R. (1956) Chorea gravidarum treated with chlorpromazine. *American Journal of Obstetrics and Gynecology,* **71**, 1353, 1354.

Wilson's Disease

Albukerk, J. N. (1973) Wilson's disease and pregnancy. A case report. *Fertility and Sterility,* **24**, 494–496.

Baldi, E. M., and Somoza, E. G. (1957) Enfermedad de Wilson y ciclo gravidopuerperal. *Obstetricia y Ginecologia latina-americanas,* **15**, 27–31.

Bearn, A. G. (1957) Wilson's disease: an inborn error of metabolism with multiple manifestations. *American Journal of Medicine,* **22**, 747–757.

Bihl, J. H. (1959) The effect of pregnancy on hepatolenticular degeneration (Wilson's disease). *American Journal of Obstetrics and Gynecology,* **78**, 1182–1188.

Crawhall, J. C., Scowen, E. F., Thompson, C. J., et al. (1967) Dissolution of cystine stones during D-penicillamine treatment of a pregnant patient with cystinuria. *British Medical Journal,* **2**, 216–218.

Dokumov, S. I. (1968) Serum copper and pregnancy. *American Journal of Obstetrics and Gynecology,* **101**, 217–222.

Dreifuss, F. E., and McKinney, W. M. (1966) Wilson's disease (hepatolenticular degeneration) and pregnancy. *Journal of the American Medical Association,* **195**, 960–962.

Geever, E. F., Youseff, S., Seifter, E., et al. (1967) Penicillamine and wound healing in young guinea pigs. *Journal of Surgical Research,* **7**, 160–167.

German, J. L., and Bearn, A. G. (1961) Effect of estrogens on copper metabolism in Wilson's disease. *Journal of Clinical Investigation,* **40**, 445–453.

Jaffe, I. A., and Altman, M. P. (1964) The antipyridoxine effect of penicillamine in man. *Journal of Clinical Investigation,* **43**, 1869–1873.

Johnson, N. C., Kheim, T., and Kountz, W. B. (1959) Influence of sex hormones on total serum copper. *Proceedings of the Society for Experimental Biology and Medicine,* **102**, 98.

Markowitz, H., Gubler, C. J., Mahoney, J. P., et al. (1955) Studies on copper metabolism: XIV. Copper, ceruloplasmin and oxidase activity in sera of normal human subjects, pregnant women, and patients with infection, hepatolenticular degeneration and the nephrotic syndrome. *Journal of Clinical Investigation,* **34**, 1498–1508.

Mjølnerød, O. K., Rasmussen, K., Dommerud, S. A., et al. (1971) Congenital connective-tissue defect probably due to D-penicillamine treatment in pregnancy. *Lancet,* **1**, 673–675.

Russ, E. M., Raymunt, J., and Pillar, S. (1957) Effect of estrogen therapy on ceruloplasmin concentration in a man with Wilson's disease. *Journal of Clinical Endocrinology,* **17**, 908, 909.

Scheinberg, I. H., Cook, C. D., and Murphy, J. A. (1954) The concentration of copper and ceruloplasmin in maternal and infant plasma at delivery. *Journal of Clinical Investigation,* **33**, 963 (Abstract).

Scheinberg, I. H., and Sternlieb, I. (1960) The long term management of hepatolenticular degeneration (Wilson's disease). *American Journal of Medicine,* **29**, 316–333.

Scheinberg, I. H., and Sternlieb, I. (1975) Pregnancy in penicillamine-treated patients with Wilson's disease. *New England Journal of Medicine,* **293**, 1300–1302.

Schenker, J. G., Jungreis, E., and Polishuk, W. Z. (1972) Oral contraceptives and correlation between serum copper and ceruloplasmin levels. *International Journal of Fertility,* **17**, 28–32.

Sherwin, A. L., Beck, I. T., and McKenna, R. D. (1960) The course of Wilson's disease (hepatolenticular degeneration) during and after delivery. *Canadian Medical Association Journal,* **83,** 160–163.

Sternlieb, I., and Scheinberg, I. H. (1964) Penicillamine therapy for hepatolenticular degeneration. *Journal of the American Medical Association,* **189**, 748–754.

Tovey, L. A. D., and Lathe, G. H. (1968) Ceruloplasmin and green plasma in women taking oral contraceptives, in pregnant women, and in patients with rheumatoid arthritis. *Lancet,* **2**, 596–600.

Walsche, J. M. (1956) Treatment of Wilson's disease with penicillamine. *Lancet,* **1,** 188–192.

Walsche, J. M. (1977) Pregnancy in Wilson's disease. *Quarterly Journal of Medicine,* **46,** 73–83.

Encephalitis Lethargica

Bland, P. B., and Goldstein, L. (1930) Pregnancy and Parkinsonism. *Journal of the American Medical Association,* **95**, 473–476.

Critchley, M. (1928) Discussion. Pregnancy and epidemic encephalitis. *Proceedings of the Royal Society of Medicine,* **21**, 1063.

Kanter, A. E., and Klawans, A. H. (1939) Postencephalitic Parkinsonism complicated by pregnancy. *American Journal of Obstetrics and Gynecology,* **38**, 334–337.

Marinesco, M. G. (1921) L'encephalite épidémique et la grossesse. *Revue Neurologique,* **37**, 1055–1061.

Roques, F. (1928a) Epidemic encephalitis in association with pregnancy, labour, and the puerperium. A review and report of twenty-one cases. *Journal of Obstetrics and Gynaecology of the British Empire,* **35**, 1–113.

Roques, F. (1928b) Pregnancy and epidemic encephalitis. *Proceedings of the Royal Society of Medicine,* **21**, 1053–1062.

Santi, E. (1920) Della cosiddetta encefalite lethargica in gravidanza. *Rassegna d'Ostetricia e Ginecologia,* **29,** 81–89.

Von Economo, C. (1917) Encephalitis lethargica. In Wilkens, R. H., and Brody, I. A. (1973) *Neurological Classics,* pp. 18–22. New York: Johnson Reprint Corp.

CHAPTER FIVE

Infections

POLIOMYELITIS

Poliomyelitis is an enteric picornavirus infection of the central nervous system with a special predilection for the motor cells of the brain stem and the anterior horn of the spinal cord. After an incubation period of from 6 to 20 days in the gut or oropharynx, a viremia occurs, producing fever, headache, malaise, and nonspecific upper respiratory or intestinal symptoms. The sudden onset of neck and back soreness, increasingly severe headache, drowsiness, and irritability herald central nervous system involvement. At this preparalytic stage the cerebrospinal fluid is always abnormal and has the pattern of a viral meningitis. Cerebrospinal fluid pressure may be increased. The cell count ranges from 25 to 500 leukocytes per cu mm, with the initial polymorphonuclear predominance shifting within 5 days to a lymphocytic response. Cerebrospinal fluid sugar concentration is normal. Protein levels in cerebrospinal fluid will be normal at first but will approach 150 mg per dl in ensuing weeks. Approximately 30 per cent of cases are nonparalytic. Recovery begins 4 to 8 weeks after onset.

Paralysis develops within 2 to 5 days of the onset of central nervous system signs and symptoms. The asymmetric flaccid paralysis with fasciculations progresses for several days and ceases independently of lysis of the fever. Approximately 15 to 20 per cent of cases involve the bulbar musculature.

The clinical diagnosis is confirmed by recovery of virus from spinal fluid or blood. If virus is found only in feces, a concomitant fourfold increase in serum polio neutralizing and complement fixation antibodies should also be demonstrated.

Epidemiology

The infection may occur separately in any season but is more common in late summer and fall. In the younger age group, males are more commonly affected than females; after adolescence the infection is found more often in females. Previous tonsillectomy at any age predisposes patients to the bulbar form. Overexertion, chilling, and recent immunization increase susceptibility. In most fertile women the onset of symptoms occurs on or near the first day of menstruation (Fig. 5.1).

Effect of Pregnancy upon Poliomyelitis

All studies show that pregnancy approximately doubles the risk of developing poliomyelitis (Aycock, 1941; Horn, 1955; Siegel and Greenberg, 1955). The mortality rate is not increased by pregnancy (Horn, 1955). An apparently higher incidence in multiparas reflects the presence of children in the household who serve as virus reservoirs (Siegel and Greenberg, 1955).

In large series more cases than expected seem to occur during the first two trimesters, but this finding is not statistically significant. The highest incidence occurs in the third month of gestation (Fig. 5.2). The number of cases reported in the first weeks of gestation may be abnormally low owing to confusion of early spontaneous abortions with late normal menses.

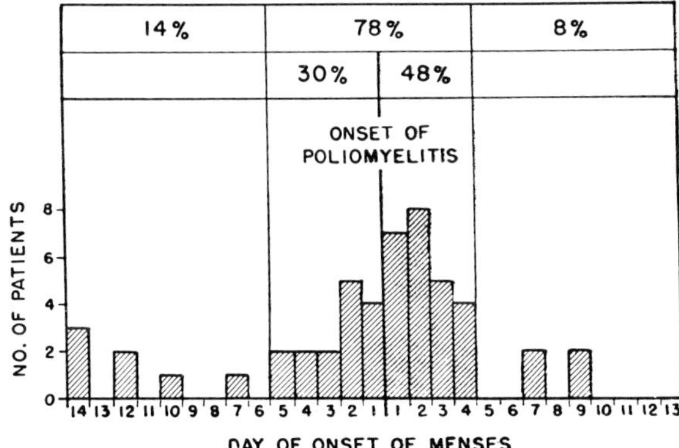

Figure 5.1. Onset of symptomatic poliomyelitis in relation to day of onset of menstruation. From Weinstein, L., Aycock, W. L., and Faemster, R. F. (1951) The relation of sex, pregnancy and menstruation to susceptibility in poliomyelitis. *New England Journal of Medicine*, **245,** 56.

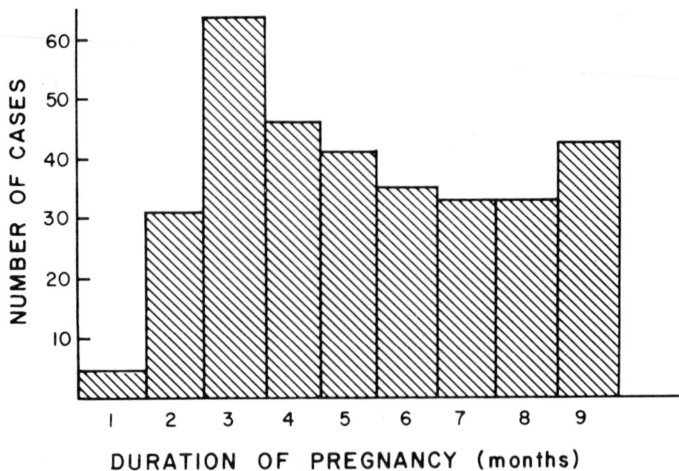

Figure 5.2. The month of gestation during which 230 pregnant women developed poliomyelitis. Compiled from Gifford and Hullinghorst (1948), Priddle et al. (1952), McCord et al. (1955), and Siegel and Greenberg (1955).

The proportion of clinical types of poliomyelitis in pregnant and nonpregnant women is almost identical (Table 5.1). Although the frequency of residual paralysis is not increased (Priddle et al., 1952), it has been observed clinically that parturition during or shortly after the onset of acute poliomyelitis is associated with paralysis of previously unaffected muscles or progressive weakness in already involved muscles (Weinstein et al., 1951).

Effect of Acute Poliomyelitis upon Pregnancy

In the first trimester, the acute febrile illness is associated with spontaneous abortion in approximately 40 per cent of pregnancies (Horn, 1958; McCord et al., 1955). This probably is a nonspecific reaction to severe illness. Maintenance of pregnancy is unimpaired in later trimesters.

Respiratory function is compromised by paralysis of the respiratory muscles, not by the enlarged uterus. Hypoventilation indicates a need for assisted respiration but not for forced termination of pregnancy by either cesarean section or induced labor (Cobb et al., 1953; Hunter and Millikan, 1954). A contrary opinion was expressed by Horn (1955), who advocated cesarean section after the 34th week of gestation for women with acute progressive bulbar poliomyelitis. She found no maternal or fetal loss associated with surgery in her ten cases.

Table 5.1. Clinical types of poliomyelitis during pregnancy of 276 women

Group	Nonparalytic Cases	Paralytic Cases		Total
		Spinal	*Bulbar*	
Pregnant women[a,b]				
First trimester	37(34%)	50(47%)	20(19%)	107(39%)
Second trimester	32(32%)	42(42%)	26(26%)	100(36%)
Third trimester	13(19%)	36(52%)	20(29%)	69(25%)
Total	82(30%)	128(46%)	66(24%)	276(100%)
Nonpregnant women[b] Ages 15 to 44 yrs.	179(28%)	326(51%)	138(21%)	643(100%)

[a]From Horn, P.: (1951) Pregnancy complicated by anterior poliomyelitis. *Annals of Western Medicine and Surgery,* **5**, 93–108.

[b]From Siegel, M., and Greenberg, M. (1955) Incidence of poliomyelitis in pregnancy: its relation to maternal age, parity, and gestational period. *New England Journal of Medicine,* **253,** 841–847.

Labor and Delivery

In the days of tank respirators the management of labor and delivery was a tour de force for the obstetrician. With modern techniques of respiratory care available, the termination of a pregnancy is only moderately complicated (Horn, 1958). The first stage of labor is normal. The second stage may be facilitated by flaccidity of the pelvic floor. However, women with acute low spinal polio are prone to retention of urine and fecal impaction which may compromise the area of the pelvic outlet.

Special precautions should be taken to prevent contamination of the infant by maternal stool or urine. Cord blood should be saved for antibody titers and virus culture. Since virus has been found in feces for weeks after acute poliomyelitis, the newborn should be isolated from its mother until 6 weeks after the onset of maternal disease.

Spinal or caudal anesthetic is contraindicated. Paracervical or pudendal blocks are effective and may be supplemented by a light inhalation anesthetic. If a cesarean section is necessary for a patient with marginal respiratory reserve, the procedure can be done after local infiltration of the abdominal wall.

Previous Poliomyelitis and Pregnancy

Previous poliomyelitis rarely has an effect upon a pregnancy unless paralysis or maldevelopment imposes a mechanical impediment to vaginal delivery. If a woman requires a chest cuirass for support of ventilation during sleep, successful pregnancy is almost impossible since each shell respirator is manufactured to fit the individual and cannot be adapted to the rapidly changing contours of a pregnant woman.

Neonatal Poliomyelitis

Although rare, neonatal poliomyelitis is invariably severe, with over 50 per cent mortality. Since the incubation period of the virus is 6 to 20 days, infants affected at birth or within the first 5 days of life are considered to have poliomyelitis secondary to transplacental transmission of the virus. Their mothers are in the early acute viremic stage of disease. Virus has been found in the infant and placenta in one case (Schaeffer et al., 1954). Neonatal infections appearing on or after the sixth day of life are considered to be caused by the intrapartum transfer of virus from maternal stool or blood.

Most children born of affected mothers are normal. Unlike rubella, polio has not been associated with a high incidence of congenital malformations.

Immunization

If the mother has had poliomyelitis long enough to produce neutralizing and complement fixation antibodies, the child will be protected by passive immunity. Antibodies readily cross the placenta after the sixth intrauterine month. At term, cord blood antibody levels equal maternal titers (Strean et al., 1957).

Pregnancy is not a contraindication to polio virus immunization in an endemic area. On theoretical grounds the *British Medical Journal* (1966) recommends the injection of Salk purified vaccine during the first 4 months of pregnancy. Oral Sabin live attenuated strains have been used elsewhere throughout pregnancy.

TUBERCULOUS MENINGITIS

Tuberculous meningitis is a subacute meningitis which presents with fever, malaise, and a progressively severe headache. Personality changes (i.e., irritability, confusion, and apathy) are often prominent. Vomiting and stiffness of the neck may be absent until later stages. Seizures and a variety of cranial nerve palsies, especially of the sixth and third nerves, develop as the patient becomes more obtunded. Untreated tuberculous meningitis results in death within 2 months.

Before 1950 and the era of readily available antituberculous chemotherapy, tuberculous meningitis was a disease of children and debilitated adults. In developing nations this is still true. In the United States, in areas where children are not immunized with Bacille Calmette-Guérin (BCG), a large segment of the population is tuberculin unreactive. Among this group of healthy adults, sporadic cases of primary tuberculosis have become an increasingly important cause of tuberculous meningitis (Barrett-Connor, 1967). Tuberculous meningitis may be the only secondary locus. The patient need not be cachectic or appear to be systemically ill. Even when chest radiographs and tuberculin skin tests may be negative, the diagnosis must be suspected.

The common denominator in all cases is the hematogenous spread of mycobacteria from the primary locus of disease, as in children, or from any location in patients with miliary tuberculosis. Neuropathologists postulate, but cannot always demonstrate, that the cerebrospinal fluid is seeded from tubercles, even minute ones, near the meninges. The subsequent inflammation is most prevalent at the base of the brain and in the sylvian fissure but can cover both cerebral hemispheres. Cranial nerve palsies are caused by fibrotic cuffing of their roots. A proliferative inflammatory vasculitis of the cerebral vessels progresses to thrombosis of these vessels and infarction of the brain.

After the diagnosis has been suspected, examination of the cerebrospinal fluid must be done properly. In tuberculous meningitis, cerebrospinal fluid can clot. As this coagulum or pellicle forms, it can sweep the collecting tube of white cells and mycobacteria. Thus it is essential that the cerebrospinal fluid be immediately examined for cells. Another tube should be spun down and the pellet stained for acid-fast bacteria. Often confirmation of the diagnosis must be delayed 6 weeks for culture results. By routine methods the cerebrospinal fluid is sterile.

The presence of infection is signaled by a low cerebrospinal fluid sugar concentration and an elevated leukocyte count. In the early stage of the disease these white cells are predominantly polymorphonuclear. By the time most patients present, the cells are chiefly lymphocytes. The protein concentration is elevated, usually over 100 mg per dl. If a subarachnoid block has developed in the high cervical–medullary region, the spinal fluid may be xanthrochromic from high protein levels (e.g., 0.4 to 3.0 g per dl).

If clinical features and spinal fluid findings are compatible with tuberculous meningitis, a therapeutic trial is indicated, at least until culture results are reported.

Pregnancy and Tuberculosis

Adequately treated pulmonary tuberculosis has no deleterious effect upon pregnancy. Hedvall in 1953 reached that conclusion after analyzing 250 of his own cases which occurred primarily in the pre-chemotherapy era. No difference has been found between pregnant and nonpregnant women with regard to sputum conversion, cavity closure, or length of hospitalization (Mehta, 1960). Fetal survival directly reflects maternal survival. With tuberculous meningitis both are in jeopardy. Abortion is not therapeutic (Schaefer et al., 1954).

Pregnancy has almost no effect upon tuberculous meningitis except to complicate its chemotherapeutic treatment. Although most studies include small numbers of patients and do not distinguish between types of cases, it appears that mortality from treated tuberculous meningitis is the same in both pregnant and nonpregnant women in either miliary or "pure" tuberculous meningitis categories.

Chemotherapy

Isoniazid (INH) is the keystone of antituberculous chemotherapy, especially tuberculous meningitis. In spite of therapy with streptomycin and para-aminosalicylic acid (PAS), the number of deaths from tuberculous meningitis did not decline until isoniazid was introduced in 1951 (Lepper and Spies, 1963). Relapses after an initial response to streptomycin were more common than cures (Brainerd and Eagle, 1950). Current treatment of nonpregnant patients with tuberculous meningitis consists of a course of isoniazid plus ethambutol or rifampin or both. Rifampin and ethambutol are effective antituberculous drugs which have replaced streptomycin as a second or third drug because they can be given orally and are less toxic. Ethambutol is recommended for pregnant patients because it has not been associated with adverse fetal effects (Weinstein and Murphy, 1974). Although rifampin has been used without ill effect, it is a potential hazard since it interferes with nucleic acid replication.

Steroids are indicated if a spinal block develops; this is manifested by low cerebrospinal fluid pressure, a rising or very high cerebrospinal fluid protein concentration, and a positive Queckenstedt test (O'Toole et al., 1969). Although steroids have reversed spinal block, they have not yet proved efficacious in diminishing the incidence of subsequent obstructive hydrocephalus.

Isoniazid

Isoniazid inhibits equally well the growth of intracellular mycobacteria and free, extracellular mycobacteria. Isoniazid easily penetrates both healthy and inflamed meninges (Elmendorf et al., 1952; Fletcher,

1953). Cord blood and maternal serum at the time of delivery contain equal concentrations of isoniazid (Bromberg, et al., 1955). Isoniazid is excreted in human milk (Bromberg et al., 1955).

In patients with tuberculous meningitis, isoniazid should be administered in daily doses of 10 mg per kg for 1 month (Clark et al., 1952). This is twice the standard dose given to tuberculin skin test converters. If the patient is comatose, isoniazid can be injected intramuscularly in three divided doses. When significant improvement is noted, the dose may be decreased to 7 mg per kg per day. Usually 2 or 3 months after onset, this dose is again decreased to the standard dose of 4 to 5 mg per kg per day (i.e., about 300 mg per day) and continued at that level for the duration of therapy—a total of 2 years.

Isoniazid causes a peripheral neuropathy by interfering with neuronal utilization of pyridoxine (vitamin B_6) (Biehl and Vitler, 1954; Ross, 1958). Development of neuropathy is dose-related. Individuals who inactivate INH slowly develop the neuropathy sooner. Concurrent administration of 100 mg of pyridoxine daily prevents this neuropathy. Much larger amounts, 200 mg per day, are needed to treat the neuropathy after it has developed. Pyridoxine deficiency or dependency can cause fetal or neonatal seizures (Bessey et al., 1957; Scriver, 1960).

Isoniazid inhibits the para-hydroxylation of phenytoin, a rate-limiting step in the excretion of phenytoin (Kutt et al., 1966). Thus, if a patient is taking phenytoin for a pre-existing seizure disorder or for convulsions symptomatic of tuberculous meningitis, the usual dose of phenytoin (300 mg per day) may be enough to produce serious toxicity (i.e., ataxia and psychosis) when isoniazid is given simultaneously.

Isoniazid is not a teratogen (Ludford et al, 1973).

Streptomycin

Streptomycin is effective against extracellular mycobacteria. When streptomycin is used alone, resistant strains of microorganisms frequently emerge, and clinical relapses are common. The customary antituberculous dose, assuming normal renal function, is 1 g intramuscularly daily for 1 month and then twice weekly for 3 to 6 months. Ototoxicity is directly related to peak plasma concentration. Thus, intravenous and large intramuscular doses are to be avoided. Smaller, more frequent injections result in a more constant and still therapeutic plasma concentration.

Streptomycin does not cross healthy meninges but does penetrate inflamed meninges to a variable extent (Hanssen and Lerche, 1950). Although therapeutic cerebrospinal fluid levels are not always achieved by intramuscular injections, the intrathecal injection of streptomycin is not indicated. When intramuscular streptomycin and isoniazid are administered together in clinical trials, no benefit from additional intrathecal streptomycin in mortality, clinical course, or residual impairment has been noted (Lepper and Spies, 1963). Besides, the intrathecal instillation of streptomycin can cause arachnoiditis, radiculitis, transverse myelitis, and even catastrophic acute encephalopathy.

At term, fetal plasma contains about half the concentration of streptomycin in maternal plasma (Woltz and Wiley, 1945; Heilman et al., 1945; Charles, 1954). Severe fetal ototoxicity has occurred (Robinson and Cambon, 1964), but disability is rare. In the most complete study of the problem, almost half of the children whose mothers had received streptomycin during pregnancy had some ototoxicity (Conway and Birt, 1965). Streptomycin is more likely to cause labyrinthine dysfunction than cochlear damage. The most sensitive indicator of streptomycin-induced vestibular injury is an abnormal caloric response to warm water (Bignall et al., 1951). Approximately one-third of children at risk showed some abnormality on caloric testing, but totally absent responses were rare. Even complete labyrinthine destruction causes little disability—only difficulty in walking in complete darkness, swimming under water, or reading while riding in a moving vehicle. Some deafness usually accompanies absent caloric responses in these circumstances. High-tone hearing loss was found in up to 25 per cent of children at risk but only rarely was a voice range impediment found. There seems to be no discernible relationship between fetal ototoxicity and the maternal daily dose, the total maternal dosage, or the trimester during which the drug was administered (Varpela et al., 1969).

In spite of potential fetal ear damage, streptomycin continues to be used in treatment of severe tuberculosis, such as tuberculous meningitis, as a third drug in addition to isoniazid and ethambutol.

Ethambutol

Ethambutol and isoniazid constitute the first-line therapy of tuberculous meningitis during pregnancy, (Weinstein and Murphy, 1974). Ethambutol achieves an inhibitory in vitro cerebrospinal fluid concentration (0.5 to 1.0 μg per ml) only when the meninges are inflamed (Bobrowitz, 1972). Ethambutol blood levels in a patient with normal renal function peak in 2 to 4 hours. An oral dose of 25 mg per kg will result in a blood level of 6 to 7 μg per ml 3 hours later. Cerebrospinal fluid obtained at approximately the same time contains 1 to 2 μg per ml. Ethambutol's serum half-life is approximately 6 hours, but the cerebrospinal fluid half-life is longer. An inhibitory cerebrospinal fluid concentration of 0.5 μg per ml has been measured only 2 hours before the patient's next daily dose.

Rifampin

Since rifampin inhibits DNA-dependent RNA polymerase (Radner, 1973), it is a potential hazard to the fetus, although adverse fetal effects have not been reported. Fetal blood and amniotic fluid contain therapeutic concentrations of rifampin after maternal ingestion of the usual doses. However, the drug is slowly cleared by the fetus. Prolonged administration can cause a fetal-maternal blood level ratio of three to one (Termine and Santuari, 1968). Rifampin should be reserved during pregnancy for cases in which there is clinical suspicion or bacteriologic proof that the mycobacterial species involved is resistant to other drugs (Weinstein and Murphy, 1974).

Rifampin crosses the blood-brain barrier in appreciable amounts only if the meninges are inflamed. A daily dose of 600 mg orally caused inhibitory spinal fluid concentrations 12 hours later but not 24 hours later (Bobrowitz, 1973). Thus, either 300 mg every 12 hours (D'Oliveira, 1972) or larger doses (25 mg per kg) (Sippel et al., 1974) have been advocated to achieve a more stable, inhibitory cerebrospinal fluid concentration.

Rifampin may interfere with the suppression of ovulation by oral contraceptives. Amenorrhea and unplanned pregnancies have been reported in women taking both rifampin and oral contraceptives (Altschuler and Valenteen, 1974).

Fetal Tuberculosis

Congenital tuberculosis is rare. It may be acquired in one of two ways. Placental foci may seed the fetal blood, causing a primary liver lesion. Or, if endometritis has developed, aspiration of infected amniotic fluid may cause the disease. Fetal infection may not be apparent at birth. Sudden death from miliary disease or a massive mycobacteremia is frequent. Maternal illness is severe.

An alarmingly high proportion of babies who have been isolated from their tuberculous mothers until the maternal infection is considered inactive still develop tuberculosis (Kendig, 1960). Temporary isolation and BCG immunization is recommended (Weinstein and Murphy, 1974).

Teratogenic Effects

There is no convincing evidence that commonly used antituberculous drugs are teratogenic (Lowe, 1964; Varpela, 1964; Marcus, 1967). In particular, isoniazid, which does cross the placenta, does not affect birth weight and is not a known teratogen (Ludford et al., 1973). Only ethionamide is a proven teratogen in humans (Potworowska and Sianożecka, 1966).

LISTERIOSIS

Listeria monocytogenes is a small, intracellular gram-positive diphtheroidlike pathogen of low virulence for man. This microorganism is more familiar to veterinarians than physicians since it produces epidemic abortions in herds of domestic animals. The peak incidence for human infection occurs in summer and early autumn (Busch, 1971). Listeria are important to obstetricians since they causes abortion, diffuse perinatal listeriosis, neonatal listerial meningitis, maternal meningitis, and asymptomatic genital infection. The serotypic distribution of the organisms causing perinatal listeriosis is different from that of those causing neonatal listerial meningitis (Albritton et al., 1976).

Perinatal Listeriosis

A prenatal transplacental infection is caused by abscesses seeded in the placenta during a maternal septicemia (Driscoll et al., 1962; Sepp and Roy, 1963). The mother develops only a nonspecific flu-like syndrome of transient low grade fever, malaise, sore throat, and headache. Fetal movements become less vigorous. Several days to 2 weeks later, gestation terminates prematurely. If fetal death has not occurred in utero, it follows within hours or days after birth. Necropsy shows the infant to be riddled with gray-white foci of necrosis approximately 1 mm in diameter, with infiltration of both mononuclear and polymorphonuclear cells (Sepp and Roy, 1963). The liver, spleen, lungs, brain, and adrenals are the most affected organs. Listeria can be cultured from these lesions and also from the placenta, amniotic fluid, uterine cavity, and maternal blood (Driscoll et al., 1962; Kelly and Gibson, 1972; Anderson, 1975).

Neonatal Listerial Meningitis

A neonatal listerial infection becomes manifest as a typical purulent meningitis within 4 weeks of birth (Nichols and Woolley, 1962). The infant's infection is presumably acquired during delivery. Although the mother is asymptomatic, cultures from her cervix, vagina, urine, or feces may grow *Listeria monocytogenes* for weeks after delivery. The yield declines after the tenth postpartum day (Gray and Killinger, 1966). Metritis may be seen in animals but is clinically insignificant in women (Gray and Killinger, 1966). Prompt treatment of the newborn with an appropriate antibiotic (e.g., ampicillin) increases its chances for survival. Even so, hydrocephalus and mental retardation may ensue.

Maternal Effects

Habitual Abortion

Repeated abortion has been reported in women from whose cervical secretions *Listeria monocytogenes* has been cultured (Rappaport et al., 1960; Kelly and Gibson, 1972). Queen Anne's failure to supply an heir for the British throne has been attributed to listerial infections (Saxbe, 1972). Serologic screening has not identified the women at risk (Bódnar et al., 1972). After treatment has eradicated the infection, a woman's subsequent pregnancies are normal. If the woman is not pregnant, oral tetracyclines are an effective mode of treatment. If pregnancy contraindicates oral tetracycline, ampicillin or tetracycline vaginal suppositories may be used.

Listeria Meningitis

Meningitis accounts for 75 per cent of all reported cases of human listeriosis. The usual maternal manifestation is an upper respiratory infection or a symptomatic genital infection which is easily overlooked. Other listerial infections include conjunctivitis, urethritis, abscesses, skin pustules, endocarditis, and pneumonia.

Listeria meningitis may present as a typical acute bacterial meningitis with fever, headache, delirium, neck stiffness, and a positive Kernig's sign. A subacute presentation similar to that of tuberculous meningitis has been reported (Simpson, 1971). Pathologically, the meninges and adjacent brain are studded with microabscesses. A purulent exudate collects at the base of the brain. The microabscesses can affect the pons, medulla, and individual cranial nerves, causing a palsy of the face, palate, or extraocular muscles (Duffy et al, 1964). This sign may supply an additional clue to the diagnosis.

Listeria monocytogenes is readily cultured from the cerebrospinal fluid but may be reported as an "unidentified diphtheroid contaminant." Gram-stained smears of the spinal fluid are often negative. Since a septicemia is often present simultaneously, blood cultures drawn early in the course of the meningitis will be positive. Cerebrospinal fluid sugar concentrations may be only minimally depressed at first. A sugar level of less than 30 mg per dl is a poor prognostic finding (Lavetter et al., 1971).

A predominantly granulocytic cerebrospinal fluid pleocytosis in the incipient meningitis soon shifts to a lymphocytic response. The peripheral blood shows a moderate granulocytosis. The monocytic response for which the pathogen is named is found in rabbits, not humans.

Treatment

Current treatment consists of ampicillin, 200 to 300 mg per kg per day. Antibiotics should be continued for 4 weeks to prevent recurrent meningitis caused by reseeding of the spinal fluid from unresolved microabscesses (Lavetter et al., 1971).

Immunity

Some listerial infections can be attributed to massive exposure (e.g., in meat packers, livestock handlers, or veterinarians). Many cases are sporadic. Other patients have defective cell-mediated (T-cell) immunity (Lane and Unanue, 1972). Mice challenged with an inoculum of *Listeria monocytogenes* are an experimental model of cell-mediated immunity (North, 1973).

Human listerial infections are associated with conditions involving defective immunity—lymphomas, Hodgkin's disease, immunosuppressive therapy, chronic alcoholism, and postoperative renal transplantation or splenectomy. Anergy may be demonstrated. Thus any mother who develops more than a transient "viral" syndrome or an asymptomatic genital infection should be suspected of having defective host responses possibly related to an underlying disease.

TETANUS

Tetanus has been known since antiquity as an affliction of soldiers, puerperal women, and neonates. Puerperal and postabortal tetanus is rarely encountered in countries where infants are routinely immunized, and a tetanus toxoid booster is an all too automatic part of emergency room visits. However, sporadic cases do crop up, usually after criminal abortions. In developing nations tetanus is a public health problem. Native childbirth customs and primitive hygiene seem designed to cause tetanus. Jelliffe and co-workers (1950) described the management of labor in Nigeria as it then existed.

> At the beginning of labour the patient is removed to the backyard or to a room in a mud house, the floor of which has been prepared by polishing with

leaves. When the contractions assume a bearing-down character the patient is placed in a squatting or kneeling position, so that her buttocks are resting on the ground or on her heels and with the vulva touching or close to the ground. She remains in this position throughout the second and third stages of labour. If labour is delayed she may stay in this position for many hours or days, to the extent that lower-limb palsies are not uncommon.

During the descent of the presenting part, a pad, which is usually a dirty cloth, is placed over the anus in order to protect the perineum, and on occasion native medicines are smeared on the vulva, especially in cases of abnormal labour. After the completion of labour the vulva is cleaned with an unsterile decoction of herbs. This is repeated on the morning and evening of the next day. A torn perineum is similarly treated.

The causative agent of tetanus is an exotoxin, tetanospasmin, produced by the strictly anaerobic gram-positive rod bacteria *Clostridium tetani.* The toxin is tightly bound to specific membrane sites in the central nervous system (Zacks and Sheff, 1970).

Clinical Signs

Local tetanus is characterized by persistent rigidity in those muscles close to the injury. Unless critical muscles are affected, local tetanus is a benign condition which disappears within several weeks.

Generalized tetanus is characterized by frequent, severe spasms of striated muscles not necessarily in the vicinity of the portal of entry. It implies spread of tetanus toxin to the central nervous system probably via the blood. The primary pathophysiologic central nervous system lesion is the blockade of inhibitory internuncial neurons (Brooks et al., 1957). Monosynaptic reflex arcs are hyperactive. The neuropathology of tetanus is scant. Chromatolysis of the Nissl substance (i.e., ribosomes) of the motor neurons may be secondary to the continual firing of anterior horn cells (Tarlov et al., 1973). Similar changes are seen in strychnine poisoning (Yates and Yates, 1966).

Generalized tetanus often presents as trismus. Persistent contraction of the masseters and facial muscles produces risus sardonicus. Splanchnic tetanus, whether secondary to abdominal wounds or an intrauterine infection, is associated with a short incubation period (less than 1 week) and early involvement of the respiratory muscles. Both are signs of a poor prognosis. A mortality rate of 50 per cent can be expected in generalized tetanus even with the use of modern respiratory care and muscle relaxants (Weinstein, 1973).

Almost any stimulus can trigger a generalized tetanic spasm. The typical posture is flexion of arms and extension of legs with the body arched in painful opisthotonus owing to contraction of the paravertebral muscles. Similar posturing may be induced by phenothiazines (Scime and Tallant, 1959). Continuous muscle contractions may cause fever and muscle breakdown with high serum "muscle enzymes," especially creatine phosphokinase. Laryngeal spasm may cause death unless an airway is maintained. Tracheostomy is routinely performed after the first generalized spasm.

Autonomic hyperreflexia coexists with somatic hyperreflexia. Constipation for weeks is the rule. Urine retention is not a problem with a spastic bladder (Kloetzel, 1963). Visceral sensory stimulation by tracheal suction, for example, can trigger dramatically labile hypertension, tachycardia, profuse sweating, blotchy erythema, and distal vasoconstriction (Kerr et al., 1968). High norepinephrine secretion has been documented (Keilty et al., 1968). Propranolol, a beta-blocking agent, prevents cardiac arrhythmias (Prys-Roberts, 1969).

Treatment

Treatment must proceed in several directions (Weinstein, 1973). Early intramuscular administration of 3000 to 6000 units of human hyperimmune globulin (human tetanus antitoxin) is essential to neutralize any circulating toxin before it is bound to a receptor. Tetanus antitoxin will bind tetanospasmin already fixed to the central nervous system but will not reverse its action (Zacks and Sheff, 1970). Active immunization with alum-precipitated tetanus toxoid should be started since tetanus itself does not initiate active immunity.

Eradication of the clostridial infection by a bactericidal antibiotic and adequate débridement is axiomatic. Procaine penicillin 1,200,000 units intramuscularly on a daily basis is sufficient. Until the advent of modern respiratory care and muscle relaxants, most authors stated that uterine débridement by dilatation and curettage was contraindicated since uncontrollable muscle spasms could be provoked (Weinstein and Beacham, 1941; Adams and Morton, 1955). This has not been true in recent experience (Adadevoh and Akinela, 1970), provided that hyperimmune globulin and antibiotics are first administered.

Numerous agents can help to control muscle spasms. A quiet, dark room, sedation, and gentle nursing were more important before effective muscle relaxants became available. Phenothiazines, intramuscular meprobamate, and diazepam are all valuable. Parenteral diazepam, sometimes over 100 mg per day in divided doses, is currently the drug of choice (Tempero, 1973). Neuromuscular blocking agents and controlled respiration must be employed in severe cases. Both curare and succinyl choline have been used.

Fetal Effects

Although tetanus itself does not appear to be a fetal hazard if the mother survives, prolonged neuromuscular blockade is a potential danger. It has not been determined whether or not tetanospasmin can pass through the human placenta, but violent intrauterine movements have not been reported in women with tetanus at various stages of pregnancy (Singleton and Witt, 1956: Holmdahl and Thoren, 1962: Januszkiewicz et al., 1973). These infants have been normal at birth.

Curare can cross the placenta. Infants born of mothers who had taken curare can also be paralyzed (Older and Harris, 1968). A mother who took curare for 12 days during the third month of her pregnancy was delivered of a child with arthrogryposis multiplex congenita (Jago, 1970). Drachman and Banker (1961) have supplied good evidence that arthrogryposis results from failure of intrauterine movement. Drachman and Coulombre (1962) have demonstrated that chicks develop clubfoot if exposed to curare before hatching.

Tetanus antitoxin crosses the placenta as do other gamma globulins (Januszkiewicz et al., 1973). Thus maternal immunization can protect an infant from neonatal tetanus unless the amount of toxin produced by the umbilical infection exceeds the infant's complement of maternal antibodies.

SYPHILIS

Syphilis during pregnancy (Holder and Knox, 1972) and congenital syphilis (Woody et al., 1964; Robinson, 1969) are increasingly prevalent problems. The special problems of women with tabes dorsalis are reviewed elsewhere (see p. 11).

Early Fetal Infection

The concept that spirochetes do not infect the fetus before the eighteenth week of intrauterine life has been disproved. *Treponema pallidum* has been demonstrated by silver and immunofluorescent stains in ninth and tenth week conceptuses (Harter and Benirschke, 1976). Bacteria are difficult to find because the fetus is as yet immunologically incapable of mounting a chronic inflammatory response (Silverstein, 1962). Dippel (1944) had failed to find an infected fetus of less than 18 weeks gestational age because he reviewed the products of spontaneous abortions. Syphilis does not cause first trimester abortions. Newer techniques applied to the products of early therapeutic abortions were necessary before the situation could be clarified.

Treatment of maternal syphilis should be instituted as soon as possible. Penicillin is the antibiotic of choice for syphilis whether or not the patient is pregnant. True penicillin allergy in a pregnant woman with syphilis is a problem. Tetracyclines should be avoided during pregnancy because of adverse fetal and maternal effects. Erythromycin is effective against maternal syphilis but will not prevent congenital syphilis (Fenton and Light, 1976). Transplacental transfer of erythromycin is minimal. Fetal blood levels of the drug are only 1 to 2 per cent of the concentration in maternal blood (Philipson and Sabath, 1973). Cephaloridine and other cephalosporins, which do cross the placenta (Arthur and Burland, 1969), are the antibiotics of second choice for syphilis in pregnancy (Holder and Knox, 1972; Thompson, 1976).

Detection of Congenital Syphilis

Serologic tests on cord blood for syphilis, which is dependent on IgG antibodies, will be unreliable due to transplacental passage of maternal antibodies. The IgM fluorescent treponemal antibody absorption test (IgM FTA–ABS test) is highly reliable in the diagnosis of congenital syphilis (Alvord et al., 1969; Rosen and Richardson, 1975). IgM, a large protein which does not cross the placenta, is a measure of the fetal immune response. Cord blood IgM levels are elevated in a number of congenital infections. The IgG FTA-ABS test specifically detects response to *Treponema pallidum.* It will not detect an early infection acquired late in gestation.

KURU

Kuru is a subacute degenerative disease of the central nervous system restricted to the cannibalistic Fore tribe of the eastern highlands of Papua, New Guinea. It is characterized by a 6- to 12-month fatal course of tremor, progressive ataxia, dysarthria, and weakness. The causative agent is a transmissible "slow" virus.

Kuru is predominantly a disease of women of childbearing age. Of 22 pregnant women with kuru who went to term, 21 were delivered of healthy babies (Zigas, 1973). One infant was stillborn. In many cases Zigas found that kuru became static during pregnancy and followed an accelerated course after childbirth. However, an unknown number of pregnant women died before term without aborting. Hornabrook (1968) did not find any influence of pregnancy upon kuru.

After the mothers' death the infants starved to death since no other nursing mother would care for them (Zigas, 1973).

REFERENCES

Poliomyelitis

Aycock, W. L. (1941) The frequency of poliomyelitis in pregnancy. *New England Journal of Medicine,* **225,** 405–408.

Aycock, W. L. (1946) Acute poliomyelitis in pregnancy. *New England Journal of Medicine,* **235,** 160, 161.

Bowers, V. M., and Danforth, D. N. (1953) The significance of poliomyelitis during pregnancy. *American Journal of Obstetrics and Gynecology,* **65,** 34–39.

Cobb, S. W., Stuart, J., and Mengert, W. F. (1953) Poliomyelitis and pregnancy. *Obstetrics and Gynecology,* **2,** 379–383.

Gifford, H., and Hullinghorst, R. L. (1948) Poliomyelitis in pregnancy. *American Journal of Obstetrics and Gynecology,* **55,** 1030–1036.

Horn, P. (1951) Pregnancy complicated by anterior poliomyelitis. *Annals of Western Medicine and Surgery,* **5,** 93–108.

Horn, P. (1955) Poliomyelitis in pregnancy: A twenty-year report from Los Angeles County, California. *Obstetrics and Gynecology,* **6,** 121–137.

Horn, P. (1958) Obstetric management of poliomyelitis complicating pregnancy. *Clinical Obstetrics and Gynecology,* **1,** 127–134.

Hunter, J. S., and Millikan, C. H. (1954) Poliomyelitis with pregnancy. *Obstetrics and Gynecology,* **4,** 147–154.

McCord, W. J., Alcock, A. J. W., and Hildes, J. A. (1955) Poliomyelitis in pregnancy. *American Journal of Obstetrics and Gynecology,* **69,** 265–276.

Priddle, H. D., Lenz, W. R., Young, D. C., et al. (1952) Poliomyelitis in pregnancy and the puerperium: experience in Detroit epidemics of 1949 and 1950. *American Journal of Obstetrics and Gynecology,* **63,** 408–413.

Rindge, M. E. (1957) Poliomyelitis in pregnancy: a report of 79 cases in Connecticut. *New England Journal of Medicine,* **256,** 281–285.

Siegel, M., and Greenberg, M. (1955) Incidence of poliomyelitis in pregnancy: its relation to maternal age, parity, and gestational period. *New England Journal of Medicine,* **253,** 841–847.

Weinstein, L., Aycock, W. L., and Feemster, R. F. (1951) The relation of sex, pregnancy and menstruation to susceptibility in poliomyelitis. *New England Journal of Medicine,* **245,** 54–57.

Poliomyelitis in the Newborn

Baskin, J. L., Soule, E. H., and Mills, S. D. (1950) Poliomyelitis of the newborn. Pathologic changes in two cases. *American Journal of Diseases of Children,* **80,** 10–21.

Bates, T. (1955) Poliomyelitis in pregnancy, fetus, and newborn. *American Journal of Diseases of Children,* **90,** 189–195.

Schaeffer, M., Fox, M. J., and Li, C. P. (1954) Intrauterine poliomyelitis infection. *Journal of the American Medical Association,* **155,** 248–250.

Wright, G. A., and Owen, T. K. (1952) Poliomyelitis in mother and newborn infant. *British Medical Journal,* **1,** 801, 802.

Maternal Immunization

British Medical Journal (1966) Immunization against poliomyelitis. *British Medical Journal,* **1,** 1314, 1315.

Gelfand, M. N., Fox, J. P., LeBlanc, D. R., et al. (1960) Studies on the development of natural immunity to poliomyelitis in Louisiana: V. Passive transfer of polio antibody from mother to fetus, and natural decline and disappearance of antibody in the infant. *Journal of Immunology,* **85,** 46–55.

Strean, G. J., Gelfand, M. M., Pavilanis, V., et al. (1957) Maternal-fetal relationships: placental transmission of poliomyclitis antibodies in newborn. *Canadian Medical Association Journal,* **77,** 315–322.

Tuberculous Meningitis

GENERAL REFERENCES

Barrett-Connor, E. (1967) Tuberculous meningitis in adults. *Southern Medical Journal,* **60**, 1061–1067.

Lepper, M. H., and Spies, H. W. (1963) The present status of the treatment of tuberculosis of the central nervous system. *Annals of the New York Academy of Science,* **106**, 106–123.

O'Toole, R. D., Thornton, G. F., Mukherjee, M. K., et al. (1969) Dexamethasone in tuberculous meningitis: relationship of cerebrospinal fluid effects to therapeutic efficacy. *Annals of Internal Medicine,* **70,** 39–48.

Udani, P. M., Parekh, U. C., and Dastur, D. K. (1971) Neurological and related syndromes in CNS tuberculosis: clinical features and pathogenesis. *Journal of the Neurological Sciences,* **14**, 341–357.

Weiss, W., and Flippin, H. F. (1961) The prognosis of tuberculous meningitis in the isoniazid era. *American Journal of Medical Science,* **242,** 423–430.

TB DURING PREGNANCY

D'Acruz, I. A., and Dandekar, A. C. (1968) Tuberculous meningitis in pregnant and puerperal women. *Obstetrics and Gynecology,* **31,** 775–778.

Golditch, I. M. (1971) Tuberculous meningitis and pregnancy. *American Journal of Obstetrics and Gynecology,* **110,** 1144–1146.

Hedvall, E. (1953) Pregnancy and tuberculosis. *Acta Medica Scandinavica,* **147** (Suppl. **286**), 1–101.

Mehta, B. R. (1961) Pregnancy and tuberculosis. *Diseases of the Chest,* **39**, 505–511.

Schaefer, G., Douglas, R. G., and Dreishpoon, I. H. (1954) Tuberculosis and abortion. *American Review of Tuberculosis,* **70**, 49–60.

Stephanopoulos, C. (1957) The development of tuberculous meningitis during pregnancy. *American Review of Tuberculosis,* **76**, 1079–1087.

Weinstein, L., and Murphy, T. (1974) The management of tuberculosis during pregnancy. *Journal of Perinatology,* **1,** 395–405.

ISONIAZID (INH)

Bessey, O. A., Adam, D. J. D., and Hansen, A. E. (1957) Intake of vitamin B_6 and infantile convulsions: a first approximation of requirements of pyridoxine in infants. *Pediatrics,* **20**, 33–44 (1957).

Biehl, J. P., and Vilter, R. W. (1954) Effect of isoniazid on vitamin B_6 metabolism: its possible significance in producing isoniazid neuritis. *Proceedings of the Society of Experimental Biology and Medicine,* **85,** 389–392.

Bromberg, Y. M., Salzberger, M., and Bruderman, I. (1955) Placental transmission of isonicotinic acid hydrazide. *Gynaecologia,* **140,** 141–144.

Clark, C. M., Elmendorf, D. F., Cawthon, W. U., et al. (1952) Isoniazid (isonicotinic acid hydrazide) in the treatment of miliary and meningeal tuberculosis. *American Review of Tuberculosis,* **66**, 391–415.

Elmendorf, D. F., Cawthon, W. U., Muschenheim, C., et al. (1952) The absorption, distribution, excretion, and short-term toxicity of isonicotinic acid hydrazide (Nydrazid) in man. *American Review of Tuberculosis,* **65**, 429–442.

Fletcher, A. P. (1953) C. S. F.-isoniazid levels in tuberculous meningitis. *Lancet,* **2**, 694–696.

Kutt, H. Winters, W., and McDowell, F. (1966) Depression of parahydroxylation of diphenylhydantoin by antituberculosis chemotherapy. *Neurology,* **16**, 591–602.

Ludford, J., Doster, B., and Woolpert, S. F. (1973) Effect of isoniazid on reproduction. *American Review of Respiratory Disease,* **108**, 1170–1174.

Ross, R. R. (1958) Use of pyridoxine hydrochloride to prevent isoniazid toxicity. *Journal of the American Medical Association,* **168,** 273–275.

Scriver, C. R. (1960) Vitamin B_6 dependency and infantile convulsions. *Pediatrics,* **26**, 62–74.

STREPTOMYCIN

Bignall, J. R., Crofton, J. W., and Thomas, J. A. B. (1951) Effect of streptomycin on vestibular function. *British Medical Journal*, **1**, 554–559.

Brainerd, H. D., and Eagle, H. R. (1950) The effect of streptomycin on tuberculous meningitis. *Annals of Internal Medicine*, **33**, 397–410.

Charles, D. (1954) Placental transmission of antibiotics. *Journal of Obstetrics and Gynaecology of the British Empire*, **61**, 750–757.

Conway, N., and Birt, B. D. (1965) Streptomycin in pregnancy: effect on the foetal ear. *British Medical Journal*, **2**, 260–263.

Hanssen, P., and Lerche, C. (1950) Streptomycinkonsentrasjonsbestemmelser i spinalvaesken ved yuberkuløs meningitt. *Nordisk Medicin*, **43**, 430–431.

Heilman, D. H., Heilman, F. R., Hinshaw, H. C., et al. (1945) Streptomycin: absorption, diffusion, excretion and toxicity. *American Journal of Medical Science*, **210**, 576–584.

Robinson, G. C., and Cambon, K. G. (1964) Hearing loss in infants of tuberculous mothers treated with streptomycin during pregnancy. *New England Journal of Medicine*, **271**, 949–951.

Sakula, A. (1954) Streptomycin and the foetus. *British Journal of Tuberculosis*, **48**, 69–72.

Varpela, E., Hietalahti, J., and Aro, M. J. T. (1969) Streptomycin and dihydrostreptomycin medication during pregnancy and their effect on the child's inner ear. *Scandinavian Journal of Respiratory Diseases*, **50**, 101–109.

Woltz, J. H. E., and Wiley, M. M. (1945) Transmission of streptomycin from maternal blood to the fetal circulation and the amniotic fluid. *Proceedings of the Society for Experimental Biology and Medicine*, **60**, 106, 107.

RIFAMPIN AND ETHAMBUTOL

Altschuler, S. L., and Valenteen, J. W. (1974) Amenorrhea following rifampin administration during oral contraceptive use. *Obstetrics and Gynecology*, **44**, 771, 772.

Bobrowitz, I. D. (1972) Ethambutol in tuberculous meningitis. *Chest*, **61**, 629–632.

Bobrowitz, I. D. (1973) Levels of rifampin in cerebrospinal fluid. *Chest*, **63**, 648, 649.

D'Oliveira, J. J. G. (1972) Cerebrospinal fluid concentrations of rifampin in meningeal tuberculosis. *American Review of the Respiratory Diseases*, **106**, 432–437.

Radner, D. B. (1973) Toxicologic and pharmacologic aspects of rifampin. *Chest*, **64**, 213–216.

Sippel, J. E., Mikhail, I. A., Girgis, N. I., et al. (1974) Rifampin concentrations in cerebrospinal fluid of patients with tuberculous meningitis. *American Review of Respiratory Diseases*, **109**, 579, 580.

Termine, A., and Santuari, E. (1968) Il passaggio transplacentare della rifampinina (dosaggio del farmaco nel siero materno e fetale e nel liquido amniotico. *Annali dell'Istituto Forlanini*, **28**. 431–439.

Weinstein, L., and Murphy, T. (1974) The management of tuberculosis during pregnancy. *Clinical Perinatology*, **1**, 395–405.

CONGENITAL TUBERCULOSIS

Horley, J. F. (1952) Congenital tuberculosis. *Archives of Diseases of Childhood*, **27**, 167–172.

Kendig, E. L. (1960) Prognosis of infants born of tuberculous mothers. *Pediatrics*, **26**, 97–100.

Ramos, A. D., Hibbard, L. T., and Craig, J. R. (1974) Congenital tuberculosis. *Obstetrics and Gynecology*, **43**, 61–64.

Voyce, M. A., and Hunt, A. C. (1966) Congenital tuberculosis. *Archives of Diseases of Childhood*, **41**, 299–300.

Weinstein, L., and Murphy, T. (1974) The management of tuberculosis during pregnancy. *Clinical Perinatology*, **1**, 395–405.

DRUG TERATOGENICITY

Lowe, C. R. (1964) Congenital defects among children born to women under supervision or treatment for pulmonary tuberculosis. *British Journal of Preventive and Social Medicine*, **18**, 14–16.

Ludford, J., Doster, B., and Woolpert, S. F. (1973) Effect of isoniazid on reproduction. *American Review of Respiratory Diseases,* **108**, 1170–1174.

Marcus, J. C. (1967) Non-teratogenicity of antituberculous drugs. *South African Medical Journal,* **41**, 758, 759.

Potworoska, M., Sianozecka, E., and Szufladowicz, R. (1966) Ethionamide treatment and pregnancy. *Polish Medical Journal,* 1152–1158.

Varpela, E. (1964) On the effect exerted by first-line tuberculosis medicines on the foetus. *Acta Tuberculosea Scandinavica,* **35,** 53–69.

Listeriosis

General References

Busch, L. A. (1971) Human listeriosis in the United States, 1969–1971. *Journal of Infectious Diseases,* **123**, 328–332.

Duffy, P. E., Sassin, J. F., Summers, D. S., et al. (1964) Rhomboencephalitis due to *Listeria monocytogenes. Neurology,* **14**, 1067–1072.

Gray, M. L., and Killinger, A. H. (1966) *Listeria monocytogenes* and Listeria infections. *Bacteriological Reviews,* **30**, 309–382.

Hoeprich, P. D. (1958) Infection due to *Listeria monocytogenes. Medicine,* **37,** 143–160.

Lane, F. C., and Unanue, E. R. (1972) Requirement of thymus (T) lymphocytes for resistance to Listeriosis. *Journal of Experimental Medicine,* **135**, 1104–1112.

Lavetter, A., Leedom, J. M., Mathies, A. W., et al. (1971) Meningitis due to *Listeria monocytogenes. New England Journal of Medicine,* **285**, 598–603.

North, R. J. (1973) Importance of thymus-derived lymphocytes in cell-mediated immunity to infection. *Cellular Immunology,* **7**, 166–176.

Sepp, A. H., and Roy, T. E. (1963) *Listeria monocytogenes* infections in metropolitan Toronto: a clinicopathological study. *Canadian Medical Association Journal,* **88**, 549–561.

Simpson, J. F. (1971) *Listeria monocytogenes* meningitis: an opportunistic infection. *Journal of Neurology, Neurosurgery, and Psychiatry,* **34**, 657–663.

Perinatal and Maternal Infections

Albritton, W. L., Wiggins, G. L., and Feeley, J. C. (1976) Neonatal listeriosis: distribution of serotypes in relation to age at onset of disease. *Journal of Pediatrics,* **88**, 481–483.

Anderson, G. D. (1975) *Listeria monocytogenes* septicemia in pregnancy. *Obstetrics and Gynecology,* **46**, 102–104.

Bodnár, L., Pap, G., and Kemenes, F. (1972) Serological screening of pregnant women for listeriosis. *Acta Microbiologica Academiae Scientiarum Hungaricae,* **19**, 389–393.

Driscoll, S. G., Gorbach, A., and Feldman, D. (1962) Congenital listeriosis: diagnosis from placental studies. *Obstetrics and Gynecology,* **20**, 216–220.

Kelly, C. S., and Gibson, J. L. (1972) Listeriosis as a cause of fetal wastage. *Obstetrics and Gynecology,* **40**, 91–97.

Nichols, W., and Woolley, P. V. (1962) *Listeria monocytogenes* meningitis: observations based on 13 case reports and a consideration of recent literature. *Journal of Pediatrics,* **61**, 337–350.

Rappaport, F., Rabinowitz, M., Toaff, R. et al. (1960) Genital listeriosis as a cause of repeated abortion. *Lancet,* **1**, 1273–1275.

Saxbe, W. B. (1972) *Listeria monocytogenes* and Queen Anne. *Pediatrics,* **49**, 97–101.

Schmid, K. O. (1956) Listeriameningitis während der Stillperiode. *Wiener Medizenische Wochenschrift,* **106**, 665–667.

Tetanus

Adadevoh, B. K., and Akinela, O. (1970) Postabortal and postpartum tetanus. *Journal of Obstetrics and Gynaecology of the British Commonwealth,* **77**, 1019–1023.

Adams, J. Q., and Morton, R. F. (1955) Puerperal tetanus. *American Journal of Obstetrics and Gynecology,* **69**, 169–173.

Brooks, V. B., Curtis, D. R., and Eccles, J. C. (1957) The action of tetanus toxin on the inhibition of motoneurons. *Journal of Physiology,* **135**, 655–672.

Drachman, D. B., and Banker, B. Q. (1961) Arthrogryposis multiplex congenita. *Archives of Neurology*, **5**, 77–93.
Drachman, D. B., and Coulombre, A. J. (1962) Experimental clubfoot and arthrogryposis multiplex congenita. *Lancet*, **2**, 523–528.
Holmdahl, M. H., and Thoren, L. (1962) Tetanus in pregnancy. *American Journal of Obstetrics and Gynecology*, **84**, 339–341.
Jago, R. H. (1970) Arthrogryposis following treatment of maternal tetanus with muscle relaxants. *Archives of Disease in Childhood*, **45**, 277–279.
Januszkiewicz, J., Galazka, A., Adamczyk, J., et al. (1973) Severe tetanus in late pregnancy. *Scandinavian Journal of Infectious Diseases*, **5**, 233–235.
Jelliffe, D. B., Walker, A. H. C., and Matthews, S. (1950) Five cases of puerperal tetanus (one associated with eclampsia). *British Medical Journal*, **2**, 814–816.
Keilty, S. R., Gray, R. C., Dundee, J. W., et al. (1968) Catecholamine levels in severe tetanus. *Lancet*, **2**, 195.
Kerr, J. H., Corbett, J. L., Prys-Roberts, C., et al. (1968) Involvement of the sympathetic nervous system in tetanus. *Lancet*, **2**, 236–241.
Kloetzel, K. (1963) Clinical patterns in severe tetanus. *Journal of the American Medical Association*, **185**, 559–567.
Older, P. O., and Harris, J. M. (1968) Placental transfer of tubocurarine. *British Journal of Anaesthesiology*, **40**, 459–463.
Prys-Roberts, C. (1969) Treatment of cardiovascular disturbances in severe tetanus. *Proceedings of the Royal Society of Medicine*, **62**, 662–664.
Scime, J. A., and Tallant, E. J. (1959) Tetanus-like reactions to prochlorperazine (Compazine). *Journal of the American Medical Association*, **171**, 1813–1817.
Singleton, A. R., and Witt, R. W. (1956) Tetanus complicating pregnancy. *Obstetrics and Gynecology*, **7**, 540, 541.
Tarlov, I. M., Ling, H., and Yamada, H. (1973) Neuronal pathology in experimental local tetanus. *Neurology*, **23**, 580–591.
Tempero, K. F. (1973) The use of diazepam in the treatment of tetanus. *American Journal of Medical Science*, **266**, 4–12.
Weinstein, B. B., and Beacham, W. D. (1941) Postabortal tetanus. *American Journal of Obstetrics and Gynecology*, **42**, 1031–1040.
Weinstein, L. (1973) Tetanus. *New England Journal of Medicine*, **289**, 1293–1296.
Yates, J. C., and Yates, R. D. (1966) An electron microscopic study of tetanus toxin on motoneurons of the rat spinal cord. *Journal of Ultrastructure Research*, **16**, 382–394.
Zacks, S. I., and Sheff, M. F. (1970) Tetanism: pathobiological aspects of the action of tetanal toxin in the nervous system and skeletal muscle. *Neurosciences Research*, **3**, 209–287.

Syphilis

Alvord, C. A., Jr., Polt, S. S., Cassady, G. E., et al. (1969) γM-fluorescent treponemal antibody in the diagnosis of congenital syphilis. *New England Journal of Medicine*, **280**, 1086–1091.
Arthur, L. J. H., and Burland, W. L. (1969) Transfer of cephaloridine from mother to fetus. *Archives of Disease in Childhood*, **44**, 82–83.
Dippel, A. L. (1944) The relationship of congenital syphilis to abortion and miscarriage, and the mechanism of intrauterine protection. *American Journal of Obstetrics and Gynecology*, **47**, 369–379.
Fenton, L. J., and Light, I. J. (1976) Congenital syphilis after maternal treatment with erythromycin. *Obstetrics and Gynecology*, **47**, 492–494.
Harter, C. A., and Benirschke, K. (1976) Fetal syphilis in the first trimester. *American Journal of Obstetrics and Gynecology*, **124**, 705–711.
Holder, W. R., and Knox, J. M. (1972) Syphilis in pregnancy. *Medical Clinics of North America*, **56**, 1151–1160.
Nicolis, G., and Loucopoulos, A. (1974) Cephalothin in the treatment of syphilis. *British Journal of Venereal Diseases*, **50**, 270, 271.
Philipson, A., Sabath, L. D., and Charles, D. (1973) Transplacental passage of erythromycin and clindamycin. *New England Journal of Medicine*, **288**, 1219–1221.
Robinson, R. C. V. (1969) Congenital syphilis. *Archives of Dermatology*, **99**, 599–610.

Rosen, E. U., and Richardson, N. J. (1975) A reappraisal of the value of the IgM fluorescent treponemal antibody absorption test in the diagnosis of congenital syphilis. *Journal of Pediatrics,* **87**, 38–42.

Silverstein, A. M. (1962) Congenital syphilis and the timing of immunogenesis in the human fetus. Nature, **194**, 196, 197.

Thompson, S. E. (1976) Treatment of syphilis in pregnancy. *Journal of the American Venereal Disease Association,* **3**, 159–167.

Woody, N. C., Sistrunk, W. F., and Platou, R. V. (1964) Congenital syphilis: a laid ghost walks. *Journal of Pediatrics,* **64**, 63–67.

Kuru

Hornabrook, R. W. (1968) Kuru—a subacute cerebellar degeneration. The natural history and clinical features. *Brain,* **91**, 53–74.

Zigas, V. (1973) Effect of kuru on pregnancy. *Tropical and Geographical Medicine,* **25**, 262–265.

CHAPTER SIX

Multiple Sclerosis

Multiple sclerosis is a patchy, demyelinating disease of the central nervous system characterized by relapses and spontaneous remissions. The lesions are disseminated and may appear over a long period of time. Manifestations include weakness, incoordination diplopia, blindness, sensory tract symptoms, and vertigo. Rarely can a gray matter symptom such as convulsions be attributed to multiple sclerosis.

The natural history of multiple sclerosis is punctuated by relapses. The relapse rate varies with geographical area, sex, age of onset, and duration of disease. Not all symptomatic relapses cause or increase disability. A relatively stationary phase can last for thirty years or more before progressive disability develops. The older the age of onset, the more likely is the course to be progressive. Patients who had retrobulbar neuritis, diplopia, sensory tract symptoms, or vertigo are least disabled and have the longest regressive stage. Motor symptoms, particularly when combined with cerebellar dysfunction, are restrictive.

The diagnosis rests upon the neurologic history, physical findings, and the exclusion of other possibilities. No specific test exists. During acute multiple sclerosis, leukocyte counts in the cerebrospinal fluid can be slightly elevated. At some point during the course of multiple sclerosis, the gamma globulin fraction of total cerebrospinal fluid proteins becomes elevated and remains elevated for the duration of the disease. Total cerebrospinal fluid protein concentration remains normal or is minimally elevated. A normal gamma globulin fraction is not helpful in diagnosis.

The cause of multiple sclerosis is unknown, although viral agents are suspected. No specific cure exists. Steroids shorten the length of relapses, probably by diminishing edema, but do not alter the course of the disease. Proper bladder care, physical therapy, and occupational therapy are of utmost importance.

Effect of Multiple Sclerosis upon Pregnancy

Uncomplicated multiple sclerosis has almost no effect upon pregnancy. The incidence of difficult delivery, premature labor, and stillbirth during 1220 pregnancies of 487 patients was almost identical to that in the general population of the same area during the same period (Kulig and Schaltenbrand, 1956). The duration of the three stages of labor is normal (Sweeney, 1953). No change in the management of delivery need be made. Toxemia is no more common than in normal pregnant women.

If a neurogenic bladder exists, a gravid uterus will interfere with bladder and bowel function. Urinary tract infection will be more frequent.

Effect of Pregnancy upon Multiple Sclerosis

The earliest comment on the influence of pregnancy upon multiple sclerosis was the following notation by Sir William Gowers (1901): "I have known it to begin during pregnancy, remain stationary until the next pregnancy, and then become progressive." German physicians found onset and relapses to be more common in the puerperium than during pregnancy itself (von Hoesslin, 1904; Dimitz, 1928). The bulk of the early literature consists of case reports and small series documenting deterioration during and after pregnancy.

To determine whether or not pregnancy or any other factor aggravates multiple sclerosis or any other fluctuating disease is a difficult statistical problem. If multiple sclerosis is already in the progressive stage, it is impossible to determine the effect of pregnancy. Relapse rates for pregnant patients in the stationary phase should be compared with those of their nonpregnant counterparts. For this purpose a pregnancy-year is defined as the 9 months of pregnancy and the 3 months postpartum. Mueller (1951) found these relapse rates to be equal. Schapira et al. (1966) found the relapse rate during a pregnancy-year to be 50 per cent higher, and Millar (1959) found it to be 100 per cent higher.

A consistent finding of all series is that half of all relapses during a pregnancy-year occur during the first 3 postpartum months. First attacks follow the same pattern (Table 6.1). One factor may be exhaustion from the chores of caring for a newborn infant. Husbands of these patients must endeavor to prevent this.

Table 6.1. Multiple sclerosis during a pregnancy year

	Onset	Relapse
Episodes	15	29
Total number of pregnancies		133
Incidence during:		
First trimester	2	5
Second trimester	1	1
Third trimester	3	7
Puerperium	9	16
Relapse rate per pregnancy year		0.22

Modified from Müller, R. (1951) Pregnancy in disseminated sclerosis. *Acta Psychiatrica et Neurologica Scandinavica,* **26**, 397–409.

Counseling

German physicians of the early twentieth century advised women with multiple sclerosis to neither marry nor have children. Beck (1913) and Fleck (1938) advocated abortion if multiple sclerosis should worsen during pregnancy even though they recognized that abortion neither resulted in remission nor altered a progressive course. These views were abandoned in light of the findings of subsequent large statistical studies. Abortion is not necessary on the sole grounds that a woman has multiple sclerosis. Marriage is not a factor. Nonpregnant married and unmarried women have the same relapse rate (Millar et al, 1959).

The desire of most couples for parenthood usually more than offsets the probably higher risk of relapse during a pregnancy-year, provided that there is a reasonable chance that the child will be unaffected by multiple sclerosis and that the mother will be able to rear and enjoy her child.

First, multiple sclerosis is more common among some families, but it is not a hereditary disease. Many patients carry the same set of histocompatibility antigens. This suggests that there is a genetic prodisposition to respond immunologically (or fail to respond) to the etiologic agent, presumably viral. Within a family, affected sibling pairs are common. Twins have the highest concordance (Cendrowski, 1973).

Affected parent-child pairs are more frequent than expected in the population at large (McAlpine, 1972). However, I can find only one affected parent-child pair in which the parent manifested multiple sclerosis *before* the birth of her subsequently affected child (Schapira, et al., 1963). The data are statistically compatible with the common exposure hypothesis of affected parent-child pairs (Cendrowski, 1969).

Second, multiple sclerosis is a chronic but intermittent disease. Few cases are fulminant. The course is unpredictable, but most young patients can expect several decades of minimal restrictions—usually long enough to rear a family. An older woman already in the progressive stage of her illness should not be encouraged to become pregnant.

REFERENCES

Beck, R. (1913) Multiple Sklerose, Schwangerschaft und Geburt. *Deutsche Zeitschrift für Nervenheilkunde,* **46,** 127.

Cendrowski, W. (1969) Multiple sclerosis in parents and children. *Acta Neurologica Scandinavica,* **45,** 380–382.

Cendrowski, W. (1973) Multiple sclerosis in twins and other relatives. *Acta Neurologica Scandinavica,* **49,** 552–556.

Dimitz, L. (1928) Über den Zusammenhang der multiplen Sklerose mit Schwangerschaft, Unfall und Kriegsdienstleistung. *Beitrage zur Gerichtlichen Medizin,* **7,** 186.

Fleck, V. (1938) Multiple Sklerose und Schwangerschaftsunterbrechung, wie Unfruchtbarmachung aus ärztlichen Grunden. *Allg. Zeitschrift für Psychiatrie,* **109,** 9–15.

Gowers, W. (1901) *Diseases of the Nervous System,* 2nd ed., Vol. 2. New York: P. Blakiston's Son & Co., p. 545.

von Hoesslin, R. (1904) Die Schwangerschaftslämung der Mutter. *Archiv fur Psychiatrie,* **38,** 732.

Kulig, K., and Schaltenbrand, G. (1956) Statistische Untersuchung zum Problem der Multiplen Skerlose. *Deutsche Zeitschrift für Nervenheilkunde,* **174,** 460–468.

Leibowitz, U., Antonovsky, A., Kats, R., et al. (1967) Does pregnancy increase the risk of multiple sclerosis? *Journal of Neurology, Neurosurgery and Psychiatry,* **30,** 354–357.

McAlpine, D. (1972) Some aspects of the natural history: Familial incidence and its significance. In *Multiple Sclerosis: A Reappraisal,* eds. McAlpine, D., Lumsden, C. E., and Acheson, E. D., 2nd ed. Edinburgh: Churchill Livingstone.

McAlpine, D., and Compston, N. (1952) Some aspects of the natural history of disseminated sclerosis. *Quarterly Journal of Medicine,* **21,** 135–167.

Millar, J. H. D. (1961) The influence of pregnancy on disseminated sclerosis. *Proceedings of the Royal Society of Medicine,* **54,** 4–7.

Millar, J. H. D., Allison, R. S., Cheeseman, E. A., et al. (1959) Pregnancy as a factor in influencing relapse in disseminated sclerosis. *Brain,* **82,** 417–426.

Müller, R. (1951) Pregnancy in disseminated sclerosis. *Acta Psychiatrica et Neurologica Scandinavica,* **26,** 397–409.

Peckham, C. H. (1945) Multiple sclerosis complicating pregnancy. *New York State Journal of Medicine,* **45,** 618–622.

Schapira, K., Poskanzer, D. C., and Miller, H. (1963) Familial and conjugal multiple sclerosis. *Brain,* **86,** 315–332.

Schapira, K., Poskanzer, D. C., and Newell, D. J., et al. (1966) Marriage, pregnancy and multiple sclerosis. *Brain,* **89,** 419–428.

Sweeney, W. J. (1953) Pregnancy and multiple sclerosis. *American Journal of Obstetrics and Gynecology,* **66,** 124–130.

Sweeney, W. J. (1958) Pregnancy and multiple sclerosis. *Clinical Obstetrics and Gynecology,* **1,** 137–145.

Tillman, A. J. B. (1949) The effect of pregnancy on multiple sclerosis and its management. *Research Publications of the Association for Research in Nervous and Mental Disease,* **28,** 548–582.

CHAPTER SEVEN

Cerebrovascular Disease

SPONTANEOUS SUBARACHNOID HEMORRHAGE

Spontaneous subarachnoid hemorrhage in a pregnant woman is a catastrophe that immediately endangers the lives of mother and fetus. A maternal mortality study in Franklin County, Ohio, found that 10 per cent of all maternal deaths occurring to women during pregnancy and the six postpartum months were caused by intracranial hemorrhage (Barnes and Abbott, 1961). In a 24-year Minnesota mortality study 4.4 per cent of maternal deaths were attributed to spontaneous subarachnoid hemorrhage, but only a few were verified by angiography or autopsy (Barno and Freeman, 1976). The exact incidence during pregnancy remains undetermined, but estimates range from 1 to 5 per 10,000 pregnancies.

The first case of cerebral hemorrhage during pregnancy was reported by Edmond Lazard in 1899.

E. D., aged 31, German, was admitted to the antepartum ward of Kings County Hospital. She had had two previous confinements, the first of which had been a difficult instrumental delivery, and the second had been a normal one. On the morning of December 18, 1898, the patient had a severe headache and the beginning of labor pains; pulse of good tension. At 10 P.M. she had a severe labor pain and from then until 10 A.M., December 19, she had at prolonged intervals long and hard pains. At this time the membranes ruptured and with the next pain a small fetus, apparently about 6 months, was rapidly expelled. The Crede method of extraction of placenta was immediately begun. While the uterus was being manipulated, the patient was noticed to sink into a semiconscious stupor, from which she could be aroused only by loud calling; breathing somewhat stertorous. [The] placenta was hastily extracted and ergot given. The pulse at this time was weak and fluttering; whisky and strichnia by hypodermic and saline solution by rectum were given. [Her] condition much improved; in about 5 minutes she again began to breath stertorously and then sank into a deeper stupor. Convulsive twitching then began in the muscles of the right hand and progressively extended to [the] right arm and right side of [the] face and then involved the whole body. Notwithstanding the previous poor condition of the pulse and the march of the convulsion, I decided the case to be one of eclampsia. Chloroform was administered, and *Veratrum viride* [was] given hypodermically. As soon as possible, the patient [was] put into a hot pack. At 6 P.M. another and less general convulsion took place. The patient remained in a comatose stage from this time until her death on December 23, 4 days and 9 hours after labor.

The autopsy showed a "ruptured artery" and intracranial hemorrhages.

Although in the late nineteenth century a massive literature on cerebral aneurysms accumulated from autopsy studies, the antemortem diagnosis of subarachnoid bleeding awaited the development of the lumbar puncture technique. Subsequently, development of cerebral angiography went hand in hand with the rational treatment of surgically amenable intracranial aneurysms and angiomas.

Clinical Presentation

Patients with spontaneous subarachnoid hemorrhage may present in one of two ways—comatose, in which state they are in immediate danger of dying, or conscious, in which case there is grave danger from rebleeding. Those who are conscious usually complain of a severe occipital headache which is described as beginning at a precisely defined moment, perhaps while straining in one manner or another. Nausea and vomiting accompany or soon follow the headache in most cases. Although muchal rigidity may be absent soon after a hemorrhage or if the patient is comatose, its presence should be sought and can be recorded as the number of finger breadths between mentum and sternum. Focal neurologic signs may be caused by an intracerebral hematoma, enlarged aneurysm, cerebral herniation, or vasospasm. Mental confusion may be further evidence of diffuse cerebral arterial spasm. The mild fever, leukocytosis, tachyarrhythmias, mild proteinuria, and fluctuating hypertension that may appear with subarachnoid hemorrhage of any cause may be ascribed to atypical eclampsia.

Cerebrospinal Fluid Examination

Examination of the cerebrospinal fluid is mandatory to make the diagnosis of subarachnoid bleeding and to rule out meningitis. Proper handling of the specimens is essential. Erythrocytes can be counted directly. If the specimen is very bloody, the concentration can be expressed as per cent of packed cell volume. Bloody or blood-tinged cerebrospinal fluid cannot be called xanthrochromic unless a centrifuged specimen has a clear amber supernatant. A traumatic tap will have a colorless supernatant. Xanthrochromic pigments from red cell destruction can appear 6 hours after the hemorrhage.

Differential Diagnosis

Once the syndrome of subarachnoid hemorrhage has been recognized, the next step is to find the causative condition. If the patient is comatose and the history inadequate, the event must be considered traumatic until promptly instituted procedures have proved otherwise. If the subarachnoid hemorrhage is spontaneous, the differential diagnosis must consider a ruptured arteriovenous malformation, a ruptured aneurysm, or one of a long list of rarer causes which collectively compose a major category.

The cooperative, multicenter "aneurysm study" collected so much

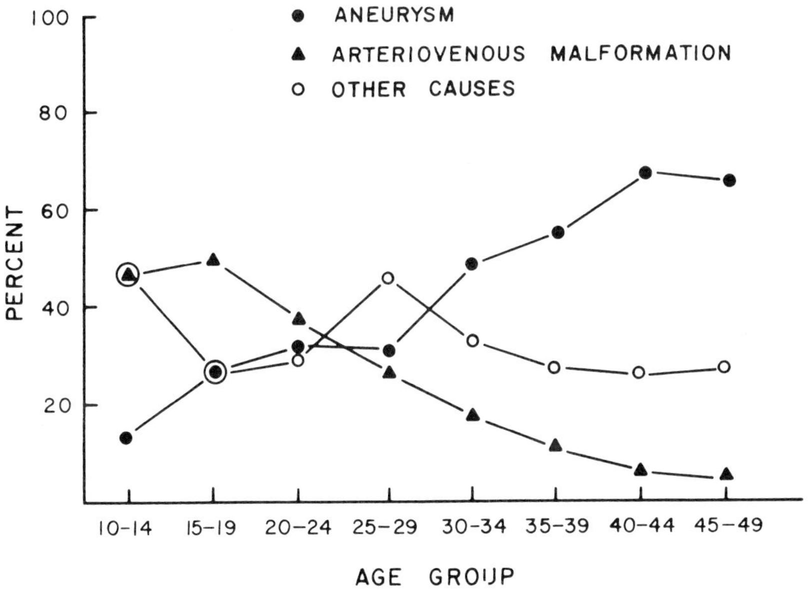

Figure 7.1. Relative probability of major causes of subarachnoid hemorrhage for women by age. From data in Locksley, H. B. (1966) Natural history of subarachnoid hemorrhage, intracranial aneurysms and arteriovenous malformations. *Journal of Neurosurgery*, 25, 219–239.

data that the probability of the various causes of subarachnoid hemorrhage can now be calculated for each sex and age range (Locksley, 1966). The probability curves show that, for women under the age of 25, arteriovenous malformations are a more common cause of subarachnoid hemorrhage than aneurysms. This is not true for men. At any age at least a third of all subarachnoid hemorrhages, including those for which no cause can be found, are caused by 'other' conditions. Robinson et al. (1974) could find no cause in only 5 per cent of their well-studied series of pregnant women. This compares favorably with the 10 to 15 per cent commonly undiagnosed in unrestricted series.

Before proceeding with angiography the physician caring for a pregnant patient with a subarachnoid hemorrhage must direct his subsequent questions, physical examination, and basic laboratory studies with the aim of excluding the rarer causes, particularly those associated with pregnancy.

Hematologic Disorders

Placental abruption with disseminated intravascular coagulation (DIC) will usually be all too obvious to the obstetrician. This condition has been associated with subarachnoid hemorrhage in two fatal cases (Heron et al., 1974). Subarachnoid hemorrhage is a well-recognized complication of anticoagulant therapy (Weigle, 1955; Hirsch et al., 1972). Since warfarin has been implicated as an agent causing congenital malformations, heparin is the anticoagulant of choice for thrombophlebitis and various cardiac problems during pregnancy. Leukemia or thrombocytopenia may be suggested by pallor, petechiae, ecchymoses, and melena. A basic battery of tests for screening purposes would include a hemoglobin determination, platelet count, and partial thromboplastin time (PTT).

Table 7.1. 'Other' causes of spontaneous subarachnoid hemorrhage during pregnancy

- Hematologic disorders
  - Anticoagulant therapy
  - Abruptio placentae with disseminated intravascular coagulation
- Mycotic aneurysm from subacute bacterial endocarditis
- Vasculitis (lupus erythematosus)
- Metastatic choriocarcinoma
- Eclampsia
  - Early—hypertensive intracerebral hematomas
  - Late—cerebral infarction and multiple petechial hemorrhages
- Postpartum cerebral phlebothrombosis
- Rupture spinal cord arteriovenous malformation
- (Ectopic endometriosis)

Cardiac Disease

A diagnosis of subacute bacterial endocarditis must always be considered. If a woman presents with subarachnoid hemorrhage from a mycotic aneurysm, a cursory examination may overlook a change in her "hemic" murmur, a spleen tip, microscopic hematuria, subungual splinter hemorrhages, Roth spots in the optic fundus, or other signs of subacute bacterial endocarditis. Even if the diagnosis is missed at first, arteriography may be characteristic.

Vasculitis

Cerebral vasculitis of various origins can cause subarachnoid hemorrhage. Systemic lupus erythematosus is often exacerbated during pregnancy, but it has not been reported as a cause of subarachnoid hemorrhage during pregnancy.

Choriocarcinoma

Choriocarcinoma may present as an intracranial hemorrhage of any description. It may accompany a normal or molar pregnancy, but more commonly it appears in the months following childbirth. It caused 3 per cent of maternal deaths in the Minnesota maternal death study (Barno and Freeman, 1976). A positive urinary pregnancy test after the hundredth day of gestation is suspect.

Eclampsia

Subarachnoid blood may be found in eclampsia due to deep hypertensive hemorrhages that are often quickly fatal. The more common cortical petechiae are less likely to produce gross bleeding until the preterminal stages.

Cerebral Venous Thromboses

Cerebral phlebothrombosis with secondary venous infarction of the brain can produce subarachnoid blood, usually when the superior sagittal sinus and cortical veins are thrombosed. Cerebral venous thromboses usually occur 3 days to 4 weeks after delivery but can happen during early pregnancy. Careful examination of the venous phase of cerebral angiograms can be diagnostic.

Spinal Subarachnoid Hemorrhage

The source of subarachnoid bleeding need not be intracranial. Hemorrhage from a spinal cord arteriovenous malformation causes sudden back pain followed by headache and a stiff neck. One patient had spinal cord subarachnoid bleeding caused by an ectopic endometrioma of the cauda equina (Lombardo et al., 1969).

Intracranial Aneurysms vs. Arteriovenous Malformations

After the clinical impression of subarachnoid hemorrhage has been confirmed by a bloody, xanthrochromic specimen of spinal fluid, and if a circumspect search for an obvious "other" cause of the bleeding has been fruitless, the differential diagnosis lies between an arteriovenous malformation and an aneurysm. A history of unilateral migraine headaches or convulsions or the presence of an ocular or cranial bruit makes an arteriovenous malformation more likely. Skull films may show a pineal shift or calcifications that are suggestive of either possibility. Computerized tomography will clearly show intracerebral hematomas and intraventricular blood if present.

Even when computerized tomography is available, the definitive diagnostic technique is angiography. Focal signs may suggest which artery should be investigated first, but unless an arteriovenous malformation is found, all four intracranial arteries (both carotid and both vertebral arteries) must be studied in these young patients. Otherwise multiple aneurysms or a posterior fossa aneurysm may be missed. If an arteriovenous malformation is demonstrated, a selective external carotid arteriogram may be needed to define all the feeding arteries completely.

The timing of angiography varies with the temperament and clinical experience of the physicians involved. Angiography should not be deferred because the patient is pregnant, as the abdomen can be shielded. Delay may create greater risk from rebleeding. Arteriography should be done early so that surgery can be performed while the cumulative percentage of rebleeding is low. In an alert patient this usually means that the study should be done during regular working hours on the day following admission to the hospital so that complications are minimized.

The treatment of an arteriovenous malformation or an aneurysm in a pregnant woman involves two basic problems: (1) the timing of an operation on a surgically approachable lesion and (2) the timing and manner of terminating the pregnancy. These questions can best be answered after an analysis of the natural history of arteriovenous malformations and aneurysms during pregnancy.

Arteriovenous Malformations During Pregnancy

During pregnancy arteriovenous malformations tend to bleed initially during the second trimester and during childbirth, although the danger exists at any stage (Table 7.2). Rebleeding during delivery may be fatal. Exactly why arteriovenous malformations should bleed frequently in the second trimester is unclear, but engorgement of the shunt is probably a factor. Intrapartum rupture is related to the strenuous Valsalva maneuver that a hard labor pain almost irresistibly produces.

There is no direct evidence of the effect of pregnancy upon cerebral arteriovenous malformations. In women with normal cerebral vasculature, total cerebral blood flow remains constant throughout pregnancy (McCall, 1949). An arteriovenous shunt deprives tissue of its normal oxygen and nutrient supply in the territory of its major feeding artery (Prosenz et al., 1971) (Fig. 7.2). An increase in shunting can cause hypoxemia, which may be clinically manifest as a seizure. No serial regional cerebral perfusion studies have been done during the pregnancy of a woman with a known, inoperable arteriovenous malformation, and no serial photographs of a retinal angioma during pregnancy have been published (Armstrong, 1937).

On indirect grounds it can be reasonably assumed that either cerebral arteriovenous malformations enlarge or shunting increases during pregnancy. Two factors support this assumption. First, vascular tumors, whether meningiomas or skin and gum tumors, enlarge during pregnancy. Second, an analogy can be drawn with the vascular spider "nevi" which appear in the majority of Caucasian woman during early pregnancy (Bean et al., 1949). These small arteriovenous fistulae increase in number and size throughout pregnancy and fade away within days after delivery. The symptoms of spinal cord arteriovenous malformations,

Table 7.2. Spontaneous subarachnoid hemorrhage during pregnancy by period of gestation

	Aneurysm	Arteriovenous malformation
Proven cases	80	38
Average age	31	27
Gestational period of first bleed		
First trimester	16%	21%
Second trimester	34%	50%
Third trimester	41%	18%
Intrapartum	5%	11%
First week postpartum	4%	Nil
Most common time	23–36 wks (18%)	16–20 wks (24%)
Rebleeding intrapartum	+	++
Rebleeding postpartum	++	±

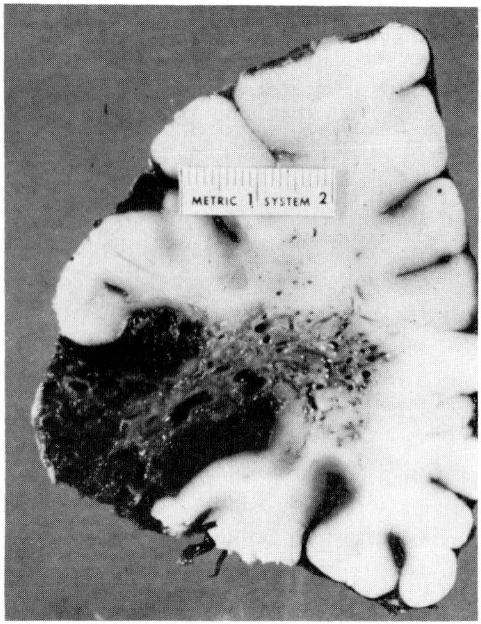

Figure 7.2. Coronal section through a typical wedge-shaped cerebral arteriovenous malformation that has ruptured. From McCormick, W. F., and Schochet, S. S. (1976) *Atlas of Cerebrovascular Disease*. Philadelphia: W. B. Saunders Company.

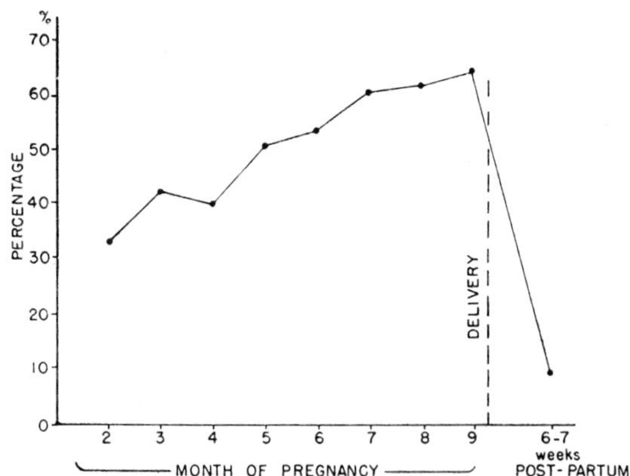

Figure 7.3. Percentage of Caucasian women exhibiting palmar erythema during the course of pregnancy and after delivery. From Bean, W. B., Cogswell, R., Dexter, M., et al. (1949) Vascular changes of the skin in pregnancy: Vascular spiders and palmar erythema. *Surgery, Gynecology and Obstetrics,* 88, 748. By permission of *Surgery, Gynecology and Obstetrics.*

meningiomas, and chorea gravidarum show the same dramatic improvement after delivery.

The cooperative aneurysm study found that at least one-third of subarachnoid hemorrhages occurred during some event involving bearing down (Locksley, 1966). Certainly the vigorous Valsalva maneuver of childbirth could cause a thin-walled aneurysm to rupture or a previously ruptured aneurysm to rebleed.

The physiology of the Valsalva maneuver has been well studied. When the glottis or mouth and nose are closed and abdominal and thoracic expiratory muscles are contracted, the intra-abdominal and intrathoracic pressure rapidly rises. The high intrathoracic pressure limits venous return to the heart. Thus after a few contractions of the heart, cardiac output and systemic blood pressure decline.

When bearing down ceases, the systemic arterial pressure drops temporarily, since the high intrathoracic pressure, which had been transmitted to the great vessels, no longer supports it. At this point the cerebral blood flow reaches its lowest point and syncope is most common. After the pump is primed by venous return, cardiac output suddenly increases, and the systemic blood pressure overshoots the resting levels before settling back to normal. In patients with autonomic neuropathy, this overshoot does not occur.

The intrathoracic pressure is transmitted to the cerebral veins and sinuses by the valveless plexus of vertebral veins. The intracranial veins, in contrast to the peripheral veins, are not stressed when intrathoracic pressure is high because the venous pressure is balanced by a concomitant increase in cerebrospinal fluid pressure. Since the cerebrospinal fluid volume is constant in a rather rigidly walled system, the pressure is transmitted across the thin veins by a simple hydraulic mechanism.

Cerebrospinal fluid pressures during labor have been measured (Hopkins et al., 1965; Marx et al., 1961, 1962; Vasicka et al., 1962). Uterine contractions without simultaneous bearing down do not alter the CSF pressure. As expected, CSF pressure rises with bearing down. It can exceed the limit of 700 mm water (about 50 mm Hg) that is measurable with the manometer (McCausland and Holmes, 1957). Intrathoracic pressures of up to 200 mm Hg have been recorded with the Valsalva maneuver (Faulkner and Sharpey-Schafer, 1959).

The exact timing of a subarachnoid hemorrhage in relation to the Valsalva maneuver has not been recorded. It seems likely that it occurs after release of straining. The sudden thrust of blood at high pressure could rupture an enlarged or weakened vessel.

Bearing down can be prevented by keeping the glottis open. Panting, a breathing exercise often taught women in antepartum courses, does just that. Adequate regional anesthesia will do the same.

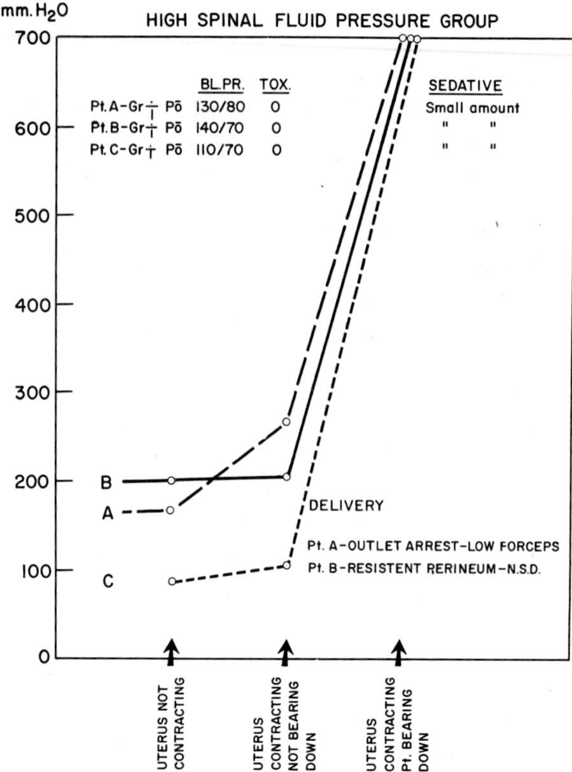

Figure 7.4. Cerebrospinal fluid pressure during labor. A contraction without bearing down does not elevate pressure. From McCausland, A. M., and Holmes, F. (1957) Spinal fluid pressures during labor. *Western Journal of Surgery,* **65,** 226.

Aneurysms During Pregnancy

Although the mechanisms by which pregnancy affects congenitally weakened arterial walls is unknown, the frequent rupture during pregnancy of aneurysms caused by cystic medial necrosis makes the existence of such factors most likely.

Cerebral Aneurysms

The chance that a cerebral aneurysm will bleed increases with each trimester of pregnancy. As in the case described by Lazard, a subarachnoid hemorrhage late in pregnancy may precipitate labor. Unlike arteriovenous malformations, aneurysms seldom rupture initially during parturition, although rebleeding frequently occurs at that time. In the weeks after delivery the woman with a cerebral aneurysm is again at greater risk. The distribution of sites of aneurysms in a group of pregnant women is approximately that expected in a nonpregnant cohort (Robinson et al., 1974).

Splenic Artery Aneurysm

Splenic artery aneurysms are the second most commonly ruptured aneurysm during pregnancy. Sixty per cent of splenic artery aneurysms are attributed to arteriosclerosis and occur in equal proportions in older individuals of both sexes (Jones and Finney, 1968). Aneurysms secondary to congenital weakness of the medial layer of the splenic artery occur in young adults, predominantly women by a margin of 2:1. The majority of these women are pregnant (MacFarlane and Thorbjarnarson, 1966). Splenic artery aneurysms have been associated with cerebral aneurysms; in one case there was spontaneous rupture at both locations (Greene and McCormick, 1968). As with cerebral aneurysms, the chance of rupture increases with duration of gestation.

Other Aneurysms

Although less common, aneurysms of the aorta (Schnitker and Bayer, 1944; Pedowitz and Perell, 1957), coronary arteries (DiMaio and DiMaio, 1971), and renal and iliac arteries (Cohen et al., 1972) due to cystic medial necrosis follow the same pattern of rupture during the third trimester. Women with Marfan's syndrome are prone to ruptured aortic aneurysms during pregnancy (Elias and Berkowitz, 1976).

Why pregnancy further weakens aneurysms can only be surmised. The direct relation between risk of bleeding and duration of pregnancy suggests a hormonal influence. The tensile strength of a healthy rabbit aorta is unaffected by pregnancy or the Pill (Johnson et al., 1965). A well-designed pathologic study from the Armed Forces Institute of Pathology found no change in the aortas of pregnant women who suffered accidental deaths (Cavanzo and Taylor, 1969). Other studies have demonstrated changes in both the elastic fibers and muscle of aortic media of women dying of a variety of diseases, including subarachnoid hemorrhage (Danforth et al, 1954; Manalo-Estrella and Barker, 1967). The effect of pregnancy may be insignificant upon normal aortas but profound upon abnormal vessels.

The relationship of aneurysmal subarachnoid hemorrhage to the puerperium is even more murky. The muscularis of arterial walls shares many histologic and pharmacologic properties with the myometrium. Perhaps there is an involution of the smooth muscle of arterial walls leading to a subarachnoid hemorrhage.

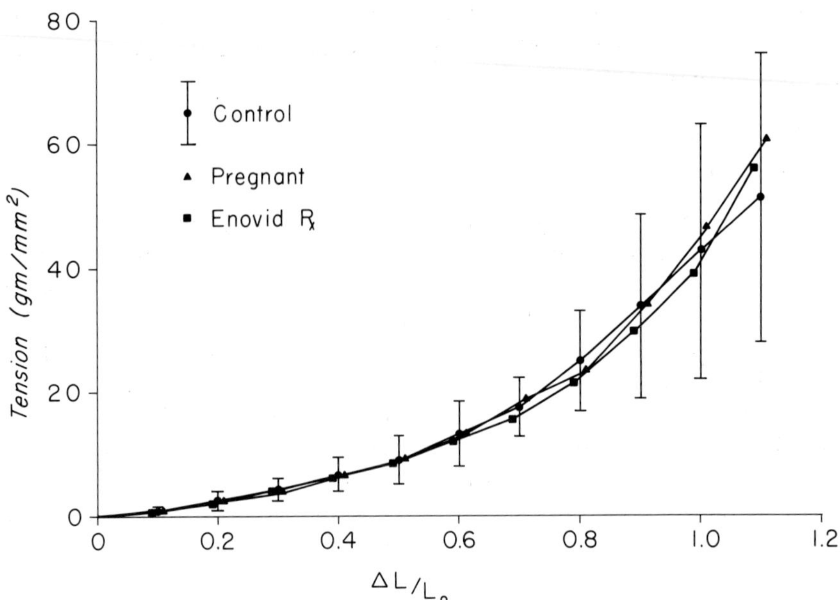

Figure 7.5. Tensile strength of aorta from nonpregnancy control and pregnant and Enovid-treated rabbits. L_0 = original length, ΔL = increase in length. From Johnson, W. L., Conrad, J. T., Whitney, D., et al. (1965) The effect of pregnancy and norethynodrel with mestranol (Enovid) on length-tension relationship in the rabbit aorta. *American Journal of Obstetrics and Gynecology,* **93,** 180. Courtesy of W. L. Johnson.

Treatment

The basic rule is that the neurosurgical evaluation and treatment of a pregnant woman with a subarachnoid hemorrhage should be the same as that for a nonpregnant patient unless she is in active labor.

The natural history of both arteriovenous malformations and aneurysms shows that both lesions can rebleed during childbirth with fatal results. The best method of preventing this risk is total excision of the arteriovenous malformation or intracranial clipping of the offending aneurysm (Pool, 1965; Robinson et al., 1974). Cumulative experience indicates that the surgery can be performed with adequate safety using hypothermia. Hypotension and the use of hyperosmolar mannitol should be avoided if possible. If multiple aneurysms are present, the one responsible for the subarachnoid hemorrhage should be clipped before childbirth. The remainder can wait.

The routine care of each patient is important but is often slighted. The patient should have a quiet room. Minor sedative drugs can be prescribed if the patient is unduly anxious. The Valsalva maneuver must be avoided by measures such as regular stool softeners, abstinence from

Table 7.3. Relation of pregnancy, form of treatment, and clinical grade to mortality in patients with aneurysms

	Group A		Group B	
	Cases	*Death Rate*	*Cases*	*Death Rate*
Pregnancy-related cases				
Conservative treatment	3	67%	12	42%
Operative management	3	Nil	25	Nil
Nonpregnancy-related cases				
Conservative treatment	4	75%	20	20%
Operative mangement	8	38%	38	5%

Group A patients were in danger of dying after their first subarachnoid hemorrhage. Group B patients were conscious initially but at risk from recurrent bleeding. Adapted from Robinson, J. L., Hall, C. S., and Sedzimir, C. B. (1974). Arteriovenous malformations, aneurysms, and pregnancy. *Journal of Neurosurgery*, **41**, 63–70.

cigarette smoking, and cough suppressives. If the patient cannot move her limbs, regular passive range-of-movement exercises will prevent muscle contractures. If she is comatose, pressure sores can be prevented by turning her every 2 hours.

Problems arise if the lesion is inoperable. Arteriovenous malformations are so prone to rebleeding during delivery that at some institutions elective cesarean sections are routinely performed at 38 weeks' gestation (Robinson et al., 1974). The average age of patients with arteriovenous malformations is less than 25 years. Most are primigravidas. If the woman is multiparous with a proven adequate pelvis, normal vaginal delivery may be possible if bearing down can be avoided by panting during severe pains or by regional anesthesia.

Women with inoperable aneurysms which are discovered early in gestation are often allowed to deliver vaginally (Hunt et al., 1974). If an aneurysm bleeds in the third trimester, most physicians elect to deliver the patient, especially if she is a primigravida, by cesarean section to avoid rebleeding. There is no way to avoid the postpartum risk.

Management of Cerebral Edema in Pregnancy

Hyperventilation. Hyperventilation reduces cerebral blood flow and decreases intracranial pressure. It is safe during pregnancy.

Hypothermia. Hypothermia may be safely used during pregnancy to decrease cerebral oxygen requirements and cerebral edema (Wilson and Sedzimir, 1959; Hehre, 1965; Kamrin and Maslin, 1965). During hypothermia uterine blood flow decreases whether or not the patient shivers. Contraction of the uterus around its arteries has been suggested as the cause (Assali and Westin, 1962). This hypothesis is supported by clinical observation of a firm uterus and a rise in intrauterine pressure. The fetus is protected since its metabolic requirements have also decreased. Hypoxia is not a problem if the mother is adequately ventilated.

Steroids. High-dose corticosteroids have been used throughout pregnancy for systemic lupus erythematosus without obvious ill effects upon the fetus (Garenstein et al., 1962). The exact effect of high-dose dexamethasone upon the fetus is unknown. It must be considered a long-term risk until more information is available.

Hyperosmolar Mannitol. If cerebral edema progresses to incipient tentorial herniation, the need to preserve the life of the living demands the use of hyperosmolar mannitol therapy. The consequences of this therapy are clear, although it has been used without reported ill effect. The hypertonic expansion of maternal extracellular space with mannitol produces osmotic forces that result in the flow of free water from the fetus and amniotic fluid to the mother. Battaglia et al. (1960) infused 1 liter of 20 per cent mannitol into normal pregnant women during the hour before delivery. A 10 per cent increase in maternal plasma osmolarity, which is in the therapeutic range for the treatment of brain swelling, was almost matched by the increase in fetal osmolarity. The physical condition of the infants was not mentioned in the report. Further studies in pregnant rabbits with a 25 per cent increase in plasma osmolarity showed profound fetal effects—severe dehydration, a 50 per cent contraction of blood volume, cyanosis, and bradycardia (Bruns et al., 1963). The amniotic fluid dried up. Thus the use of hyperosmolar mannitol should be avoided during pregnancy if possible.

ARTERIAL CEREBROVASCULAR DISEASE

The sudden onset of motor and sensory deficits is characteristic of cerebral infarction. Signs and symptoms vary with the site of the lesion. Headache, vomiting, and seizures can occur but are not typical. The cerebrospinal fluid is bloodless. Improvement rather than worsening should be expected. Edema surrounding a large infarction may initially simulate a mass lesion, but a slowly progressive course suggests tumor, abscess, or hematoma. Additional occlusions, often embolic, can add deficits in sudden stages.

Nonhemorrhagic stroke is infrequent in young women. The risk increases with age, pregnancy, and the Pill. Most nonhemorrhagic strokes during pregnancy and the first postpartum week are caused by arterial occlusions rather than by cerebral venous thromboses as once believed (Cross et al., 1968; Amias, 1970). Venous occlusions occur usually 1 to 4 weeks after childbirth.

Incidence

In a well-studied series of ischemic strokes in young patients from Glasgow, 35 per cent of the 65 women of childbearing age were pregnant or puerperal (Cross et al., 1968). This is at least 3 or 4 times the normal pregnancy rate for this population. A sampling error large enough to account for this difference was deemed unlikely. The number of arterial occlusions occurring in the puerperium was as high as the number occurring during the second and third trimesters of pregnancy (Cross et al., 1968).

The incidence of ischemic stroke in young women taking the Pill is similarly increased. Estimates range from sixfold (Vessey and Doll, 1968) to ninefold the normal number (Collaborative Study, 1973). Incidence cannot be correlated to duration of usage of contraceptives. Most women affected are parous (Bickerstaff, 1975). Cigarette smoking is an associated risk factor (Collaborative Study, 1973), but surprisingly, hypertension is not (Bickerstaff, 1975). Low doses of estrogen preparations are associated with a lower incidence of thromboembolism (Inman, 1970).

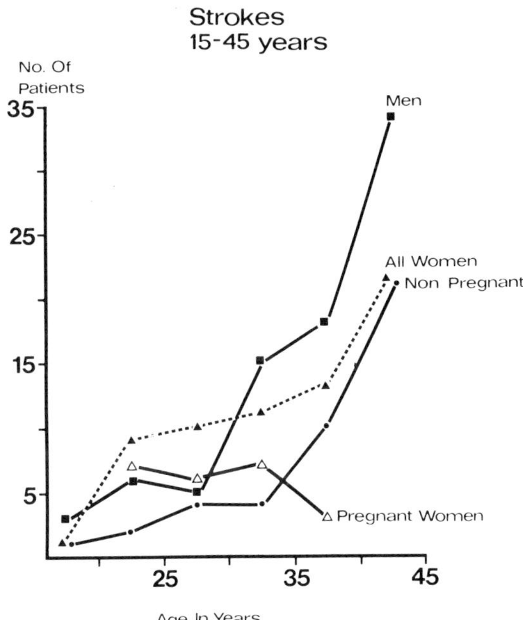

Figure 7.6. Ischemic carotid strokes in 146 young adults, aged 15 to 45 years. Sixty-five per cent of the women under 35 years of age who suffered a stroke were pregnant or puerperal. From Jennett, W. B., and Cross, J. N. (1967) Influence of pregnancy and oral contraception on the incidence of strokes in women of childbearing age. *Lancet*, **1**, 1020. Courtesy of Prof. W. B. Jennett.

Site of Lesion

The majority of strokes in the young involve the carotid territory. A significant fraction, about one-quarter, will not have an angiographically demonstrable occlusion of either the internal carotid or the middle cerebral arteries. This is attributed to clot lysis. In pregnancy-associated strokes, middle cerebral artery occlusions are twice as common as those in a nonpregnant cohort (Cross et al., 1968).

An unusually high frequency—25 to 40 per cent—of strokes associated with the Pill are vertebral-basilar artery occlusions (Salmon et al., 1968; Bickerstaff, 1975). Bickerstaff demonstrated that these occlusions occur just below the juncture of the vertebral arteries. Transient cortical phenomena (e.g., limb weakness, aphasia, dyscalculia, apraxia) occurring in women taking the Pill can be attributed to thromboembolic transient ischemia.

Etiology

Exactly why vascular diseases is more common in women who are pregnant or are taking the Pill is unknown. The literature on this subject is such a quagmire that I shall not attempt to review it. It is enough to say here that the physician treating such a patient should institute a search for other disease.

There are four etiologic categories of arterial occlusive disease—thrombosis, embolism, vasculitis, and spasm. Thrombosis is the most common cause. Spasm is least likely but occurs with migraine and eclampsia. A search for a source of emboli or the presence of vasculitis must be conducted since proper treatment can limit further damage. A search is especially important in the presence of an unusual factor such as a heart murmur, carotid bruit, unequal brachial blood pressures, cardiac arrhythmia, abnormal optic fundi, fever, purpura, or signs of systemic disease. A work-up is outlined in Table 7.4, but a careful history and physical examination will eliminate many possibilities. Unless an obvious source of emboli is found, angiography is indicated for pregnant and puerperal stroke patients in order to rule out cerebral venous thrombosis. In addition, it may show an arterial occlusion or the beaded arteries characteristic of vasculitis. If available, computerized tomography of the brain can be helpful, but in this instance it is not diagnostic.

Unusual Emboli During Pregnancy

Several unusual sources of emboli exist in pregnant and puerperal women.

Table 7.4. Laboratory evaluation of nonhemorrhagic stroke in pregnant and puerperal women

Tests	Conditions considered
Hemogram	Erythrocytemia
Platelet count	Thrombotic thrombocytopenic purpura
Blood smear	Thrombocytosis
Blood sugar	Hypoglycemia
Urinalysis for	Vasculitis
Red cells/red cell casts	Lupus erythematosus
Proteinuria	Heart disease
Sedimentation rate, serologic test for syphilis	Subacute bacterial endocarditis, valvular disease
Chest x-ray	Cardiomyopathy
Electrocardiogram	Atrial myxoma
?Echocardiogram	Neoplasm (metastatic choriocarcinoma)
Pregnancy test	Focal status epilepticus
Skull x-rays	Subarachnoid hemorrhage
Electroencephalogram	Cerebral venous thrombosis
Computerized tomography	
Spinal fluid examination	
?Arteriography	

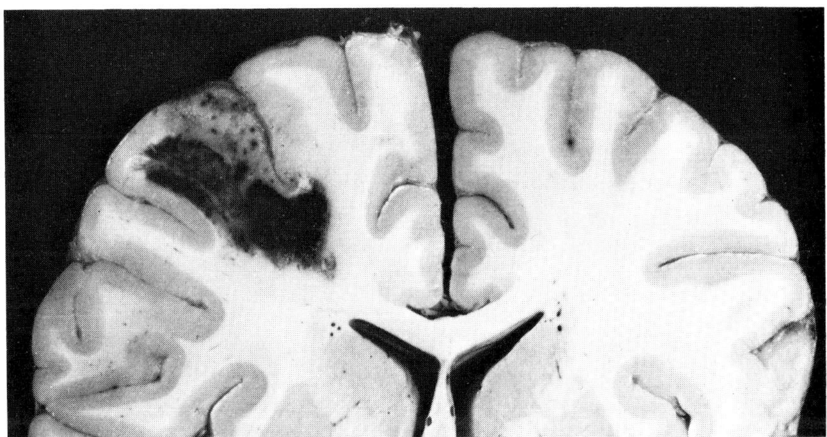

Figure 7.7. A wedge-shaped, focally hemorrhagic cerebral infarct in the left middle frontal gyrus from the brain of a 27 year old woman who died in the twentieth week of gestation with cardiomyopathy. Border zone or watershed infarctions are due to inadequate perfusion of terminal arterial beds secondary to severe hypotension. This infarction occurred in the boundary zone between the left anterior and the middle cerebral arteries. From Connor, R. C. R., and Adams, J. H. (1966) Importance of cardiomyopathy and cerebral ischemia in the diagnosis of fatal coma in pregnancy. *Journal of Clinical Pathology*, **19**, 245. Courtesy of Prof. J. Hume Adams.

Peripartum Cardiomyopathy

Postpartum cardiomyopathy presents as congestive failure during the third trimester as well as after childbirth. In this, as in any other cardiomyopathy, fragments of mural thrombi can lodge in cerebral vessels (Connor and Adams, 1966).

Paradoxical Emboli

Paradoxical emboli move from right heart to left heart chambers via an abnormal communication, usually a patent foramen ovale. An anatomically patent foramen ovale of varing caliber persists beyond neonatal life in 30 per cent of persons. Higher pressure in the left atrium keeps this potential valvelike orifice closed. Pulmonary hypertension from a massive pulmonary embolus or from multiple small emboli, including amniotic emboli, can allow subsequent emboli to cross into the systemic circulation.

Amniotic Fluid Emboli

Amniotic fluid embolism is characterized by sudden dyspnea, cyanosis, shock, and often death occurring during or just after childbirth. Any woman is susceptible, especially multiparas over 30 years of age. Labor can be tumultuous or prolonged. Uterine, cervical, or vaginal tears are common portals of entry. Postpartum hemorrhage from uterine laceration or associated disseminated intravascular coagulopathy aggravates shock. The antemortem diagnosis can be proved by demonstrating fetal epithelial squamous cells just above the buffy coat of settled blood withdrawn from the right atrium while placing a central venous pressure catheter (Resnik et al., 1976).

Ten per cent of any large series of patients with amniotic fluid emboli experience convulsions, usually within minutes of the onset of dyspnea and shock (Aguillon et al., 1962; Smibert, 1967; Peterson and Taylor, 1970). Probably this occurs on a hypoxic basis. Paradoxical cerebral amniotic fluid emboli do occur (Smibert, 1967) and could induce seizures. The true incidence of this phenomenon is unknown. Careful pathology is infrequently mentioned, and the extent of search surely is variable. Fetal epithelial squamous cells and mucus are difficult enough to detect in the lung. Multiple tissue blocks and special stains are desirable (Attwood, 1972; Roche and Norris, 1974).

Fat Emboli

Two obese women with a clinical course typical of amniotic fluid embolism were shown to have pulmonary and cerebral fat emboli

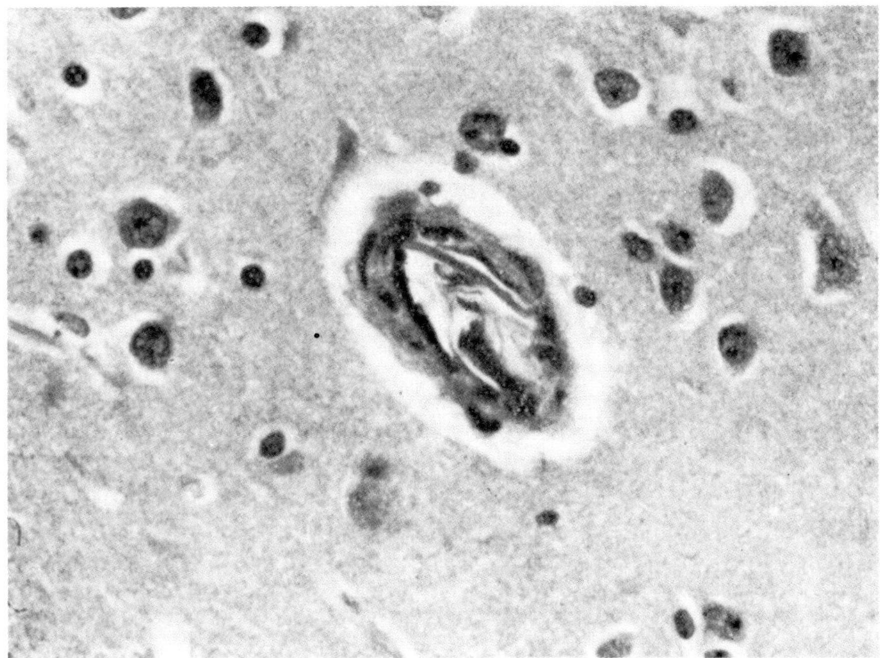

Figure 7.8. Clump of squames in a cerebral vessel of a woman with a patent foramen ovale who died after a convulsion of amniotic fluid embolism (Alcian phloxin, × 400). From Smibert, J. (1967) Amniotic fluid embolism: A clinical review of twenty cases. *Australian and New Zealand Journal of Obstetrics and Gynaecology,* 7:7. Courtesy of J. Smibert.

(Lillian et al., 1955; Jonas, 1961). Fat from the vernix caseosa is one of the components of amniotic fluid (Steiner and Tushbaugh, 1949), but in neither of these cases could squames be found. Cerebral fat emboli can occur after crises of sickle cell disease and hemoglobin S/C disease. In one case this occurred after a crisis induced by childbirth (Chmel and Bertles, 1975). This woman had a latent interval which is commonly observed in systemic fat embolization (Thomas and Ayyar, 1972).

Air Emboli

Air emboli cause sudden death in women during pregnancy and in the early puerperium. The signs and symptoms of air emboli are dramatic: sudden apprehension, tachycardia, dyspnea, cyanosis, and shock. Sometimes a hypoxic convulsion precedes coma and death. An early case reported by May (1857) is typical. A 30 year old woman was in normal labor with her third child until shortly after her membranes ruptured. She exclaimed, "Oh! How faint I feel," convulsed, and died. At

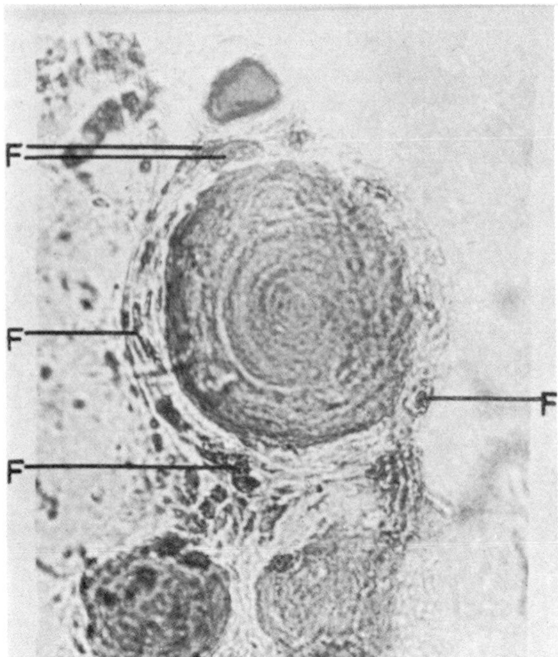

Figure 7.9. Fat in the choroid plexus of a woman who died during labor after a convulsion (hematoxylin and Sudan 4, × 400). Multiple fat emboli were demonstrated in the lungs. (F= fat) From Jonas, E. G. (1961) Maternal death due to fat embolism. *Journal of Obstetrics and Gynaecology of the British Commonwealth,* **68,** 481. Courtesy of E. G. Jonas.

postmortem examination the inferior vena cava was empty, and the right atrium was distended by air.

Treatment depends upon instantaneous recognition of the cause. A diagnostic feature is the gurgling, churning heart sound attributed to frothy blood. The patient must be turned on her left side to trap air in the right heart chambers, from which it must be promptly aspirated.

A special procedure must be followed for pathologic proof of a suspected case of fatal air embolism. Before removing the heart from the thorax, the great vessels must be ligated to contain any air within the heart. The heart is then opened under water so that escaping bubbles will demonstrate the existence of intracardiac air. Sudden death is characteristic of cardiopulmonary deaths but not brain deaths.

Venous air emboli cause almost 1 per cent of maternal deaths, according to the Ohio State Maternal Mortality Survey (1972). Nearly one-half of reported cases are induced during criminal abortion (Nelson, 1960). Accidental air embolization can occur during cesarean section and complicated vaginal delivery. Avoidable deaths have happened dur-

Table 7.5. Causes of air emboli during pregnancy and the puerperium

Causes
Abortion
Cesarean section
Complicated vaginal delivery
Air insufflation of the vagina during:
Douches
Powder instillation
Cunnilinctus
Puerperal knee-chest exercises

ing douching (Cooke, 1950) and powder insufflation as a treatment for vaginal infections (Martland, 1945). Forceful vaginal insufflation as a variant of sexual activity is not safe during pregnancy and the early puerperium (Aronson and Nelson, 1967).

Air embolization can follow knee-chest exercises in the puerperium. Redfield and Bodine (1939) drew an analogy to a bellows when he described the following mechanism. Air could flow into a patulent vagina while the woman assumed the knee-chest position. After lying down the closed vagina and labia would trap air within. Neurologic symptoms while in the knee-chest position could be caused by hyperextension and rotation of the neck (Schwarz, 1966). This extreme position can reduce cerebral circulation by kinking a vertebral or carotid artery (Toole and Tucker, 1960).

CEREBRAL VENOUS THROMBOSIS

Cerebral venous thrombosis is now an uncommon form of cerebrovascular disease. In the pre-antibiotic era septic cerebral thrombophlebitis was a feared and well-recognized complication of any infection of the face, scalp, nasal sinuses, tonsils, skull, ear or mastoids. Aseptic cerebral venous thrombosis occurs in children and accompanies dehydration, polycythemia, leukemia, and sickle cell crises. During active adult life aseptic cerebral venous thrombosis is either idiopathic or associated with trauma, pregnancy, the puerperium, or the Pill.

Clinical Syndromes

The anatomy of the cerebral venous system and the pathogenesis of venous cerebrovascular disease are ill-understood by most physicians. The best analogy to a cortical vein thrombosis is a retinal vein occlusion, which produces retinal hemorrhages and edema that can be easily seen and followed. Cerebral venous drainage is much more complex. The

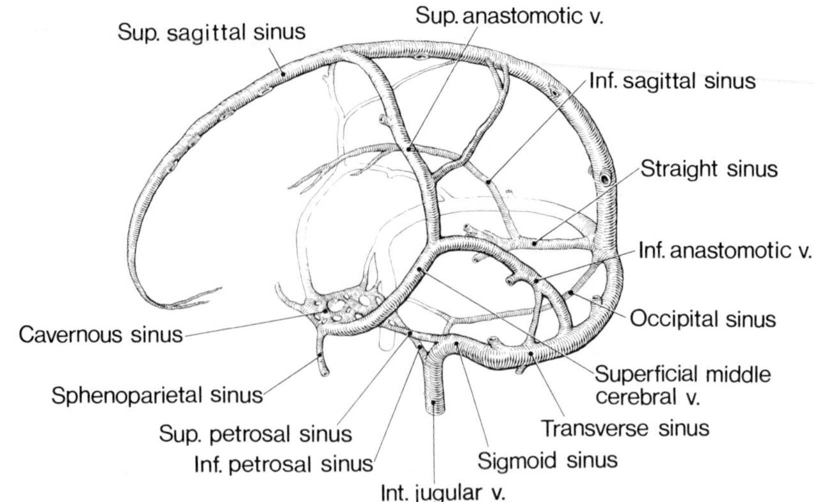

Figure 7.10. Venous drainage of the cerebral hemispheres. From Dunkerley, G. B. (1975) *A Basic Atlas of the Human Nervous System.* Philadelphia, F. A. Davis Company. Courtesy of G. B. Dunkerley.

symptoms of four major clinical syndromes differ according to the sinus and adjacent veins involved.

Cavernous Sinus Thrombosis

Cavernous sinus thrombosis is caused by local infection of the face, orbit, or nasal sinuses. Incidence is unrelated to childbirth. In addition to signs of local infection and exophthalmos, ophthalmoplegia and hyperalgesia in the ophthalmic division of the trigeminal nerve are evident, caused by the involvement of the cranial nerves that course through the cavernous sinus (cranial nerves III, IV, V(1), and VI). Bilateral involvement occurs via the circular sinus. Visual impairment varies.

Lateral Sinus Thrombosis

Lateral sinus thrombosis almost always follows otitis or mastoiditis. One case of extensive cerebral venous thrombosis due to otitis has been associated with pregnancy (Deane, 1908). Since the right transverse sinus drains the superior sagittal sinus, cerebrospinal fluid reabsorption can decrease with no extension of the clot into the superior sagittal sinus, as usually occurs. In either instance intracranial pressure increases, causing the so-called otitic hydrocephalus. Obstruction of the left transverse sinus, which drains the straight sinus and the inferior sagittal sinus, usually does not cause intracranial hypertension. Propagation of the clot from the lateral sinus into the adjacent cortical veins causes seizures and contralateral weakness of the face and arm.

The two syndromes associated with the puerperium, pregnancy, and the Pill are (1) primary aseptic superior sagittal sinus thrombosis, sometimes with extension into the cortical veins, and (2) primary cortical vein thrombosis, sometimes with extension into the sagittal sinus. The clinical and pathologic distinction is real, as appreciated by Ducrest (1847) and by Martin and Sir Charles Symonds a century later.

Primary Sagittal Sinus Thrombosis

Primary longitudinal sinus thrombosis presents in one of two patterns—intracranial hypertension and paraplegia after alternating Jacksonian seizures. Both cause headache. Intracranial hypertension is caused by the obstruction of reabsorption of cerebrospinal fluid by the arachnoid villi which stud the dural walls of the sinus. Spread of the clot into the superior cortical veins can be asynchronous and asymmetrical. Thus, focal convulsions may be seen at first in one leg and later in the other. Paralysis usually follows the seizures but may develop without preceding convulsions. Primary aseptic sagittal sinus thrombosis has been ascribed to seemingly insignificant head trauma, grazing of the skull by a bullet, sepsis, dehydration, hyperviscosity syndromes, and sickle cell crises. One case with maternal hypernatremia followed intrauterine instillation of hypertonic saline solution in an attempt to induce abortion (Goldman and Eckerling, 1972).

Primary Cortical Vein Thrombosis

Primary cortical vein thrombosis is the more common variety of cerebral phlebothrombosis seen by obstetricians. Headache is the most common prodrome and may occur at any site. It may vary in intensity but is usually intense, progressive, and resistant to simple analgesics. Presumably the headache is caused by inflammation of pain-sensitive veins and dura. Transient aphasia, weakness, or numbness may be experienced. These symptoms are similar to the transient cortical phenomenon that occurs with the use of oral contraceptives.

The onset of seizures rings the alarm. When the headache is most

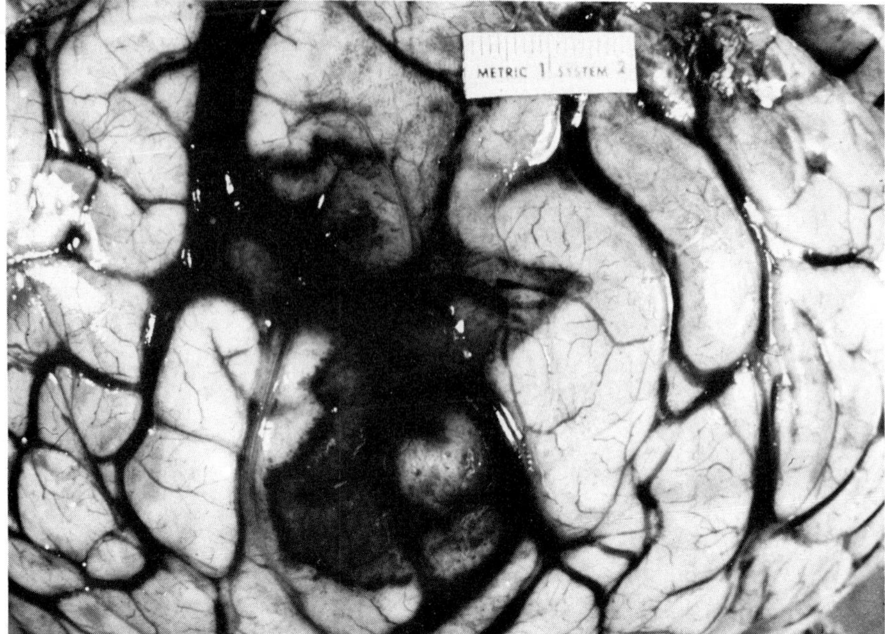

Figure 7.11. Cortical vein thrombosis in a 25 year old woman who had taken the Pill for 3 months. The dilated thrombosed cortical veins of the right parietal lobe are surrounded by focal subarachnoid and subpial hemorrhages. From McCormick, W. F., and Schochet, S. S. (1976) *Atlas of Cerebrovascular Disease*. Philadelphia: W. B. Saunders Company.

intense, the fits begin and probably coincide with the rapid filling of a cortical vein with red thrombus after its occlusion at a branch point (Martin, 1941). The fits are routinely focal or are generalized seizures with focal or aversive features. After occlusion of the vein, small hemorrhages form, dotting the softened swollen patch of cortex like a retinal vein occlusion. Paralysis or aphasia results.

Recurrence of convulsions, often followed by deepening stupor, implies spreading of the clot. If it reaches the superior sagittal sinus, the intracranial pressure increases by the mechanism previously mentioned. The thrombus need not reach a dural sinus to produce increased intracranial pressure, provided the cortical infarction and concomitant cerebral edema are great enough to act as an expanding mass lesion, thereby producing a shift of the midline structures, papilledema, and coma.

Cerebellar veins as well as cerebral veins can be involved (Hunt, 1917). Subsequent cerebellar infarction and edema act like an expanding posterior fossa mass and may require emergency surgical decompression.

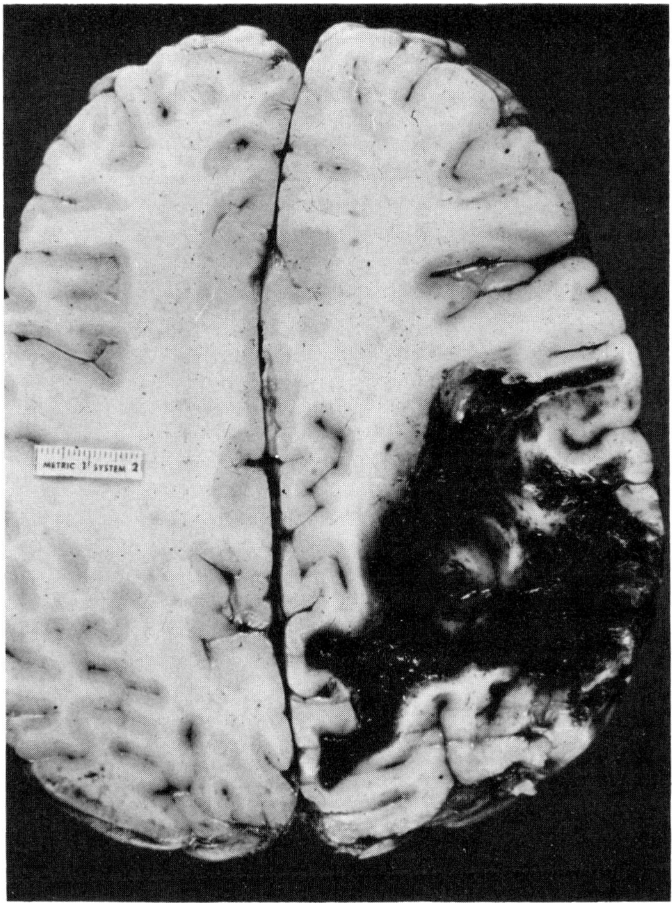

Figure 7.12. Massive hemorrhagic infarction and hematoma deep to the thrombosed veins shown in Figure 7.11. From McCormick, W. F., and Schochet, S. S. (1976) *Atlas of Cerebrovascular Disease*. Philadelphia: W. B. Saunders Company.

History

The long history of puerperal cerebral phlebothrombosis is replete with names of famous physicians who have rediscovered the entity. In 1828, John Abercrombie of Scotland wrote the following clinicopathologic description.

A lady, aged 24, had long been liable to severe attacks of headache, which occurred at regular intervals and were excited by various causes, such as warm rooms and bodily exertions, and for which she had had a variety of treatment with little benefit. They had not, however, affected her general health, and she was recovering favourably from her second accouchement under the care of Dr.

Mackintosh, when about the beginning of the second week, she was seized with severe headache, and considerable oppression. She was bled with relief and continued tolerably well for several days, although with occasional complaint of headache. On Sunday 14th January, 1827, after a disturbed night with some delirium, she complained in the course of the day of slight uneasiness in her head, and a peculiar feeling of numbness in the back of her head and neck; but she was otherwise well and in good spirits, till about ten o'clock at night, when she suddenly complained of numbness and loss of power of the right hand. These feelings spread rapidly along the arm, which very soon became entirely paralytic, and this was speedily followed by loss of speech, and twisting of the mouth. She was immediately bled, and when I saw her soon after bleeding, I found her with a look of intelligence, but without any attempt at speech; the pulse quick and feeble, the right arm entirely powerless, and with a degree of spasmodic rigidity. She continued without any further change till about three o'clock in the morning, when she was seized with severe and general convulsion, affecting both sides of the body, but strongest on the left side. The convulsion returned three times betwixt this and mid-day of the 15th, after which the attacks became much more frequent; and from this time she showed no appearance of sensibility. She had from the first swallowed with difficulty, but every attempt to make her swallow now excited general convusions. During the attacks, the face was much distorted, and equally so on both sides; the limbs on the left side were violently convulsed, while the right arm was affected chiefly with a spasmodic contraction and a tremulous motion. The convulsions now returned with great violence and frequency, sometimes every half hour, and each attack continued for ten or fifteen minutes. The pulse was generally rapid, sometimes extremely feeble, and sometimes of tolerable strength. The breath was sometimes frequent and convulsive, and sometimes slow and oppressed, as if she were moribund; and on many occasions she was considered as being within a few minutes of death; but she continued to live in this state till the evening of the 16th, being forty-eight hours from the attack. On the second day, the rigid contraction of the right arm had disappeared, and it continued entirely paralytic, except when it was affected by the convulsions.

Inspection. On the upper surface of the left hemisphere, and between the convulsions (sic), there was a considerable ecchymosis produced by a very thin layer of extravasated blood betwixt the arachnoid and pia mater. The veins on the upper part of this hemisphere were remarkably turgid, and were found to be distended with dark blood in a perfectly firm fleshy state, mixed with some firm white matter; and their coats appeared to be thickened. Where these veins entered the longitudinal sinus, there was a remarkable diminution of its area, arising partly from the thickening of its coats, and partly from deposition of firm white matter on its inner surface. In the substance of the left hemisphere about the centre of its long diameter towards the outer side, and rather above the level of the ventricle, there was a distinctly defined portion about the size of a small walnut in a state of complete ramollissement, but retaining entirely the natural white colour; and immediately bordering upon the part, there was a considerable portion in a state of the deep redness described in the former cases; the brain in other respects was healthy, except a small softened spot in the right hemisphere.

This was the last case on autopsy material reported in the English language until William Collier presented a case to his colleagues in the London Pathological Society in 1891. Both Prosper Meniere (1828) and Fleetwood Churchill (1854) collected reports of postpartum paralysis.

Some cases of each series are probably examples of cerebral venous thromboses, but neither author appreciated the entity or presented enough clinical or pathologic information to make a secure retrospective diagnosis. Sporadic reports of puerperal hemiplegia or puerperal aphasia (Sinclair, 1902) with pathologic evidence of cerebral phlebothrombosis appeared so irregularly in the continental literature that the clinical syndrome was not included in a textbook until Sir William Gowers' *Diseases of the Nervous System* was published in 1893. It was not until about 1940 with the observations of J. Purdon Martin, H. L. Sheehan, and Sir Charles Symonds that the syndrome gained enough widespread recognition that the diagnosis could be made antemortem. Many cases had been labeled atypical or late eclampsia (Sheehan and Lynch, 1973). Survival became recognized. Since 1965 several cases have been reported among women taking the Pill.

Epidemiology

Of all kinds of aseptic cerebral vein thrombosis occurring during active adult life, the puerperal and idiopathic categories are the most common (Kalbag and Woolf, 1967). All other kinds are rare. Retrospective series at several major institutions show an average incidence of one case per 2500 deliveries at each hospital (Carroll et al., 1966). Since some cases would probably be referred to these centers, the true incidence is doubtless lower. One well-investigated series of strokes during and after pregnancy found the incidence to be less than one case per 10,000 deliveries (Cross et al., 1968).

Postpartum cerebral phlebothrombosis usually occurs from 3 days to 4 weeks after childbirth. Eighty per cent of cases begin in the second or third postpartum weeks. In one case associated with postpartum uterine hemorrhage and shock the symptoms occurred immediately after delivery (Burt et al., 1957). A few cases of cerebral phlebothrombosis occurring 4 or 5 months after childbirth are tenuously included in the postpartum category by some authors.

Age and parity are apparently indeterminant factors. Of 31 pathologically or clinically proven cases in the English-language literature, the age distribution forms a bell-shaped curve, with the most numerous cases occurring between ages 25 and 29 years. The distribution among primigravidas, secundigravidas, and multigravidas for the same series is 13:7:7 (gravidity is not mentioned in all reports). Labor and delivery are characteristically normal. Recurrence after subsequent pregnancies has been reported (Carroll et al., 1966). The exact risk is unknown but is probably low as judged by the paucity of reports.

Although a clear relationship exists between cerebral venous thrombosis and the puerperium, a relationship either to pregnancy itself or to use of the Pill has not been proved, although it is suspected. Cases occurring in all stages of pregnancy have been reported, although only a cluster of cases in the first trimester are well substantiated (Fishman et al., 1957; Stevens and Ammerman, 1959; Eckerling et al., 1963). One-half of the 12 cases reported in women taking oral contraceptives have occurred within 2 months of its inception, but the range extends to 2 years. Whether or not the incidence of cerebral phlebothrombosis in these circumstances exceeds the occurrence of idiopathic cases is unknown.

Differential Diagnosis

The constellation of prodromal headache, focal or generalized fits followed by paralysis, aphasia, progressive obtundation, and papilledema occurring from the third day to the fourth week after childbirth defines the clinical syndrome of puerperal cerebral venous thrombosis. The differential diagnosis in puerperal women is somewhat easier if the influence of pregnancy upon the other possibilities is known.

Mild fever and leukocytosis may be present, as can be expected with any inflammatory process or after a seizure. A local infection of the face, nasal sinuses, ear, and mastoids must be excluded by examination and skull radiographs. The possibility of thrombosis elsewhere must be reasonably eliminated by a careful examination of the legs and pelvis.

A lumbar puncture is indicated to rule out meningitis and gross subarachnoid hemorrhage. Usually the cerebrospinal fluid is normal, although sometimes increased tension is noted. Red cells or frank blood may be seen, especially late in the course of the disease when venous infarction is widespread. If gross blood is seen immediately after the onset of disease, another cause for the subarachnoid hemorrhage is more likely. In a puerperal woman this would most likely be a ruptured aneurysm.

Serial electroencephalograms (EEG) are valuable diagnostic aids, since improvement occurs more rapidly than expected in arterial strokes but will not occur if an untreated abscess or tumor is present. The EEG in subarachnoid hemorrhage without intracerebral bleeding should be almost normal. Rolling, high amplitude, slow waves may appear ominous, but resolution within 2 weeks parallels the sometimes dramatic clinical improvement. Spike waves and paroxysmal discharges are unusual unless the patient is having convulsions.

Special studies are needed to rule out other possibilities. Computerized tomography can demonstrate infarction, intracerebral hematomas, abscess, or tumor. Since tumors usually shrink significantly after childbirth, the presentation of a tumor during the puerperium but not during pregnancy is, with the exception of metastatic choriocarcinoma, unlikely. In spite of computerized tomography, critical scrutiny of the venous phase of cerebral angiograms may be needed to demonstrate venous obstruction (Morris, 1960; Askenasy et al., 1962; Gettelfinger and Kokmen, 1977).

Prognosis

The prognosis is good if the patient doesn't die. A survey of the literature, which by its very nature includes many autopsied cases, shows a 30 per cent mortality rate. How much lower the mortality rate really is remains unknown. Poor prognostic factors are coma, rapid progression of symptoms, and subarachnoid blood. The level of consciousness is the most important determinant, as in almost all neurologic conditions. The rapid progression of symptoms implies rapid progression of the thrombosis and usually serious cerebral edema. The rapidity of the process allows less time for anastomotic channels to enlarge and drain the region. Thus the area of venous infarction is presumably enlarged. Subarachnoid hemorrhage is another sign of significant cerebral infarction as the red cells from the cortical hemorrhages seep into the cerebrospinal fluid in proportionately greater numbers. Gross subarachnoid hemorrhage occurs only with bilateral or massive unilateral lesions. The very fact that the abnormality is on the venous side is a favorable factor, as the normal arterial supply of oxygen allows healing to proceed more swiftly than with arterial lesions. Residual disability will vary with the extent and site of the original insult, but a great handicap is less likely with a venous infarction than with an arterial stroke in the same area. The involved cortical vein becomes a fibrotic ribbon. The sagittal sinus is recanalized.

Treatment

The rational treatment consists of antibiotics if needed, anticoagulants if possible, and anticonvulsants. The need for appropriate antibiotics in the presence of an infection is evident. Anticonvulsants may not prevent the occurrence of more focal seizures if another cortical vein becomes obstructed, but generalized convulsions can be limited.

Anticoagulation with heparin was first suggested for this circumstance by Stansfield in 1942. It is still controversial (Gettelfinger and Kakmen, 1977). If the diagnosis is made early, administration of heparin to inhibit the propagation of the clot is reasonable. If there is concomitant phlebitis in the pelvis or legs, the argument for heparin is stronger. Deaths due to pulmonary emboli are not uncommon. However, if an intracerebral hematoma or gross subarachnoid hemorrhage has developed, the prognosis is already grave and the risk of anticoagulation too great. Anticoagulation in the early puerperium also carries the risk of profuse uterine bleeding (Kendall, 1948).

Etiology

The reasons for the occurrence of cerebral phlebothrombosis after pregnancy are still unknown. One theory that now seems improbable is the suggestion that emboli from the pelvis pass through the paravertebral venous plexus to reach the cerebral veins. Higher concentrations of some clotting factors are found during pregnancy, and more changes occur at delivery and during uterine involution. But higher concentrations of clotting factors do not necessarily mean that clots will form spontaneously.

SHEEHAN'S SYNDROME

Sheehan's syndrome is the name given to postpartum hypopituitarism secondary to pituitary infarction during severe shock at or near the time of delivery. The pituitary enlarges during pregnancy because the prolactin-secreting chromophobe cells are stimulated. This enlarged gland is vulnerable to ischemia or infarction should shock occur. Infarction occurs primarily in the region supplied by the hypophyseal artery (Sheehan and Stanfield, 1961). In half of the cases coming to autopsy, the necrosis involved more than 95 per cent of the anterior lobe but spared the stalk and posterior lobe. Sheehan (1954) estimates that 70 per cent of the anterior lobe must be lost before the remnant loses the ability to maintain normal endocrine function. Rarely, postpartum pituitary necrosis is associated with diabetes insipidus secondary to infarction of or hemorrhage into the posterior lobe (Spain and Geoghegan, 1946; Beernick and McKay, 1962). Even more rare is blindness due to infarction of the optic nerves or optic chiasm, which is supplied by a more proximal twig of the superior hypophyseal artery (Stewart, 1936; Lee et al., 1975).

If a woman survives whatever peripartum catastrophe occurred, hypopituitarism may be evident by failure to lactate and by rapid mammary involution. This early sign may be overlooked if suppression of lactation is desired.

Hypopituitarism is a chronic disease. The first sign is failure to

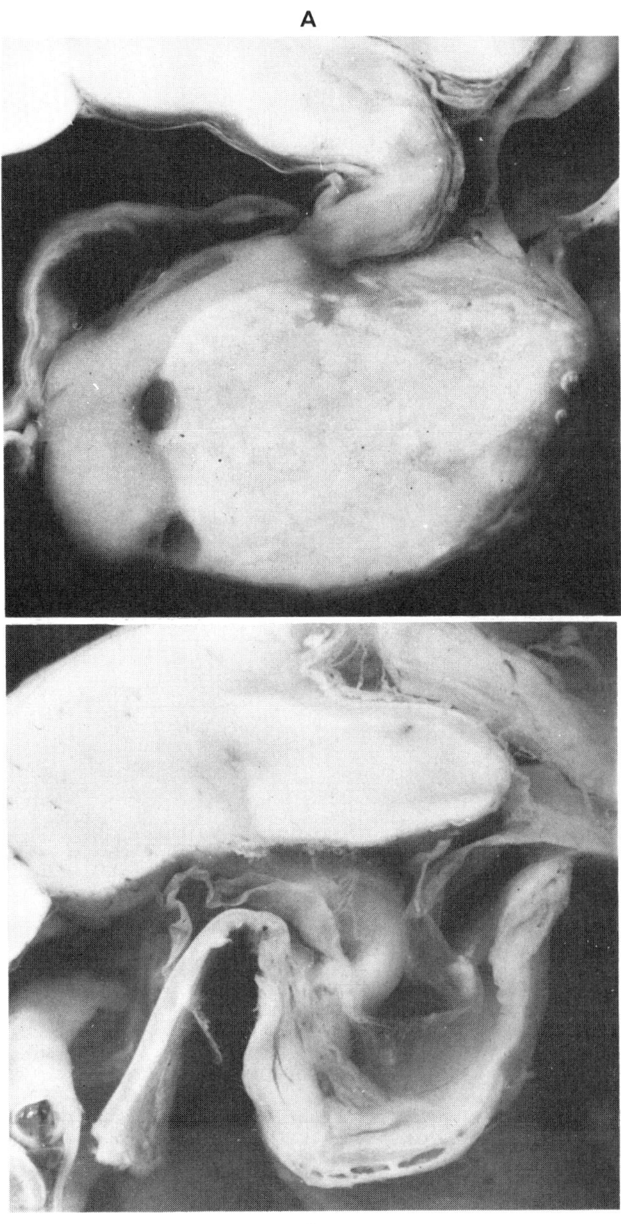

Figure 7.13. Sheehan's postpartum pituitary necrosis. *A*, Normal pituitary. *B*, Healed postpartum necrosis, with the anterior lobe consisting of loose fibrous tissue. From Sheehan, H. L. (1954) The incidence of postpartum hypopituitarism. *American Journal of Obstetrics and Gynecology*, **68**, 203. Courtesy of Prof. H. L. Sheehan.

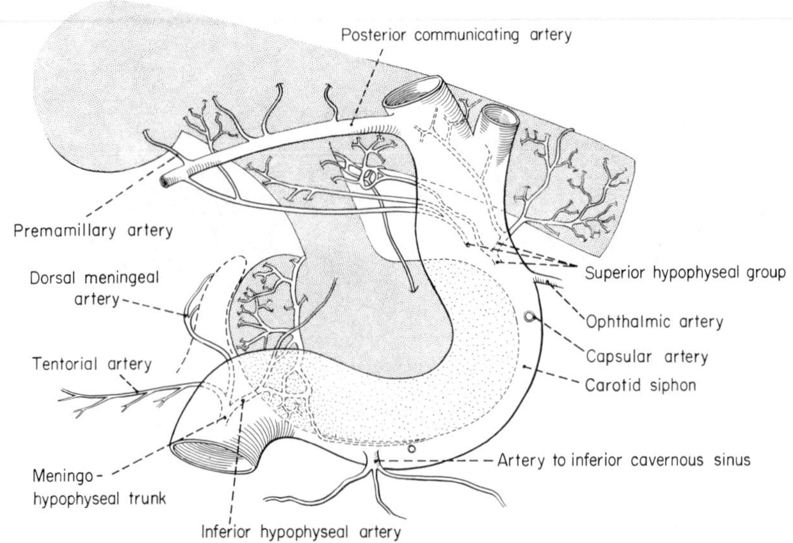

Figure 7.14. Arterial blood supply to the hypophysis, optic nerve, and parasellar structures. From Powell, D. F., Baker, H. L., Jr., Laws, E. R., Jr., et al. (1974) The primary angiographic findings in pituitary adenomas. *Radiology,* **110,** 589. Courtesy of D. F. Powell and the Publications Department, Mayo Foundation.

regain the vigor enjoyed before delivery. During subsequent years the patient may drift into a state of torpor subject at any time to sudden collapse, coma, and death if challenged by stress or infection. These patients reach medical attention in many ways. A gynecologist may be consulted for premature amenorrhea or dyspareunia secondary to atrophic genitalia. Hot flashes are not a complaint. Axillary and pubic hair is lost or does not regrow after shaving. The areolae lose pigmentation and exposed skin does not tan. The signs and symptoms of myxedema are present.

Rarely, a neurologist may be asked to evaluate the mental dullness, forgetfulness, and depression characteristic of the disease. Hyponatremic and hypoglycemic convulsions can occur (Farmer and Flowers, 1955).

Treatment consists of slowly instituted steroid and thyroid hormone replacement.

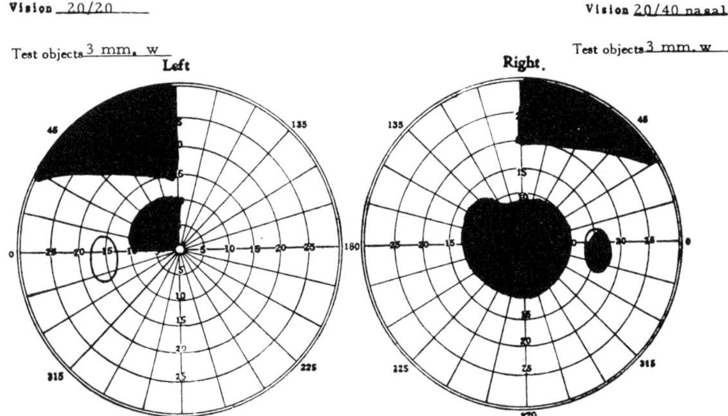

Figure 7.15. Visual fields of a 27 year old woman with postpartum pituitary necrosis demonstrating a central scotoma in the right eye and a superior bitemporal field defect. Pneumoencephalography showed an empty sella turcica. From Lee, K. F., Schatz, N. J., and Savine, P. J. (1975) Ischemic chiasmal syndrome. In *Neuro-ophthalmology,* Vol. 8, ed. Glaser, J. S., and Smith, J. L., St. Louis: C. V. Mosby Company.

SPONTANEOUS CAROTID–CAVERNOUS SINUS FISTULAE

Spontaneous carotid–cavernous sinus fistulae are shunts between the tiny meningeal branches of the internal carotid artery and the cavernous sinus or the dural veins in its vicinity. A large medical center will see about one such case yearly, but the diagnosis may be obscured by the absence of clinical features commonly associated with the more dramatic post-traumatic variety. Post-traumatic carotid–cavernous fistulae are fast flow systems with prominent, pulsating exophthalmos and an orbital bruit that is easily appreciated by the patient and his physician. In contrast, spontaneous shunts involve small vessels, are low pressure—low flow fistulae, and may not have a bruit.

The most common presenting symptom is unilateral frontal headache, often with ipsilateral conjunctival injection which may have been mistaken for conjunctivitis or episcleritis. Diplopia may occur at the outset or weeks later (Newton and Hoyt, 1970).

Physical signs are a lateral rectus palsy with ipsilateral conjunctival injection, mild proptosis, mildly elevated intraocular tension, and occasionally an orbital bruit. Monocular dimmed vision and even blindness secondary to ocular hypoxia have been described (Sanders and Hoyt, 1969).

These fistulae are believed to be formed by the rupture of an aneurysm of the small meningeal and meningohypophyseal branches of the intracavernous portion of the internal carotid artery (Obrador et al., 1974). Many patients have noted the onset of symptoms while straining in some manner.

Women of all ages outnumber men in any series by a 3:1 margin. Approximately 25 per cent of all affected women and almost all of those under 40 develop the syndrome during the second half of pregnancy or during the puerperium. It is very unusual for men under 40 to develop a spontaneous carotid–cavernous fistula.

The diagnosis is established by selective internal carotid angiography using magnification and subtraction techniques. The treatment consists of observation and reassurance. Symptoms often abate over a period of months, although mild lateral rectus paresis may persist. Progressive impairment of vision indicates a need for a neurosurgical opinion.

REFERENCES

Subarachnoid Hemorrhage

INTRACRANIAL ANEURYSMS AND ARTERIOVENOUS MALFORMATIONS

Amias, A. G. (1970) Cerebral vascular disease in pregnancy: I. Haemorrhage. *Journal of Obstetrics and Gynaecology of the British Empire,* **77,** 100–120.

Armstrong, M. V. (1937) Angiomatosis retinae (von Hippel's disease, Lindau's disease) complicated by pregnancy. *American Journal of Obstetrics and Gynecology,* **34,** 494–496.

Barnes, J. E., and Abbott, K. H. (1961) Cerebral complications incurred during pregnancy and the puerperium. *American Journal of Obstetrics and Gynecology,* **82,** 192–207.

Barno, A., and Freeman, D. W. (1976) Maternal deaths due to spontaneous subarachnoid hemorrhage. *American Journal of Obstetrics and Gynecology,* **125,** 384–392.

Bean, W. B., Cogswell, R., Dexter, M. et al. (1949) Vascular changes of the skin in pregnancy: Vascular spiders and palmar erythema. *Surgery, Gynecology and Obstetrics,* **88,** 739–752.

Cannell, D. E., and Botterell, E. H. (1956) Subarachnoid hemorrhage and pregnancy. *American Journal of Obstetrics and Gynecology,* **72,** 844–855.

Conley, J. W., and Rand, C. W. (1951) Spontaneous subarachnoid hemorrhage occurring in noneclamptic pregnancy. *Archives of Neurology and Psychiatry,* **66,** 443–463.

Copelan, E. L., and Mabon, R. F. (1962) Spontaneous intracranial bleeding in pregnancy. *Obstetrics and Gynecology,* **20,** 373–378.

Daane, T. A., and Tandy, R. W. (1960) Rupture of congenital intracranial aneurysm in pregnancy. *Obstetrics and Gynecology,* **15,** 305–314.

Dunn, J. M., and Raskind, R. (1967) Rupture of a cerebral arteriovenous malformation during pregnancy. *Obstetrics and Gynecology,* **30,** 423–426.

Fliegner, J. R. H., Hooper, R. S., and Kloss, M. (1969) Subarachnoid haemorrhage and pregnancy. *Journal of Obstetrics and Gynaecology of the British Commonwealth,* **76,** 912–917.

Henderson, W. R., and Gomez, R. R. L. (1967) Natural history of cerebral angiomas. *British Medical Journal,* **1,** 571–574.

Hunt, H. B., Schifrin, B. S., and Suzuki, K. (1974) Ruptured berry aneurysms and pregnancy. *Obstetrics and Gynecology,* **43,** 827–837.

Lazard, E. Y. (1899) A case of cerebral hemorrhage following labor. *Philadelphia Medical Journal,* **4,** 1091, 1092.

Locksley, H. B. (1966) Natural history of subarachnoid hemorrhage, intracranial aneurysms and arteriovenous malformations. *Journal of Neurosurgery,* **25,** 219–239.

McCall, M. L. (1949) Cerebral blood flow and metabolism in toxemias of pregnancy. *Surgery, Obstetrics and Gynecology,* **89,** 715–721.

McCormick, W. F. (1966) The pathology of vascular ("arteriovenous") malformations. *Journal of Neurosurgery,* **24,** 807–816.

Pedowitz, P., and Perell, A. (1957) Aneurysms complicated by pregnancy: Part II. Aneurysms of the cerebral vessels. *American Journal of Obstetrics and Gynecology,* **73,** 736–749.

Perret, G., and Nishioka, H. (1966) Arteriovenous malformations. An analysis of 545 cases of cranio-cerebral arteriovenous malformations and fistulae reported to the cooperative study. *Journal of Neurosurgery,* **25,** 467–490.

Pool, J. L. (1965) Treatment of intracranial aneurysms during pregnancy. *Journal of the American Medical Association,* **192,** 209–214.

Prosenz, P., Heiss, W-D., and Kvicala, V. et al. (1971) Contribution to the hemodynamics of arterial venous malformations. *Stroke,* **2,** 279–289.

Robinson, J. L., Hall, C. J., and Sedzimir, C. B. (1972) Subarachnoid hemorrhage in pregnancy. *Journal of Neurosurgery,* **36,** 27–33.

Robinson, J. L., Hall, C. S., and Sedzimir, C. B. (1974) Arteriovenous malformations, aneurysms, and pregnancy. *Journal of Neurosurgery,* **41,** 63–70.

Walton, J. N. (1953) Subarachnoid haemorrhage in pregnancy. *British Medical Journal,* **1,** 869–871.

Valsalva Maneuver

Alman, R. W., and Fazekas, J. F. (1962) Cerebral physiology of the augmented Valsalva maneuver. *American Journal of Medical Science,* **244,** 202–209.

Faulkner, M., and Sharpey-Schafer, E. P. (1959) Circulatory effects of trumpet playing. *British Medical Journal,* **1,** 685, 686.

Hamilton, W. F., Woodbury, R. A., and Harper, H. T. (1936) Physiologic relationships between intrathoracic, intraspinal and arterial pressures. *Journal of the American Medical Association,* **107,** 853–856.

Hamilton, W. F. (1944) Arterial, cerebrospinal and venous pressures in man during cough and strain. *American Journal of Physiology,* **141,** 42–50.

Hopkins, E. L., Hendricks, C. H., and Cibils, L. A. (1965) Cerebrospinal fluid pressure in labor. *American Journal of Obstetrics and Gynecology,* **93,** 907–916.

Klein, L. J., Saltzman, H. A., Heyman, A. et al. (1964) Syncope induced by the Valsalva maneuver: A study of the effects of arterial blood gas tensions, glucose concentration and blood pressure. *American Journal of Medicine,* **37,** 263–268.

Marx, G. F., Oka, Y., and Orkin, L. R. (1962) Cerebrospinal fluid pressures during labor. *American Journal of Obstetrics and Gynecology,* **84,** 213–219.

Marx, G. F., Zematis, M. T., and Orkin, L. R. (1961) Cerebrospinal fluid pressures during labor and obstetric anesthesia. *Anesthesiology,* **22,** 348–354.

McCausland, A. M., and Holmes, F. (1957) Spinal fluid pressures during labor. *Western Journal of Surgery,* **65,** 220–233.

McHenry, L. C., Fazekas, J. F., and Sullivan, J. F. (1961) Cerebral hemodynamics of syncope. *American Journal of Medical Science,* **241,** 173–178.

Vasicka, A., Kretchmer, H., and Lawas, F. (1962) Cerebrospinal fluid pressures during labor. *American Journal of Obstetrics and Gynecology,* **84,** 206–212.

ANEURYSMS: EXTRACRANIAL

Cohen, S. G., Cashdan, A., and Burger, R. (1972) Spontaneous rupture of a renal artery aneurysm during pregnancy. *Obstetrics and Gynecology,* **39,** 897–902.

Di Maio, V. J. M., and Di Maio, D. J. (1971) Postpartum dissecting coronary aneurysm. *New York State Journal of Medicine,* **71,** 767–769.

Elias, S., and Berkowitz, R. L. (1976) The Marfan syndrome and pregnancy. *Obstetrics and Gynecology,* **47,** 358–361.

Greene, J. L., and McCormick, W. F. (1968) Concurrent rupture of intracranial and intra-abdominal aneurysms. *Journal of Neurosurgery,* **29,** 545–550.

Jones, E. L., and Finney, G. G. (1968) Splenic artery aneurysms: A reappraisal. *Archives of Surgery,* **97,** 640–647.

MacFarlane, J. R., and Thorbjarnarson, B. (1966) Rupture of splenic artery aneurysm during pregnancy. *American Journal of Obstetrics and Gynecology,* **95,** 1025–1037.

Pedowitz, P., and Perell, A. (1957) Aneurysms complicated by pregnancy: Part I. Aneurysms of the aorta and its major branches. *American Journal of Obstetrics and Gynecology,* **73,** 720–735.

Schnitker, M. A., and Bayer, C. A. (1944) Dissecting aneurysm of the aorta in young individuals, particularly in association with pregnancy with report of a case. *Annals of Internal Medicine,* **20,** 486–511.

ANEURYSMS: HISTOPATHOLOGY

Cavanzo, F. J., and Taylor, H. B. (1969) Effect of pregnancy on the human aorta and its relationship to dissecting aneurysms. *American Journal of Obstetrics and Gynecology,* **105,** 567, 568.

Danforth, D. N., Manalo-Estrella, P., and Buckingham, J. C. (1964) The effect of pregnancy and of "Enovid" on the rabbit vasculature. *American Journal of Obstetrics and Gynecology,* **88,** 952–962.

Johnson, W. L., Conrad, J. T., Whitney, D., et al. (1965) The effect of pregnancy and norethynodrel with mestranol (Enovid) on length-tension relationship in the rabbit aorta. *American Journal of Obstetrics and Gynecology,* **93,** 179, 180.

Manalo-Estrella, P., and Barker, A. E. (1967) Histopathologic findings in human aortic media associated with pregnancy. *Archives of Pathology,* **83,** 336–341.

OTHER CAUSES

Heron, J. R., Hutchinson, E. C., Boyd, W. N., and Aber, G. M. (1974) Pregnancy, subarachnoid hemorrhage, and the intravascular coagulation syndrome. *Journal of Neurology, Neurosurgery and Psychiatry,* **37,** 521–525.

Hirsh, J., Cade, J. F., and Gallus, A. S. (1972) Anticoagulants in pregnancy: A review of indications and complications. *American Heart Journal,* **83,** 301–305.

Lombardo, L., Mateos, J. H., and Barroeta, F. F., (1969) Subarachnoid hemorrhage due to endometriosis of the spinal canal. *Neurology,* **18,** 423–428.

Weigle, E. H. (1955) Pregnancy complicated by subarachnoid hemorrhage following anticoagulant therapy of subacute bacterial endocarditis. *American Journal of Obstetrics and Gynecology,* **69,** 888–891.

OBSTETRIC MANAGEMENT

Hunt, H. B., Schifrin, B. S., and Suzuki, K. (1974) Ruptured berry aneurysms and pregnancy. *Obstetrics and Gynecology,* **43,** 827–837.

Laubstein, M. B., Kotz, H. L., and Hehre, F. W. (1962) Obstetric and anesthetic management following spontaneous subarachnoid hemorrhage. *Obstetrics and Gynecology,* **20,** 661–667.

McGinty, L. B. (1956) A study of the vasopressor effects of oxytocics when used intravenously in the third stage of labor. *Western Journal of Surgery,* **64,** 22–28.

Miller, F. C., Petrie, R. H., Arce, J. J., et al. (1974) Hyperventilation during labor. *American Journal of Obstetrics and Gynecology,* **120,** 489–495.

NEUROSURGICAL TREATMENT

Carmel, P. W. (1974) Neurologic surgery in pregnancy. In *Surgical Disease in Pregnancy,* ed. Barber, H. R. K., and Graber, E. A., Ch. 13, pp. 203–224. Philadelphia: W. B. Saunders Co.

Pool, J. L. (1965) Treatment of intracranial aneurysms during pregnancy. *Journal of the American Medical Association,* **192,** 209–214.

Robinson, J. L., Hall, C. J., and Sedzimir, C. B. (1972) Subarachnoid hemorrhage in pregnancy. *Journal of Neurosurgery,* **36,** 27–33.

NEUROSURGICAL TREATMENT DURING PREGNANCY

Hypothermia

Assali, N. S., and Westin, B. (1962) Effects of hypothermia on uterine circulation and on the fetus. *Proceedings of the Society for Experimental Biology,* **109,** 485–488.

Burstein, P. N., Perese, D. M., and Kaminski, C. J. (1964) Ruptured berry aneurysm during pregnancy: Successful repair under hypothermia. *Obstetrics and Gynecology,* **24,** 463–467.

Davey, L. M., Fiorito, J. A., and Hehre, F. W. (1965) Intracranial aneurysm in late pregnancy. Report of a successful operation utilizing hypothermia. *Journal of Neurosurgery,* **23,** 542–546.

Hehre, F. W. (1965) Hypothermia for operations during pregnancy. *Anesthesia and Analgesia,* **44,** 424–428.

Jensen, F. (1962) Hypothermia and controlled hypotension employed in an operation during pregnancy. *Danish Medical Bulletin,* **9,** 250–252.

Kamrin, R. P., and Masland, W. (1965) Intracranial surgery under hypothermia during pregnancy. *Archives of Neurology,* **13,** 70–76.

Pool, J. L. (1965) Treatment of intracranial aneurysms during pregnancy. *Journal of the American Medical Association,* **192,** 209–214.

Wilson, F., and Sedzimir, C. B. (1959) Hypothermia and hypotension during craniotomy in a pregnant woman. *Lancet,* **2,** 947–949.

Hypertonic Mannitol

Battaglia, F., Prystowsky, H., Smisson, C., et al. (1960) The effect of the administration of fluids intravenously to mothers upon the concentrations of water and electrolytes in plasma of human fetuses. *Pediatrics,* **25,** 2–10.

Bruns, P. D., Linder, R. O., Drose, V. E., et al. (1963) The placental transfer of water from fetus to mother following the intravenous infusion of hypertonic mannitol to the maternal rabbit. *American Journal of Obstetrics and Gynecology,* **86,** 160–169.

Fishman, R. A. (1975) Brain edema. *New England Journal of Medicine,* **293,** 706–711.

Corticosteroids

Beitins, I. Z., Bayard, F., Ances, I. G., et al. (1972) The transplacental passage of prednisone and prednisolone in pregnancy near term. *Journal of Pediatrics,* **81,** 936–945.

Bongiovanni, A. M., and McPadden, A. J. (1960) Steroids during pregnancy and possible fetal consequences. *Fertility and Sterility,* **11,** 181–189.

Garenstein, M., Pollak, V. E., and Kark, R. M. (1962) Systemic lupus erythematosus and pregnancy. *New England Journal of Medicine,* **267,** 165–169.

Arterial Cerebrovascular Disease

STROKE IN YOUNG ADULTS

Berlin, L., Tumarkin, B., and Martin, H. L. (1955) Cerebral thrombosis in young adults. *New England Journal of Medicine,* **252,** 162–166.

Humphrey, J. G., and Newton, T. H. (1960) Internal carotid artery occlusion in young adults. *Brain,* **83,** 617.

Louis, S., and McDowell, F. (1967) Stroke in young adults. *Annals of Internal Medicine,* **66,** 932.

Schoenberg, B. S., Whisnant, J. P., Taylor, W. F. et al. (1970) Strokes in women of childbearing age: A population study. *Neurology,* **20,** 181–189.

STROKE DURING PREGNANCY

Amias, A. G. (1970) Cerebral vascular disease in pregnancy: II. Occlusion. *Journal of Obstetrics and Gynecology of the British Commonwealth,* **77,** 312–325.

Cross, J. N., Castro, P. O., and Jennett, W. B. (1968) Cerebral strokes associated with pregnancy and the puerperium. *British Medical Journal,* **3,** 214–218.

Fisher, C. M. (1971) Cerebral ischemia—less familiar types. *Clinical Neurosurgery,* **18,** 267–336.

Fite, J. M., and Gould, P. L. (1959) Thrombosis of the middle cerebral artery during pregnancy. *Obstetrics and Gynecology,* **14,** 371–373.

Gibbs, C. E. (1974) Maternal death due to stroke. *American Journal of Obstetrics and Gynecology,* **119,** 69–75.

Jennett, W. B., and Cross, J. N. (1967) Influence of pregnancy and oral contraception on the incidence of strokes in women of childbearing age. *Lancet,* **1,** 1019–1023.

STROKE AND THE PILL

Bergeron, R. T., and Wood, E. H. (1969) Oral contraceptives and cerebrovascular complications. *Radiology,* **92,** 231–238.

Bickerstaff, E. R., and Holmes, J. M. (1967) Cerebral arterial insufficiency and oral contraceptives. *British Medical Journal,* **1,** 726–729.

Bickerstaff, E. R. (1975) *Neurological Complications of Oral Contraceptives.* Oxford: Clarendon Press.

Cole, M. (1967) Strokes in young women using oral contraceptives. *Archives of Internal Medicine,* **120,** 551–555.

Collaborative Group for the Study of Stroke in Young Women, (1973) Oral contraception and increased risk of cerebral ischemia or thrombosis. *New England Journal of Medicine,* **288,** 871–878.

Enzell, K., and Lindemalm, G. (1973) Cryptogenic cerebral embolism in women taking oral contraceptives. *British Medical Journal,* **4,** 507–512.

Goldzieher, J. W., and Dozier, T. S. (1975) Oral contraceptives and thromboembolism: A reassessment. *American Journal of Obstetrics and Gynecology,* **123,** 878–914.

Heyman, A., and Hurtig, H. (1975) Clinical complications of oral contraceptives. *Disease-a-Month,* August, 1975.

Illis, L., Kocen, R. S., McDonald, W. I., et al. (1965) Oral contraceptives and cerebral arterial occlusion. *British Medical Journal,* **2,** 1164–1166.

Inman, W. H. W., and Vessey, M. P. (1968) Investigation of deaths from pulmonary, coronary, and cerebral thrombosis and embolism in women of child-bearing age. *British Medical Journal,* **2,** 193–199.

Jennett, W. B., and Cross, J. N. (1967) Influence of pregnancy and oral contraception on the incidence of strokes in women of childbearing age. *Lancet,* **1,** 1019–1023.

Lorentz, I. T. (1962) Parietal lesion and "Enavid." *British Medical Journal,* **2,** 1191.

Masi, A. T., and Dugdale, M. (1970) Cerebrovascular diseases associated with the use of oral contraceptives: A review of the English-language literature. *Annals of Internal Medicine,* **72,** 111–121.

Nevin, N. C., Elmes, P. C., and Weaver, J. A. (1965) Three cases of intravascular thrombosis occurring in patients receiving oral contraceptives. *British Medical Journal,* **1,** 1586–1589.

Salmon, M. L., Winkelman, J. Z., and Gay, A. J. (1968) Neuro-ophthalmic sequelae in users of oral contraceptives. *Journal of the American Medical Association,* **206,** 85–91.

Sanchez Longo, L. P. (1968) Transitory vascular-like phenomena with the use of oral contraceptives. *Vascular Disease,* **5,** 194–198.

Shafey, S., and Schedinberg, P. (1966) Neurological syndromes occurring in patients receiving synthetic steroids (oral contraceptives). *Neurology,* **16,** 205–211.

Vessey, M. P., and Doll, R. (1968) Investigation of relation between use of oral contraceptives and thromboembolic disease. *British Medical Journal,* **2,** 199–205.

Vessey, M. P. (1973) Oral contraceptives and stroke. *New England Journal of Medicine,* **288,** 906–907.

CARDIOMYOPATHY OF PREGNANCY

Becker, F. F., and Taube, H. (1962) Myocarditis of obscure etiology associated with pregnancy. *New England Journal of Medicine,* **266,** 62–67.

Connor, R. C. R., and Adams, J. H. (1966) Importance of cardiomyopathy and cerebral ischemia in the diagnosis of fatal coma in pregnancy. *Journal of Clinical Pathology*, **19**, 244–249.

PUERPERAL PARADOXICAL EMBOLI

DeSwiet, J. (1962) Puerperal paradoxical embolism. *Lancet*, **2**, 1197, 1198.

Sauer, H. H. A. (1955) Paradoxical embolism in pregnancy: Review of the literature and report of a case. *Journal of Obstetrics and Gynecology of the British Empire*, **62**, 906–908.

AMNIOTIC FLUID EMBOLI

Aguillon, A., Andjus, T., Grayson, A., et al. (1962) Amniotic fluid embolism: A review. *Obstetric and Gynecological Survey*, **17**, 619–636.

Attwood, H. D. (1972) Amniotic fluid embolism. *Pathology Annual*, **7**, 145–172.

Olcott, C., Robinson, A. J., and Griffin, H. A. (1973) Amniotic fluid embolism and disseminated intravascular coagulation after blunt abdominal trauma. *Journal of Trauma*, **13**, 737–740.

Peterson, E. P., and Taylor, H. B. (1970) Amniotic fluid embolism: An analysis of 40 cases. *Obstetrics and Gynecology*, **35**, 787–793.

Reis, R. L., Pierce, W. S., and Behrendt, D. M. (1969) Hemodynamic effects of amniotic fluid embolism. *Surgery, Gynecology and Obstetrics*, **129**, 45–48.

Resnik, R., Swartz, W. H., Plumer, M. H., et al. (1976) Amniotic fluid embolism with survival. *Obstetrics and Gynecology*, **47**, 295–298.

Roche, W. D., and Norris, H. J. (1974) Detection and significance of maternal pulmonary amniotic fluid embolism. *Obstetrics and Gynecology*, **43**, 729–732.

Smibert, J. (1967) Amniotic fluid embolism: A clinical review of twenty cases. *Australian and New Zealand Journal of Obstetrics and Gynecology*, **7**, 1–12.

Steiner, P. E., and Lushbaugh, C. C. (1941) Maternal pulmonary embolism by amniotic fluid as a cause of obstetric shock and unexpected deaths in obstetrics. *Journal of the American Medical Association*, **117**, 1245–1254, 1340–1345.

FAT EMBOLI

Chmel, H., and Bertles, J. F. (1975) Hemoglobin S/C disease in a pregnant woman with crisis and fat embolization syndrome. *American Journal of Medicine*, **58**, 563–566.

Huaman, A., Nice, W., Merkel, R. L., et al. (1972) Amniotic fat embolism. *Journal of the Kansas Medical Society*, **73**, 441–443.

Jonas, E. G. (1961) Maternal death due to fat-embolism. *Journal of Obstetrics and Gynecology of the British Commonwealth*, **68**, 479–483.

Lillian, M., Pope, R. H., and Elliott, F. G. (1955) Puerperal fat embolism. *New England Journal of Medicine*, **253**, 143–144.

Pritchard, R. W. (1965) Generalized fat embolism: A complication of rupture of a dermoid cyst during labor. *Medical Times*, **93**, 1359–1362.

Ross, A. P. J. (1970) The fat embolism syndrome: With special reference to the importance of hypoxia in the syndrome. *Annals of the Royal College of Surgeons of England*, **46**, 159–171.

Sevitt, S. (1960) The significance and classification of fat-embolism. *Lancet*, **2**, 825–828.

Thomas, J. E., and Ayyar, D. R. (1972) Systemic fat embolism: A diagnostic profile in 24 patients. *Archives of Neurology*, **26**, 517–523.

AIR EMBOLI

Aronson, M. E., and Nelson, P. K. (1967) Fatal air embolism in pregnancy resulting from an unusual sex act. *Obstetrics and Gynecology*, **30**, 127–130.

Cooke, R. T. (1950) Fatal air embolism due to vaginal douching in pregnancy. *British Medical Journal*, **1**, 1241.

Martland, H. S. (1945) Air embolism: Fatal air embolism due to powder insufflators used in gynecologic treatment. *American Journal of Surgery*, **130**, 164–169.

May, G. (1857) Sudden death after parturition with air in veins. *British Medical Journal*, **1**, 477.

Nelson, P. K. (1960) Pulmonary gas embolism in pregnancy and the puerperium. *Obstetric and Gynecological Survey,* **15,** 449–481.
Ohio State Medical Association Committee on Maternal Health, (1972). Maternal deaths due to air embolism. *Ohio State Medical Journal,* **68,** 1105–1107.
Redfield, R. L., and Bodine, H. R. (1939) Air embolism following knee-chest position. *Journal of the American Medical Association,* **113,** 671–673.
Schwarz, G. A. (1966) Pathogenesis of certain neurologic complications following knee-chest position in the puerperium. *Obstetrics and Gynecology,* **27,** 536–540.
Toole, J. F., and Tucker, S. H. (1960) Influence of head position upon cerebral circulation. *Archives of Neurology,* **2,** 616–623.
Waldrop, G. S. (1953) Fatal air embolism during term labor and the puerperium. *Obstetrics and Gynecology,* **1,** 454–459.

Cerebral Venous Thrombosis

History

Abercrombie, J. (1828) *Pathological and Practical Researches on Diseases of the Brain and Spinal Cord,* pp. 83–85. Edinburgh.
Churchill, F. (1854) On paralysis occurring during gestation and in childbed. *Dublin Journal of Medical Science,* **1,** 257–296.
Collier, W. (1891) Thrombosis of cerebral veins. *British Medical Journal,* **1,** 521, 522.
Ducrest, F. M. (1847) De la phlébite cérébrale et méningée chez les femmes en couches. *Archives Gen. Med.* **15,** 1–39.
Meniere, P. (1829) Observations et reflexions sur l'hémorrhagie cérébrale, considérée pendant la grossesse, pendant et après l'accouchement. *Archives Générales de Medecine,* **16,** 491–522.
Sinclair, M. A. M. (1902) On puerperal aphasia, with an analysis of 18 cases. *Lancet,* **2,** 204–207.

With the Pill

Atkinson, E. A., Fairburn, B., and Heathfield, K. W. G. (1970) Intracranial venous thrombosis as complication of oral contraception. *Lancet,* **1,** 914–918.
Buchanan, D. S., and Brazinsky, J. H. (1970) Dural sinus and cerebral venous thrombosis: Incidence in young women receiving oral contraceptives. *Archives of Neurology,* **22,** 440–444.
Dindar, F., and Platts, M. E. (1974) Intracranial venous thrombosis complicating oral contraception. *Canadian Medical Association Journal,* **111,** 545–548.
Fairburn, B. (1973) Intracranial venous thrombosis complicating oral contraception: Treatment by anticoagulant drugs. *British Medical Journal,* **2,** 647.
Shende, M. C., and Lourie, H. (1970) Sagittal sinus thrombosis related to oral contraceptives. *Journal of Neurosurgery,* **33,** 714–717.

During Pregnancy

Dowie, R. (1952) Cerebral thrombosis complicating pregnancy. *British Medical Journal,* **2,** 547.
Eckerling, B., Goldman, J. A., and Gans, B. (1963) Intracranial sinus thrombosis, a rare complication of early pregnancy. *Obstetrics and Gynecology,* **21,** 368–371.
Fishman, R. A., Cowen, D., and Silbermann, M. (1957) Intracranial venous thrombosis during the first trimester of pregnancy. *Neurology,* **7,** 217–220.
Goldman, J. A., and Eckerling, B. (1972) Intracranial dural sinus thrombosis following intrauterine instillation of hypertonic saline. *American Journal of Obstetrics and Gynecology,* **112,** 1132, 1133.
McNairn, J. (1948) Cerebral venous thrombosis in pregnancy; A report of two possible cases. *Journal of Obstetrics and Gynaecology of the British Empire,* **55,** 630–634.
Stevens, H., and Ammerman, H. H. (1959) Intracranial venous thrombosis in early pregnancy. *American Journal of Obstetrics and Gynecology,* **78,** 104–108.

PUERPERAL

Barnett, H. J. M., and Hyland, H. H. (1953) Non-infective intracranial venous thrombosis. *Brain,* **76,** 36–49.

Biback, S. M., Franklin, A., and Sata, W. K. (1962) Puerperal hemiplegia: Case report and review of primary puerperal cerebral venous thrombosis. *American Journal of Obstetrics and Gynecology,* **83,** 45–53.

Burt, R. L., Donnelly, J. F., and Whitener, D. L. (1951) Cerebral venous thrombosis in the puerperium: Report of two cases with necropsy findings. *American Journal of Obstetrics and Gynecology,* **62,** 639–643.

Cairns, D. R., and Melton, G. (1942) Primary thrombosis of cerebral veins in the puerperium. *British Medical Journal,* **1,** 439.

Carroll, J. D., Leak, D., and Lee, H. A. (1966) Cerebral thrombophlebitis in pregnancy and the puerperium. *Quarterly Journal of Medicine,* **35,** 347–368.

Cross, J. N., Castro, P. O., and Jennett, W. B. (1968) Cerebral strokes associated with pregnancy and the puerperium. *British Medical Journal,* **3,** 214–218.

Deane, L. C. (1908) Thrombosis of superior longitudinal and lateral sinuses complicated by pregnancy. *Journal of the American Medical Association,* **51,** 997–1000.

Goldman, J. A., Eckerling, B., and Gans, B. (1964) Intracranial venous sinus thrombosis in pregnancy and puerperium. *Journal of Obstetrics and Gynaecology of the British Commonwealth,* **71,** 791–796.

Hunt, J. R. (1917) Thrombosis of the cerebral sinuses and veins as complication of the puerperium. *Bulletin of the Lying-in Hospital, New York,* **11,** 73–80.

Hyland, H. H. (1950) Intracranial venous thrombosis in the puerperium. *Journal of the American Medical Association,* **142,** 707–710.

Kalbag, R. M., and Woolf, A. L. (1967) *Cerebral Venous Thrombosis.* London: Oxford University Press.

Kendall, D. (1948) Thrombosis of intracranial veins. *Brain,* **71,** 386–402.

Lorincz, A. B., and Moore, R. Y. (1962) Puerperal cerebral venous thrombosis. *American Journal of Obstetrics and Gynecology,* **83,** 311–319.

Martin, J. P. (1941) Thrombosis in the superior longitudinal sinus following childbirth. *British Medical Journal,* **2,** 537–540.

Martin, J. P. (1944) Venous thrombosis in the central nervous system. *Proceedings of the Royal Society of Medicine,* **37,** 383–386.

Martin, J. P., and Sheehan, H. L. (1941) Primary thrombosis of cerebral veins (following childbirth). *British Medical Journal,* **1,** 349–353.

Myrick, H. G. (1910) Some cases of sudden death during pregnancy and the puerperium. *Boston Medical and Surgical Journal,* **163,** 764–767.

Prakash, C., and Singh, S. (1960) Cerebral venous and sinus thrombosis in the puerperium. *Journal of the Association of Physicians of India,* **8,** 363–366.

Sheehan, H. L., and Lynch, J. B. (1973) *Pathology of Toxaemia of Pregnancy.* Baltimore: The Williams & Wilkins Co.

Stevens, H. (1954) Puerperal hemiplegia. *Neurology,* **4,** 723–738.

Symonds, C. P. (1940) Cerebral thrombophlebitis. *British Medical Journal,* **2,** 348–352.

RADIOGRAPHIC DEMONSTRATION

Askenasy, H. M., Kosary, I. Z., and Braham, J. (1962) Thrombosis of the longitudinal sinus: Diagnosis by carotid angiography. *Neurology,* **12,** 288–292.

Gettelfinger, D. M., and Kokmen, E. (1977) Superior sagittal sinus thrombosis. *Archives of Neurology,* **34,** 2–6.

Morris, L. (1960) Angiography of the superior sagittal and transverse sinuses. *British Journal of Radiology,* **33,** 606–613.

Raskind, R., and Weiss, S. R. (1969) Postpartum cortical venous thrombosis with unusual angiographic and operative findings. *Angiology,* **20,** 102–106.

Ray, B. S., Dunbar, H. S., and Dotter, C. T. (1951) Dural sinus venography as an aid to diagnosis in intracranial disease. *Journal of Neurosurgery,* **8,** 23–37.

ANTICOAGULATION

Gettelfinger, D. M., and Kokmen, E. (1977) Superior sagittal sinus thrombosis. *Archives of Neurology,* **34,** 2–6.

Kalbag, R. M., and Woolf, A. L. (1967) *Cerebral Venous Thrombosis.* London: Oxford University Press.

Krayenbühl, H. A. (1967) Cerebral venous and sinus thrombosis. *Clinical Neurosurgery,* **14,** 1–24.

Stansfield, F. R. (1942) Puerperal cerebral thrombophlebitis treated by heparin. *British Medical Journal,* **1,** 436–439.

Sheehan's Syndrome

Beernink, F. J., and McKay, D. G. (1962) Pituitary insufficiency associated with pregnancy, panhypopituitarism, and diabetes insipidus. *American Journal of Obstetrics and Gynecology,* **84,** 318–338.

Farmer, T. W., and Flowers, C. A. (1955) Neurologic manifestations of postpartum pituitary insufficiency. *Neurology,* **5,** 212–214.

Lee, K. F., Schatz, N. J., and Savino, P. J., (1975) Ischemic chiasmal syndrome. *In Neuro-Ophthalmology,* Vol. 8, pp. 115–130, ed. Glaser, J. S., and Smith, J. L. St. Louis: C. V. Mosby Co.

Sheehan, H. L. (1937) Postpartum necrosis of anterior pituitary. *Journal of Pathology and Bacteriology,* **45,** 189–214.

Sheehan, H. L. (1954) The incidence of postpartum hypopituitarism. *American Journal of Obstetrics and Gynecology,* **68,** 202–223.

Sheehan, H. L., and Murdoch, R. (1938) Postpartum necrosis of the anterior pituitary: pathological and clinical aspects. *Journal of Obstetrics and Gynaecology of the British Empire,* **45,** 456–489.

Sheehan, H. L., and Stanfield, J. P. (1961) The pathogenesis of postpartum necrosis of the anterior lobe of the pituitary gland. *Acta Endocrinologica,* **37,** 479–510.

Spain, A. W., and Geoghegan, F. (1946) Diabetes insipidus in association with postpartum pituitary necrosis. *Journal of Obstetrics and Gynaecology of the British Empire,* **53,** 223–227.

Stewart, A. (1936) A case of Simmonds' disease. *Lancet,* **2,** 1391, 1392.

Spontaneous Carotid-Cavernous Fistulae

Dandy, W. E. (1937) Carotid-cavernous aneurysms (pulsating exophthalmos). *Zentralblatt für Neurochirurgie,* **2,** 165–204.

Dandy, W. E., and Follis, R. H. (1941) On the pathology of carotid-cavernous aneurysms (pulsating exophthalmos). *American Journal of Ophthalmology,* **24,** 365–385.

Hamby, W. B. (1962) *Carotid-Cavernous Fistula.* Springfield, Illinois: Charles C Thomas, Publishers.

Newton, T. H., and Hoyt, W. F. (1970) Dural arteriovenous shunts in the region of the cavernous sinus. *Neuroradiology,* **1,** 71–81.

Obrador, S., Gomez-Bueno, J., and Silvela, J. (1974) Spontaneous carotid-cavernous fistula produced by ruptured aneurysm of the meningohypophyseal branch of the internal carotid artery. *Journal of Neurosurgery,* **40,** 539–543.

Sanders, M. D., and Hoyt, W. F. (1969) Hypoxic ocular sequelae of carotid-cavernous fistulae: Study of the causes of visual failure before and after neurosurgical treatment in a series of 25 cases. *British Journal of Ophthalmology,* **53,** 82–97.

Taniguchi, R. M., Goree, J. A., and Odom, G. L. (1971) Spontaneous carotid-cavernous shunts presenting diagnostic problems. *Journal of Neurosurgery,* **35,** 384–391.

Walker, A. E., and Allegre, G. E. (1956) Carotid-cavernous fistulas. *Surgery,* **39,** 411–422.

CHAPTER EIGHT

Tumors

BRAIN TUMORS

The coexistence of brain tumors and pregnancy appears to be coincidental, judged by the paucity of cases reported since Bernard first noted the combination in 1898. Every category of tumor has been reported. No tumor category in any large series is more common than would be expected in a young female population. Pituitary tumors are more frequently reported in small series owing to the interesting relationship among sellar tumors, visual fields, and pregnancy.

Mortality

The Franklin County [Ohio] Maternal Mortality Study (Barnes and Abbott, 1961) found that brain tumors caused one death during pregnancy or in the 6-month postpartum period for each 2500 live births. Brain tumors accounted for 8 per cent of all maternal deaths. A high mortality rate occurs with malignant or intraventricular supratentorial tumors and almost all infratentorial tumors except acoustic neuromas (Tarnow, 1960) (Table 8.1). Among survivors there is significant morbidity secondary to direct pressure or invasion. Pituitary adenomas and parasellar meningiomas can cause irreversible visual field defects. Sphenoid ridge meningiomas can encase the carotid artery, making later excision impossible. Acoustic neuromas cause unilateral hearing loss and encroach upon the brain stem (Fig. 8.1).

The second half of pregnancy is more dangerous than the first. Divry and Babon (1949) found that 80 per cent of tumors appear or progress more rapidly in the second half of pregnancy. Forty per cent of

Table 8.1. Prognosis of brain tumors during pregnancy by location and histologic category

	Symptomatic	Deaths
Supratentorial tumors		
Pituitary adenomas	10	0
Meningiomas	23	2
Gliomas		
"Benign" astrocytomas	15	0
Oligodendrogliomas	5	0
Glioblastoma	7	4
Unclassified	8	6
Metastases	8	5
Choroid plexus papillomas	3	3
Infratentorial tumors		
Acoustic neuromas	15	1
Hemangioblastomas	6	2
Medulloblastomas	2	1
Chordomas	2	2
Gliomas		
Spongioblastomas	4	3
Glioblastomas	2	2
Unclassified	4	4

Data from Tarnow (1960), Kempers and Miller (1963), and Toakley (1965).

deaths occur during the second half of pregnancy, and an equal percentage occur after childbirth (Tarnow, 1960). Herniation and death have occurred during childbirth, but the details of contributing factors are unknown. All tumors may show remission after parturition, but the malignant tumors soon progress toward death. Small acoustic neuromas (Allen et al., 1974), meningiomas (Bickerstaff et al., 1958), and cerebellar hemangioblastomas (Robinson, 1965) may be only symptomatic in the third trimester. Symptoms can dramatically decrease postpartum only to reappear years later or during subsequent pregnancies. Unfortunately, the problem may not be investigated until symptoms and deficits have become persistent.

Effect of Pregnancy

Brain tumors are larger during pregnancy than before or (usually) after it. Radiographic proof of this fact was supplied by Michelsen and New (Fig. 8.2) (1969). A grade I frontal lobe astrocytoma produced a 12 mm shift of midline structures in the sixth month of pregnancy. Seven weeks after an elective cesarean section later in the pregnancy, angiography showed less stretching of vessels and only a 9 or 10 mm shift.

Clinical evidence of the effect of pregnancy upon brain tumors is available from sequential visual field determinations during many years and from several pregnancies in women who had pituitary adenomas and

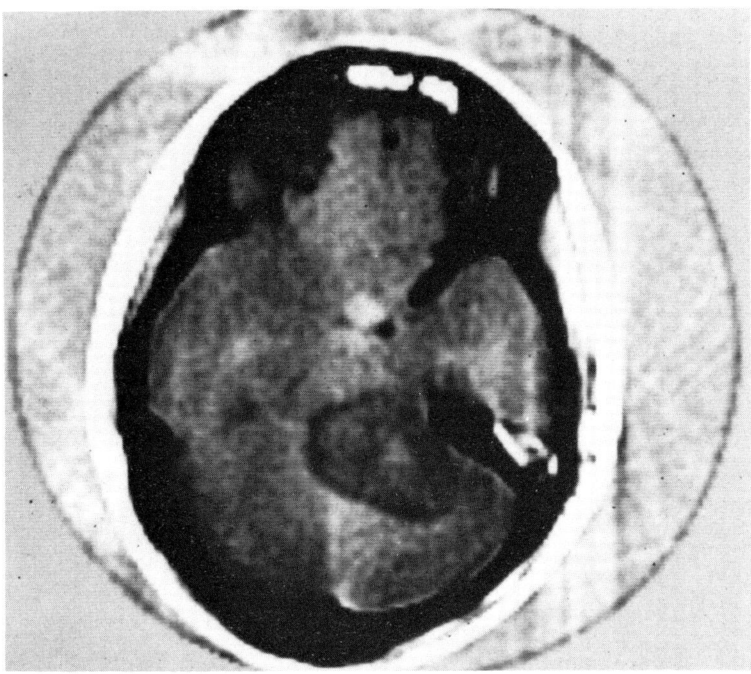

Figure 8.1. Computerized tomogram after contrast enhancement showing a huge acoustic neuroma that became symptomatic during each of two pregnancies 3 years apart but was asymptomatic between pregnancies except for unilateral deafness which the patient ignored. During the last month of her first pregnancy she was unable to stand with her feet together on her obstetrician's scales. Balance returned postpartum. During the last 4 to 6 weeks of her second pregnancy, the imbalance returned, preceding facial weakness, spastic paraparesis, and an inane effect. About the time of delivery she became almost anarthric and was unable to swallow. Computerized tomography showed this large tumor distorting the brain stem and causing hydrocephalus. Surgery was performed 3 weeks after childbirth when the recovery that was expected after childbirth and from high-dose steroids had reached a plateau.

tuberculum sella meningiomas. Hagedoorn (1937) described a woman who first noted blurred vision in the fifth month of her tenth pregnancy (Fig. 8.3). In the seventh month vision in the right eye had deteriorated, and a temporal field cut was noted. The sella was normal. By the ninth month, vision in the previously normal left eye was one-fourth of normal. One month after childbirth, vision had improved in both eyes. Six months later, now once again 2 months pregnant, vision in the left eye was normal, but acuity in the right eye was still reduced (to one-half), and some pallor of the optic disc was noted. By the fourth month of pregnancy, vision in the right eye was again failing and there was an almost complete right temporal hemianopsia. Within 2 weeks a left temporal hemianopsia began to develop and was complete by the seventh month. As vision ap-

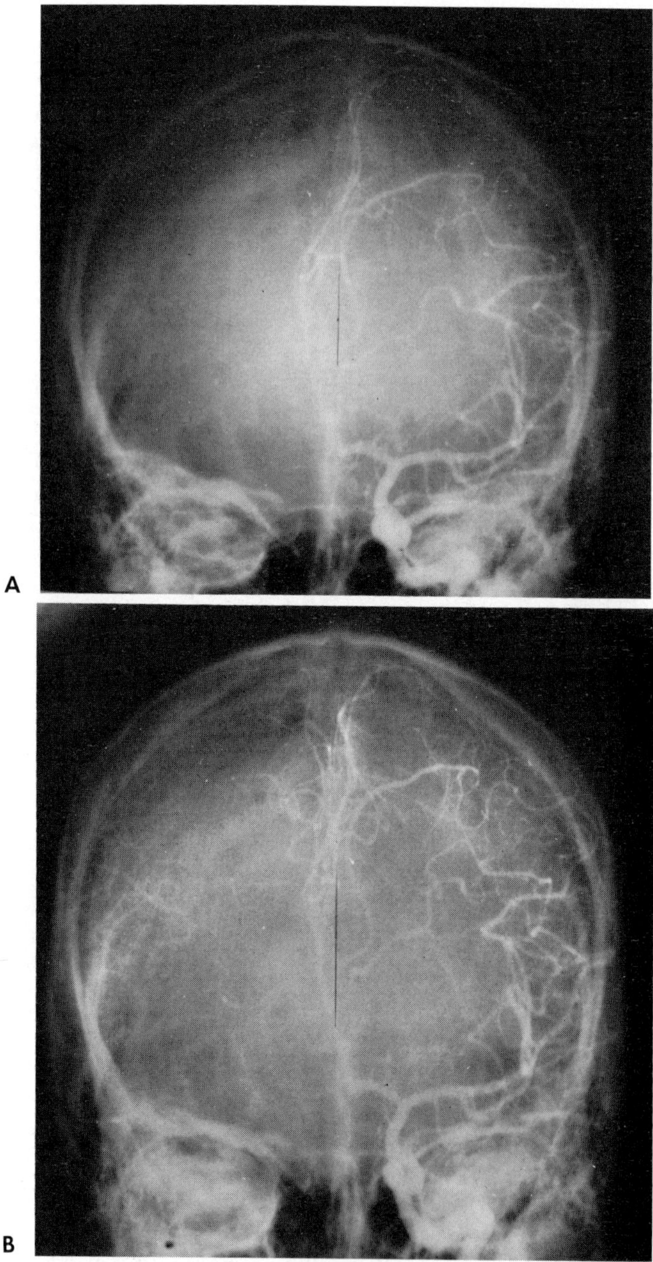

Figure 8.2. Angiographic demonstration of reduction in size of brain tumor after childbirth. Bowing and displacement of the left pericallosal artery due to a left frontal lobe astrocytoma decreased from (*A*) a 12 mm shift during the sixth month of pregnancy to (*B*) a 9 or 10 mm shift 7 weeks postpartum. Reproduced from Michelsen, J. J., and New, P. F. J. (1969). Brain tumour and pregnancy. *Journal of Neurology, Neurosurgery and Psychiatry*, **32,** 306. Courtesy of the authors.

proached light perception, labor was induced. Subsequently, visual acuity in the left eye improved to almost normal with a full field of sight. The right temporal hemianopsia persisted. Fifteen months later the bitemporal hemianopsia had returned. At operation the optic nerves were found to be embedded in a large meningioma. Postoperative bleeding caused death.

A similar case caused by a chromophobe adenoma was followed through two pregnancies (Enoksson et al. 1961) (Fig. 8.4). Pneumoencephalography 3 days after the first delivery showed that the third ventricle was normal. The same procedure during the second pregnancy demonstrated suprasellar extension of tumor which was distorting the anterior third ventricle. Progressive visual failure in late pregnancy prompted induction of labor. Both times visual acuity returned within a month.

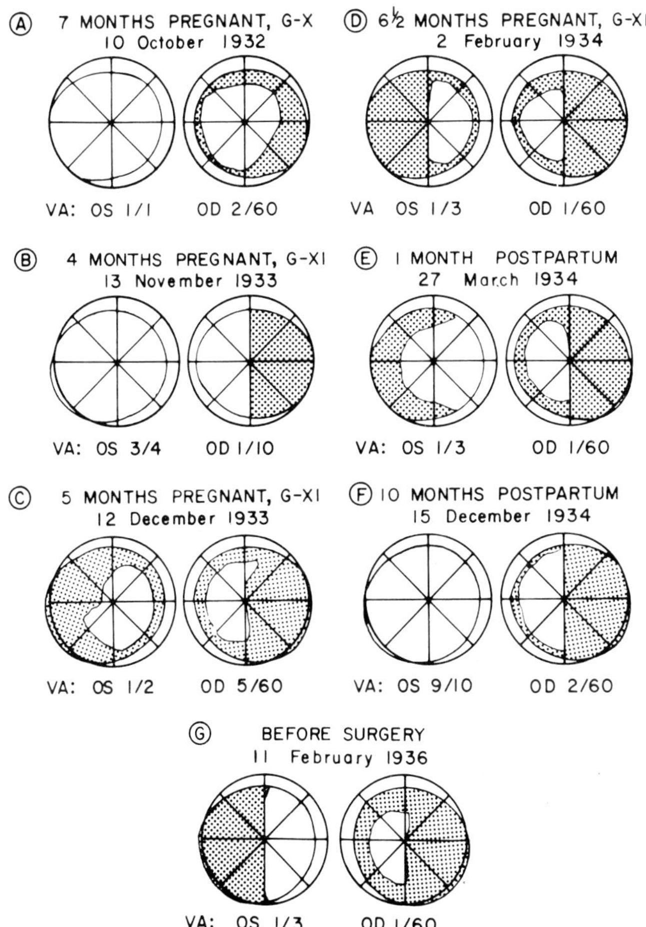

Figure 8.3. Relapsing visual failure during pregnancy due to suprasellar meningioma. Adapted from Hagedoorn, A. (1937). The chiasinal syndrome and retrobulbar neuritis in pregnancy. *American Journal of Ophthalmology,* **20,** 691.

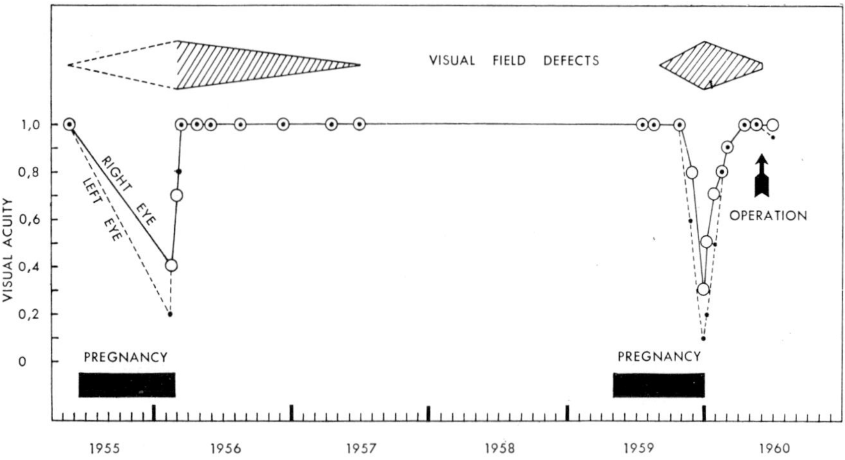

Figure 8.4. Relapsing visual failure during pregnancy due to a pituitary adenoma. From Enoksson, P., Lundberg, N., Sjöstedt, S., et al. (1961). Influence of pregnancy on visual fields in suprasellar tumours. *Acta Psychiatrica et Neurologica Scandinavica.*, **36,** 531.

The exact mechanism by which pregnancy affects brain tumors is debatable. Weyand and co-workers (1951) felt that the volume of individual tumor cells increased, since the cells of two meningiomas excised during pregnancy appeared to be swollen (Fig. 8.5). Two cases which showed premenstrual exacerbations over a period of years support this idea (Bickerstaff et al., 1958). However, hormones may directly stimulate the growth cycle of tumor cells as in breast cancer (Jensen, 1974). The blood volume of vascular tumors may increase.

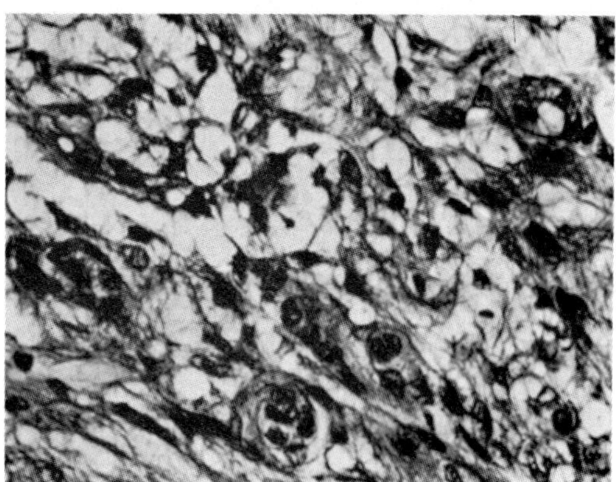

Figure 8.5. A meningiotheliomatous meningioma of the tuberculum sellae removed from a woman in the first trimester of gestation who had previously noted blurred vision at the beginning of her menses. Note cells with an increased amount of cytoplasm (hemotoxylin and eosin, × 435). From Weyand, R. D., MacCarty, C. S., and Wilson, R. B. (1951). The effect of pregnancy on intracranial meningiomas occurring about the optic chiasin. *Surgical Clinics of North America,* **31,** 1231.

Pituitary Tumors

Pituitary tumors are somewhat different. The normal pituitary increases in size (about 0.5 g) and vascularity during pregnancy. Erdheim and Strumme (1909) examined the hypophyses of 150 pregnant women and found all to be enlarged; the size was proportional to parity. This enlargement is probably due to an increase in the prolactin-secreting cells (Gobuloff and Ezrin, 1969). Some authors have attributed dimmed vision and loss of a sector of sight to this physiologic growth, but the likelihood of this is improbable at best. Almost all cases so ascribed either were poorly investigated, had no long-term follow-up care, or actually showed radiographic changes of a pituitary tumor.

Small pituitary adenomas that produce primary or secondary amenorrhea cause a real problem, since methods to induce ovulation are now available. Even if galactorrhea may point to a prolactin-secreting chromophobe adenoma, the tumor may not be detected (Boyar et al., 1976). If ovulation is induced by human menopausal gonadotropin, clomiphene, or a prolactin-suppressing drug such as bromocriptine, the resulting pregnancy causes expansion of the tumor. At some point fulminant visual loss and constriction of the visual field may develop, forcing intervention. Pituitary surgery can be managed during any trimester of pregnancy. If gestation has reached the thirty-fourth week, induction of labor is often elected, since these tumors rapidly shrink after parturition.

Before fertility drugs are prescribed, the physician should do a careful neurologic evaluation, check vision and visual fields, and be certain that the sella turcica is normal. Computerized tomography with contrast enhancement can detect some otherwise subclinical microadenomas. Although headaches may alert the physician to a problem, sequential ophthalmologic evaluations should be done throughout pregnancy if a pituitary tumor is suspected or known to exist.

If a pituitary microadenoma is found and the patient desires to become pregnant, the next questions are whether to treat and how to treat. There is no commonly accepted approach to either question. Experience indicates that pituitary irradiation before inducing ovulation will prevent visual failure and is still compatible with successful gestation (Child et al., 1975; Thorner et al., 1975). Surgery also has had its advocates (Falconer and Stafford-Bell, 1975). Trans-sphenoidal surgery before induction of pregnancy will probably prove to be the best approach.

Management of Pregnancy

It is impossible to lay down absolute rules for the conduct of the pregnancy of a woman with a brain tumor. Each case must be well studied so that informed judgments can be made. The possibility of an abscess or of a metastatic tumor from the breast or lung should not be overlooked. The numerous presentations of choriocarcinoma metastatic to brain are discussed later as a separate entity (see p. 165). Routine skull radiographs and angiographs can be done using abdominal shielding. Computerized tomography will usually define the situation well with minimal radiation exposure. Serial studies are now possible without significant risk.

With current techniques of neurosurgery, an attack upon a brain tumor is possible during pregnancy. Hypothermia is utilized to decrease cerebral metabolism and edema, since the use of mannitol should be restricted during pregnancy (see p. 128). Tumors with a high mortality rate—supratentorial malignant gliomas and many posterior fossa tumors—are best managed by prompt surgery. If a patient can be carefully followed, surgery for a meningioma or a pituitary adenoma may be delayed until after a normal term delivery or at least until the fetus has a reasonable chance for survival should the pregnancy need to be interrupted. Although intracranial surgery has been performed as early as 3 days postpartum, a delay of 2 or 3 weeks, if the clinical course permits, allows partial remission of benign tumors and a drier operating field.

Interruption of early pregnancy is seldom medically indicated, although some women faced with the diagnosis of a glioblastoma multiforme may elect an abortion. Toakley (1965) recommends therapeutic abortion during early gestation for any woman with a malignant brain tumor. One commonly recognized medical indication for therapeutic abortion is the presence of uncontrollable seizures after incomplete excision of a malignant tumor. Indications for interruption of a pregnancy in the last 2 months include increasing intracranial pressure and visual failure.

Cesarean section was once the routine method of delivery in this situation (Reeves, 1952). However, this method can be reserved for primagravidas. In multiparous women induced labor and a vaginal delivery through a proven pelvis is practical (Kempers and Miller, 1963). Adequate regional anesthesia prevents Valsalva maneuver, which elevates cerebrospinal fluid pressure. Low forceps shorten the second stage of labor.

CHORIOCARCINOMA

Choriocarcinoma is a highly invasive tumor of trophoblastic origin which is unusual in Western countries but occurs more frequently in the tropics and the Orient. Its incidence is unrelated to parity or age within the childbearing age range. Most choriocarcinomas present with irregular vaginal bleeding and sometimes an enlarged uterus in the months following a molar pregnancy or an abortion. About 15 per cent follow or accompany a normal term pregnancy (Van der Werf et al., 1970). The initial complaint may be referable to metastases, such as hemoptysis after hematogenous spread to the lungs. In 10 per cent of cases brought to autopsy, a primary choriocarcinoma could not be found in the uterus (Novak and Seah, 1954).

Neurologic Manifestations

Cerebral metastases are a frequent manifestation of this rare tumor. In 1901 Inglis and Bruce reported a case with cerebral hemorrhage that caused death 6 months after expulsion of a hydatid mole. Since that time the literature in Western countries has consisted of case reports and small series. The best statistical studies of neurologic manifestations of choriocarcinoma come from Nigeria and the Philippines. Nigerian investigations found that choriocarcinoma was the seventh most common cause of malignancy and the leading cause of cerebral metastases, which occurred in 12 per cent of all choriocarcinomas (Adeloye et al., 1972). In the Philippine Islands, 28 per cent of all metastatic choriocarcinomas involved the brain (Acosta-Sison, 1958). Cerebral metastases are secondary seedings from lung tumors which may not be apparent on chest radiographs or by gross inspection at autopsy. Although the disease usually becomes apparent during or following a pregnancy, central nervous system manifestations have occurred as the initial complaint as much as 3 years later (Russell et al., 1961) and 4 years (Dockerty and Craig, 1942) after molar pregnancies.

Cerebral metastases of choriocarcinoma may present as single or multiple "strokes," intracranial hemorrhage, or solitary mass lesions (Table 8.2). The pathogenesis of all these lesions is easily understood. Trophoblastic tissue, even when not malignant, penetrates vascular walls

Table 8.2. Neurologic manifestations of metastatic choriocarcinoma

Cerebral metastases
Single or multiple arterial occlusions
Intracerebral hematomas
Subarachnoid hemorrhage
Subdural hematoma
Solitary mass lesion
Vertebral metastases
Spinal cord compression
Cauda equina compression
Nerve root entrapment
Sacral plexus invasion

and proliferates. The artery involved may be a large carotid artery (Collomb et al., 1969) or a small branch of a cerebral or meningeal vessel. Multiple small lesions may present as multiple strokes or as inability to pay attention and changes in personality (Aguilar and Rabinovitch, 1964; Gurwitt et al., 1975). Occlusion of the artery and cerebral infarction can result. On the other hand, the weakened dilated artery may rupture with extensive bleeding, causing an intracerebral hematoma, a subarachnoid hemorrhage, or a subdural hematoma. At necropsy or operation the offending vessel can be easily overlooked if the basic pathology is not suspected.

Solitary large masses are heralded by ipsilateral, unilateral headaches and seizures, usually with Jacksonian or other focal features (Adeloye et al., 1972). Hemiplegia may appear and develop within days or can persist after a Jacksonian seizure. Radioisotopic brain scans show localized increased uptake if the mass is large enough. Arteriograms demonstrate localized distortion and widening of the affected artery by tumor, which is usually large enough to cause a mass effect.

Other neurologic manifestations are caused by local invasion of the sacral plexus as with any pelvic malignancy (Tupasi et al., 1968). Further extension of tumor about and into the vertebrae may compromise the canal and compress the cauda equina (Cary, 1913; Patterson, 1956). Rarely, metastases to the vertebrae via the paravertebral venous plexus have caused paraplegia from extradural cord compression as high as T_8 (Tupasi et al., 1968).

CSF Chorionic Gonadotropin

Serum chorionic gonadotropin assays are important both for the diagnosis of a molar pregnancy and for follow-up treatment of a patient with choriocarcinoma. Several articles on metastatic brain choriocarcinoma have recommended obtaining spinal fluid gonadotropin levels, implying they are useful in the diagnosis of cerebral involvement. In almost all cases these authors had failed to obtain such assays in their own patients.

Bernhard Zondek (1937) was the first to determine spinal fluid chorionic gonadotropin qualitatively in an attempt to distinguish between choriocarcinoma in any site and pregnancy. Using the mouse assay system he did not find gonadotropin in the spinal fluid of pregnant women. Eleanor Delfs (1957) found chorionic gonadotropin in the cerebrospinal fluid of women with normal pregnancies, molar pregnancies, and choriocarcinomas. Spinal fluid levels averaged 0.5 per cent of serum concentrations. In one case of choriocarcinoma with cerebral spread, this percentage was 2 per cent, but this is insignificant since in one molar pregnancy it reached 3 per cent. Until further study proves conclusive, it can be said that determination of spinal fluid gonadotropin has no diagnostic value in the detection of cerebral metastases. Cytologic examination of cerebrospinal fluid after millipore filtration would be far more valuable.

Treatment

Before chemotherapy cerebral metastases indicated impending death. Recent success has been reported using a combination of evacuation of any intracranial hematoma, whole brain irradiation, and chemotherapy (Bucy and Stilip, 1972; Stilip et al., 1972; Javaheri and Sall, 1975). Craniotomy is not necessary unless an expanding hematoma has formed. Regression of cerebral metastases has been observed using only irradiation and chemotherapy (Stilip et al., 1972).

Infantile Choriocarcinoma

Infantile choriocarcinoma is exceedingly rare. In the six published cases the children presented with acute anemia and hepatomegaly during the first year of life (Witzleben and Bruninga, 1968). Breast enlargement and pubic hair may be present. Chest radiographs show multiple metastatic tumors. The mother may or may not have choriocarcinoma, and the infants may show signs of disease before or after the mother becomes symptomatic from her tumor.

SPINAL CORD DISEASE

Spinal Cord Tumors

Spinal cord tumors are uncommon, and coexistence with pregnancy is rare. In most cases the "tumor" is an arteriovenous malformation. Georg Glaser (1885) recorded the first spinal cord tumor during gestation – an angiosarcoma. Since then meningiomas (Bailey and Bucy, 1930; Rath et al., 1967; Mealey and Carter, 1968; O'Connell, 1962), ependymomas (Rogers, 1955; Mealey and Carter, 1968), sarcomas (Taylor, 1906; Smolik et al., 1957), and a melanoma (Smolik et al. 1957) have been documented. In these cases there was a rapid worsening after the signs presented, usually in the second half of gestation. Only in a patient with a very slow growing oligodendroglioma were symptoms provoked during each of two pregnancies, with a remission between pregnancies (Slooff et al. 1964).

Neurofibromas are common extramedullary tumors, but they have not yet been reported to cause spinal cord compression during pregnancy. This can be expected to occur, since cutaneous neurofibromas grow after puberty and during pregnancy (Sharpe and Young, 1937; Swapp and Main, 1973). Pelvic neurofibromas may obstruct vaginal delivery (Messina and Strauss, 1976).

Sudden spinal cord compression during pregnancy caused by spontaneous epidural hematoma has been observed twice, but there was no evidence of a pre-existing vascular anomaly (Bidzinski, 1966; Yonekawa et al., 1975). One spinal epidural abscess developed shortly after childbirth, during which no spinal anesthesia had been used (Male and Martin, 1973). A cauda equina cyst in another patient presumably enlarged to become symptomatic during pregnancy (O'Connell, 1962). Rupture of an intrapelvic anterior sacral meningocele during delivery resulted in maternal death from meningitis in one patient (Silvis et al., 1956), but this is not always the case (Fujimoto et al., 1973).

Arteriovenous Malformations

Arteriovenous malformations account for 75 per cent of all spinal cord "tumors" associated with pregnancy. An initial diagnosis of multiple sclerosis may have been made due to the relapsing and remitting course of the disease, which is exacerbated during pregnancies and sometimes during menses. A prone myelogram may be normal, since the arteriovenous malformation develops on the dorsal aspect of the spinal cord from small radicular arteries. These anomalies may be intradural arteriovenous malformations, extradural hemangiomas, vertebral vascular anomalies, or any combination of the three. Sometimes a cutaneous angioma which flushes during the Valsalva maneuver is found in the affected segment (Fig. 8.6).

There are two basic clinical presentations. By a 3 to 1 margin, men over 40 years of age slowly develop a spastic paraparesis with early bladder dysfunction. Approximately one-third complain of claudication with exercise, but peripheral pulses are strong. One-quarter find that symptoms are aggravated by specific postures. Under 40 years of age, both sexes are equally affected. In the younger age group an abrupt onset (i.e., hematomyelia, transverse myelopathy, or subarachnoid hemorrhage) is more common. The condition usually progresses without remission except when associated with pregnancy. One woman was symptomatic during three pregnancies but experienced complete remission after each one (Aminoff and Logue, 1974a). Transient exacerbations with menstruation have been documented but are rare (Epstein, 1949; Tobin, 1976).

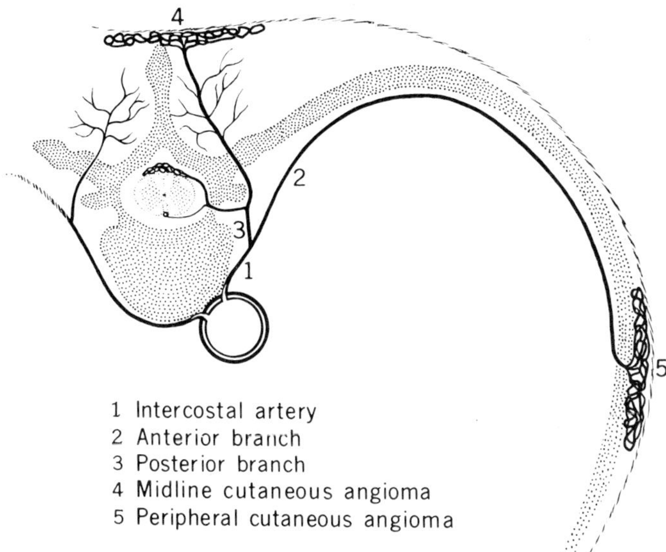

Figure 8.6. Cutaneous angiomas as a clue to the presence and location of a spinal cord arteriovenous malformation. Diagrammatic cross section shows common origin of multiple angiomas from one segmental artery. From Doppman, J. L., Wirth, F. P., DiChiro, G., et al. (1969). Value of cutaneous angiomas in the arteriographic localization of spinal-cord arteriovenous malformations. *New England Journal of Medicine,* **281,** 1443.

Extradural angiomatous compression of the spinal cord can also follow a waxing and waning course. Balado and Morea (1928) reported a case which still holds the record for the most relapses with pregnancy. A 36 year old woman presented with a 10 year history of intermittent paraplegia associated with seven of eight pregnancies. At unspecified times while carrying each of her first five children she developed spastic paraparesis which necessitated the use of a cane. Usually urinary incontinence accompanied the weakness. All symptoms quickly abated after the first four pregnancies, but after the fifth the weakness lasted for 1 month. The sixth pregnancy provoked no neurologic symptoms. The seventh was uneventful until 8 days before term, when paraplegia developed. This time the weakness lasted for 5 months. In the fourth month of her eighth pregnancy, spastic paraplegia affecting the midthoracic sensory level returned permanently. At autopsy an extradural hemangioma extending from the second to the seventh thoracic segments was found.

Pathogenesis of Exacerbations During Pregnancy

Arteriovenous malformations are direct shunts from a feeding artery to veins without an intervening capillary bed (Fig. 8.6). The fast flow of blood through the shunt deprives the adjacent areas of oxygen and nutrients. The result with spinal cord arteriovenous malformations is a progressive ischemic myelomalacia.

Several mechanisms have been postulated to explain the intermittent course characteristic of pregnancy. First, a bulky uterus impedes venous return via the vena cava. Flow shifted to the vertebral and epidural veins could engorge the venous side of the malformation. This may contribute to enlargement of an extradural angioma, but it would not increase flow through a spinal cord arteriovenous malformation. Nor can it explain the appearance of symptoms in the first trimester.

Second, increased uterine perfusion could be analogous to exercise. However, acute deterioration has not been noted during labor when uterine flow is high.

Third, hormones (probably estrogens) acting directly upon the abnormal blood vessels could dilate the shunt, thereby increasing blood flow and subsequent symptoms. The hyperestrogenic state of cirrhosis results in gynecomastia, spider "nevi," and liver palms. Spider nevi are actually small arteriovenous shunts that quickly blanch if the central arteriole is occluded by a pencil point. Spider nevi and palmar erythema become manifest as early as the third month of gestation; they last throughout the pregnancy and promptly abate after parturition (Bean et al., 1949). This is clearly analogous to the course of a spinal cord arteriovenous malformation.

Diagnostic Tests

If a spinal cord or caudal equinal mass is suspected, all necessary radiographic studies must be done despite any radiation risk to the fetus. Spinal radiographs may show the widened interpeduncular distances characteristic of intramedullary tumors, the enlarged foramina typical of neurofibromas, bone erosion due to tumors or osteomyelitis, or the vertical trabeculations associated with vertebral angiomas. Myelography presents the highest radiation exposure to the fetus of any neuroradiologic procedure. Use of television image intensifiers will keep the radiation dose as low as possible. If the prone myelogram is normal, a supine view must be done to detect an arteriovenous malformation.

If myelography and the spinal fluid are both normal, there is an increased possibility of multiple sclerosis or a viral transverse myelitis. With foresight spinal fluid will have been saved for protein electrophoresis and viral studies.

BENIGN INTRACRANIAL HYPERTENSION

Benign intracranial hypertension (pseudotumor cerebri) is characterized by increased intracranial pressure not caused by an intracranial space-occupying lesion. Headache is its universal symptom and is the presenting complaint in 90 per cent of patients (Weisberg, 1975a). The remainder seek a physician because of visual symptoms—blurred vision, transient obscured vision, or horizontal diplopia on lateral gaze. Abducens palsy is a common false localizing sign of intracranial hypertension. The diagnosis is likely to be missed unless the examiner looks for papilledema, because the patient is usually alert and otherwise healthy.

Diagnosis

The diagnosis of benign intracranial hypertension is made by excluding other causes. Lumbar cerebrospinal fluid pressure must be abnormally elevated, and CSF composition should be normal. About 60 per cent of patients will have a concentration of protein in the cerebrospinal fluid of less than 20 mg/dl (Weisberg, 1975b). An intracranial mass can now be ruled out by computerized tomography; formerly, arteriography followed by pneumoencephalography was needed. (Some physicians relied upon ventriculography, but this was hazardous, as the small ventricles characteristic of this disease were often difficult to find.) Arteriography or, strictly speaking, cerebral venography is still needed to detect a cerebral venous thrombosis, which may be caused by an ear infection or seemingly minor head trauma, or may spontaneously occur during pregnancy or the puerperium. A careful medical history and a few blood studies can eliminate other known causes (Table 8.3).

The idiopathic category remains. Interestingly, about 80 per cent of

Table 8.3. Postulated mechanisms of pathogenesis of benign intracranial hypertension

Diffuse brain swelling	↑ Vascular volume	↓ CSF reabsorption	Unknown
Encephalitides	Extracranial venous occlusions	Dural sinus thrombosis	Addison's disease
Poliomyelitis	Radial neck dissections	↑ CSF protein	Scurvy
Coxsackie virus B encephalitis	Superior vena cava thrombosis	Guillain-Barré syndrome	Steroid treatment
Reye's syndrome	Mediastinal tumor	Spinal cord tumor	Steroid withdrawal
Lead poisoning	Congestive failure	Hypervitaminosis A	Hypoparathyroidism
Hypertensive encephalopathy (eclampsia)	Polycythemia	? Tetracycline	Obesity
Status epilepticus	Chronic pulmonary hypoventilation	? Nalidixic acid	Menarche
	? Dural sinus thrombosis		Menstrual dysfunction
			Pregnancy
			The Pill

this group are women of childbearing age (Johnston and Paterson, 1974a; Weisberg, 1975a). Ninety per cent are obese (Weisberg, 1975a). Not infrequently, these women are passing through menarche, have menstrual irregularities, are taking the Pill, or are pregnant.

Effect of Menarche

Benign intracranial hypertension at menarche is short-lived. Typically, patients become asymptomatic within 3 weeks after onset (Greer, 1964a). Recurrence during subsequent menses has not been reported.

Effect of Menses

Headache and papilledema may be associated with significant generalized premenstrual edema (Thomas, 1933; McCullagh, 1941), but this is not common. Usually the menses are irregular and vary in character (Paterson et al., 1961; Greer, 1964b). Total amenorrhea is unexpected. These women are generally fat and some are hirsute (Greer, 1964b). Galactorrhea can occur (Paterson et al., 1961). Symptoms frequently last several months to a year or more.

Effect of the Pill

A small group of women have developed benign intracranial hypertension while taking the Pill (Arbenz and Wormser, 1965; Walsh et al., 1965; Mumenthaler et al., 1970). This may be coincidental. Unlike many conditions ascribed to the Pill, benign intracranial hypertension in most of these women occurs some time after the patient has begun to take the Pill. These women are slim (Bickerstaff, 1975).

Effect of Pregnancy

Benign intracranial hypertension commonly begins in the third, fourth, or fifth month of gestation. Unlike papilledema from a brain tumor, symptoms usually disappear in a month or two (Paterson et al., 1961; Greer, 1963). Pseudotumor cerebri can persist throughout pregnancy before a remission occurs after childbirth (Foley, 1955). Recurrent benign intracranial hypertension, which occurs in 5 to 10 per cent of all cases (Weisberg, 1975a), has been reported in one woman in two successive pregnancies (Elian et al., 1968). After benign intracranial hypertension occurred in a nongravid patient, pregnancy did not trigger a second episode (Johnston and Paterson, 1974a).

Labor and delivery are normal. A healthy baby can be expected.

Treatment

The natural course of the syndrome improvement occurs, but the disease may not be as "benign" as its name implies. Chronic high intracranial pressure causes optic atrophy and an enlarged "empty" sella turcica (Foley and Posner, 1975). Treatment is aimed at preserving vision. The efficacy of any treatment can be followed by serial determinations of visual acuity, the size of the blind spot, and the ability to distinguish colors in the Ishihara charts.

The traditional treatment consists of draining the cerebrospinal fluid by repeated lumbar punctures. This treatment also allows sequential measurements of CSF pressure to be made. High-dose steroids are now the treatment of first choice even though steroid withdrawal can provoke the syndrome. A lumbar-peritoneal shunt is effective in chronic cases. A ventricular shunt is not needed, since the cerebrospinal fluid flows freely to the lumbar sac. The lumbar and ventricular pressures are almost equal (Johnston and Paterson, 1974b). Since the ventricles are of normal size in this condition, placement of a ventricular shunt can be difficult and dangerous. Few neurosurgeons still do a suboccipital decompression.

Weight reduction is a neglected part of the overall treatment of these obese patients. Weight loss has been associated with dramatic decreases in the high intracranial pressure of pseudotumor cerebri (Greer, 1965; Newborg, 1974).

Pathogenesis

Intracranial pressure can be increased by a localized mass, diffuse brain swelling, increased vascular volume, or impaired reabsorption of cerebrospinal fluid but relatively unimpaired formation of cerebrospinal fluid. Encephalitis, lead poisoning, and eclampsia produced diffuse cerebral swelling. Intracranial and extracranial venous obstructions and polycythemia increase the vascular volume.

Reabsorption of cerebrospinal fluid can be blocked in syndromes with high cerebrospinal fluid protein concentrations—the Guillain-Barré syndrome and lower spinal cord tumors (Gardner et al., 1954). Raynor (1969) points out that although spinal cord tumors are almost equally divided between the sexes, over 60 per cent of spinal cord tumors with papilledema occur in women. Sixty-four per cent of those women are under 40 years of age.

Any theory of the pathogenesis of benign intracranial hypertension must account for:

1. its association with endocrinologic conditions (e.g., Addison's disease, steroid withdrawal, hypoparathyroidism)
2. its prevalence in women of childbearing age
3. transient symptoms at menarche
4. the correlated signs of obesity, menstrual dysfunction, hirsutism, and galactorrhea
5. its association with oral progestational agents
6. its association with pregnancy—primarily the midtrimester.

Something must link obesity and steroid/estrogen metabolism with intracranial pressure (probably via arachnoid villus function). Although I cannot diagram a cause and effect relationship between extraglandular estrogen production and increased intracranial pressure, I feel that there is circumstantial evidence for its existence.

Estrogens can be synthesized *de novo* from acetate by the ovary. Estrogens can also arise from extraglandular aromatization of C_{19} steroid precursors—primarily androstenedione but also testosterone (Siiteri and MacDonald, 1973). Placental production of estrogens from circulating C_{19} steroids is a well-established concept familiar to obstetricians if not

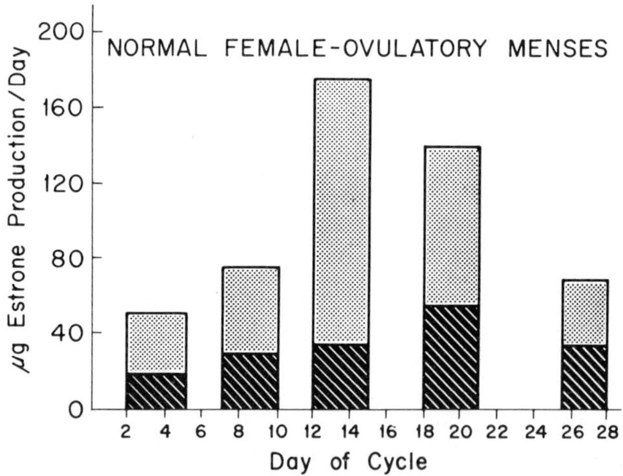

Figure 8.7. Sources of estrogen production during a normal ovulatory menstrual cycle. Total height of bars represents sum of estrone and estradiol production. Hatched portion is amount derived from plasma androstenedione. From Siiteri, P. K., and MacDonald, P. C. (1973) Role of extraglandular estrogen in human endocrinology. In *Handbook of Physiology,* Section 7: Endocrinology; Vol. II. *The Female Reproductive System,* Part I, Washington, D.C., American Physiological Society.

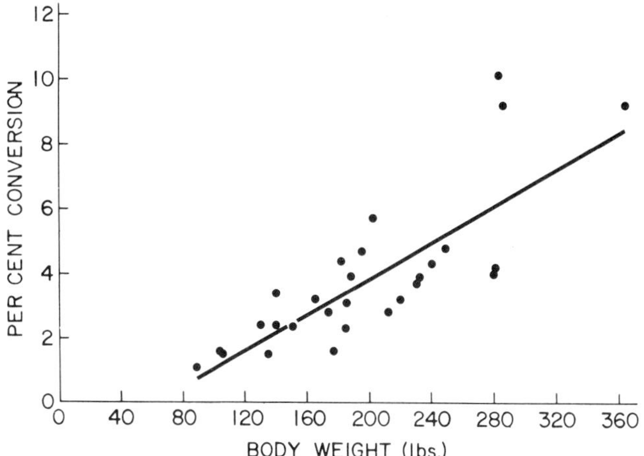

Figure 8.8. Correlation of extent of conversion of androstenedione to estrone with body weight in postmenopausal women. From Sitteri, P. K., and MacDonald, P. C. (1973). Role of extraglandular estrogen in human endocrinology. In *Handbook of Physiology,* Section 7: Endocrinology; Vol. II, *The Female Reproductive System,* Part I. Washington, D.C., American Physiological Society.

neurologists (Siiteri and MacDonald, 1966). During the normal ovulatory menstrual cycle, 10 to 50 per cent of the total estrone production is derived from circulating androstenedione (Fig. 8.7). The extent of conversion of androstenedione to estrogens increases with age, liver disease, and body weight (Fig. 8.8). Obese, elderly, postmenopausal women can be hyperestrogenic. The implications of extraglandular estrogen production from testosterone and inert precursors are tremendous. Our concepts of postmenopausal bleeding, endometrial hyperplasia, endometrial carcinoma, precursor-secreting ovarian and adrenal tumors, and male gynecomastia must all be re-evaluated. I would add benign intracranial hypertension to that list.

Benign intracranial hypertension occurring at or near the time of menarche may actually be a manifestation of adrenarche and rising production of adrenal steroids, including androstenedione.

The treatment of benign intracranial hypertension associated with obesity by weight reduction may have a sound pathophysiologic basis.

REFERENCES

Brain Tumor

Allen, J., Eldrige, R., and Koerber, T. (1974) Acoustic neuroma in the last months of pregnancy. *American Journal of Obstetrics and Gynecology,* **119,** 516–520.

Barnes, J. E., and Abbott, K. H. (1961) Cerebral complications incurred during pregnancy and the puerperium. *American Journal of Obstetrics and Gynecology,* **82,** 192–207.

Bernard, M. H. (1898) Sarcome cérébral à évolution rapide au cours de la grossesse et pendant les suites de couches. *Bulletin de la Société d'Obstétrique et Gynécologie de Paris,* **1,** 196–198.

Bickerstaff, E. R., Small, J. M., and Guest, I. A. (1958) The relapsing course of certain meningiomas in relation to pregnancy and menstruation. *Journal of Neurology, Neurosurgery and Psychiatry,* **21,** 89–91.

Carmel, P. W. (1974) Neurologic surgery in pregnancy. In *Surgical Disease in Pregnancy,* Chap. 13, pp. 203–224. ed. Barber, H. R. K., and Graber, E. A., Philadelphia: W. B. Saunders Co.

Cushing, H., and Bailey, P. (1928) Case XXIV: Cerebellar hemangioblastoma. In *Tumors Arising from the Blood Vessels of the Brain,* pp. 167–178. Springfield, Illinois: Charles C Thomas, Publishers.

Divry, P., and Bobon, J. (1949) Tumeurs encéphalique et gravidité. *Acta Neurologica Belgica,* **49,** 59–80.

Goldstein, P. J., Rosenberg, S., and Smith, R. W. (1972) Maternal death and brain tumor: Case report. *American Journal of Obstetrics and Gynecology,* **112,** 297, 298.

Jensen, E. V. (1974) Some newer endocrine aspects of breast cancer. *New England Journal of Medicine,* **291,** 1252–1254.

Kempers, R. D., and Miller, R. H. (1963) Management of pregnancy associated with brain tumors. *American Journal of Obstetrics and Gynecology,* **87,** 858–864.

Lorenz, R. (1968) Der Einfluss der Schwangerschaft auf drücksteigernde intrakranielle Prozesse. *Deutsche Medizinische Wochenschrift,* **93,** 1787–1791.

Michelsen, J. J., and New, P. F. J. (1969) Brain tumour and pregnancy. *Journal of Neurology, Neurosurgery and Psychiatry,* **32,** 305–307.

Rand, C. W., and Andler, M. (1950) Tumors of the brain complicating pregnancy. *Archives of Neurology and Psychiatry,* **63,** 1–41.

Reeves, D. L. (1952) Tumors of the brain complicating pregnancy. *Western Journal of Surgery,* **60,** 211–219.

Robinson, R. G. (1965) Aspects of the natural history of cerebellar haemangiomas. *Acta Neurologica Scandinavica,* **41,** 372–380.

Scarcella, G., Allen, M. B., and Andy, O. J. (1961) Vascular lesions of the posterior fossa during pregnancy. *American Journal of Obstetrics and Gynecology,* **82,** 836–840.

Tarnow, G. (1960) Hirntumor und Schwangerschaft. *Zentralblatt Neurochirurgie,* **20,** 134–158.

Toakley, G. (1965) Brain tumors in pregnancy. *Australian and New Zealand Journal of Surgery,* **35,** 148–154.

Weyand, R. D., MacCarty, C. S., and Wilson, R. B. (1951) The effect of pregnancy on intracranial meningiomas occurring about the optic chiasm. *Surgical Clinics of North America,* **31,** 1225–1333.

Pituitary Tumors

Boyar, R. M., Kapen, S., Wetizman, E. D., et al. (1976) Pituitary microadenoma and hyperprolactinemia. A cause of unexplained secondary amenorrhea. *New England Journal of Medicine,* **294,** 236–265.

Bringle, C. G. (1937) Pregnancy in an acromegalic following removal of pituitary tumor. *Memphis Medical Journal,* **12,** 72, 73.

British Medical Journal (1975) Bromocriptine—a changing scene. *British Medical Journal,* **4,** 667, 668.

Burke, C. W., and Joplin, G. F. (1972) Pituitary tumour treated by pituitary implantation of yttrium 90 during or before pregnancy. *Proceedings of the Royal Society of Medicine,* **65,** 486–488.

Carvill, M. (1923) Bitemporal contraction of the fields of vision in pregnancy. *American Journal of Ophthalmology,* **6,** 885–891.

Child, D. F., Gordon, H., Mashiter, K., et al. (1975) Pregnancy, prolactin and pituitary tumours. *British Medical Journal,* **4,** 87–89.

Enoksson, P., Lundberg, N., Sjöstedt, S., et al. (1961) Influence of pregnancy on visual fields in suprasellar tumours. *Acta Psychiatrica et Neurologica Scandinavica,* **36,** 524–538.

Erdheim, J., and Stumme, E. (1909) Über die Schwangerschaftsveränderung der Hypophyse. *Beitraege zur Pathologische Anatomie und Allgemeinen Pathologie,* **46,** 1–132.

Falconer, M. A., and Stafford-Bell, M. A. (1975) Visual failure from pituitary and parasellar tumours occurring with favourable outcome in pregnant women. *Journal of Neurology, Neurosurgery and Psychiatry,* **38,** 919–930.

Finaly, C. E. (1923) Bitemporal contraction of visual fields in pregnancy. *Archives of Ophthalmology,* **52,** 50–55.

Gemzell, C. (1973) Induction of ovulation in patients following removal of a pituitary adenoma. *American Journal of Obstetrics and Gynecology,* **117,** 955–961.

Goluboff, L. G., and Ezrin, C. (1969) Effect of pregnancy on the somatotrophic and prolactic cells of the human adenohypophysis. *Journal of Clinical Endocrinology,* **29,** 1533–1538.

Hagedoorn, A. (1937) The chiasmal syndrome and retrobulbar neuritis in pregnancy. *American Journal of Ophthalmology,* **20,** 690–699.

Johns, J. P. (1930) The influence of pregnancy on the visual field. *American Journal of Ophthalmology,* **13,** 956–967.

Kajtar, T., and Tomkin, G. H. (1971) Emergency hypophysectomy in pregnancy after induction of ovulation. *British Medical Journal,* **4,** 88–90.

Malarkey, W. B., and Johnson, J. C. (1976) Pituitary tumors and hyperprolactinemia. *Archives of Internal Medicine,* **136,** 40–44.

Pearce, H. M. (1963) Physiologic bitemporal hemianopsia in pregnancy. *Obstetrics and Gynecology,* **22,** 612–614.

Swyer, G. I. M., Little, V., and Harries, B. J. (1971) Visual disturbance in pregnancy after induction of ovulation. *British Medical Journal,* **4,** 90, 91.

Thorner, M. O., Besser, G. M., Jones, A. M., et al. (1975) Bromocriptine treatment of female infertility: Report of 13 pregnancies. *British Medical Journal,* **4,** 694–697.

Varga, L., Wenner, R., and del Pozo, E. (1973) Treatment of galactorrhea-amenorrhea syndrome with Br-ergocryptine (CB 154): Restoration of ovulatory function and fertility. *American Journal of Obstetrics and Gynecology,* **117,** 75–79.

Choriocarcinoma

Acosta-Sison, H. (1956) Extensive cerebral hemorrhage caused by the rupture of a cerebral blood vessel due to a chorionepithelioma embolus. *American Journal of Obstetrics and Gynecology,* **71,** 1119–1121.

Acosta-Sison, H. (1958) The relative frequency of various anatomic sites as the point of first metastasis in 32 cases of chorionepithelioma. *American Journal of Obstetrics and Gynecology,* **75,** 1149–1152.

Adeloye, A., Osuntokun, B. O., Hendrickse, J. P. DeV., et al. (1972) The neurology of metastatic chorion carcinoma of the uterus. *Journal of the Neurological Sciences,* **16,** 315–329.

Aguilar, M. J., and Rabinovitch, R. (1964) Metastatic chorionepithelioma simulating multiple strokes. *Neurology,* **14,** 933–937.

Beasley, W. H., and Williams, D. M. (1962) Chorioncarcinoma causing cerebral haemorrhage. *Journal of Pathology and Bacteriology,* **84,** 215–217.

Bucy, P. C., and Stilip, T. J. (1972) Metastatic choriocarcinoma of the brain: Its recognition, treatment and cure; and other matters. *Schweizer Archiv für Neurologic und Psychiatrie,* **111,** 237–242.

Cary, E. (1913) Chorio-epithelioma: Recurrence after three years; invasion of the spinal cord; villi in secondary growth. *Surgery, Gynecology and Obstetrics,* **16,** 362–368.

Collomb, H., Girard, P.-L., Lemercier, G., et al. (1969) Thrombose carotidenne à partir d'embol métastatique d'un chorioépithéliome. *Bulletin de la Societe Medicale d'Afrique Noire de Langue Francaise,* **14,** 326–333.

Delfs, E. (1975) Hydatidiform mole, an editorial comment. *Obstetrics and Gynecology,* **45,** 95, 96.

Dockerty, M. B., and Craig, W. M. (1942) Chorionepithelioma: An unusual case in which cerebral metastasis occurred four years after hysterectomy. *American Journal of Obstetrics and Gynecology,* **44,** 497–501.

Gurwitt, L. J., Long, J. M., and Clark, R. E. (1975) Cerebral metastatic choriocarcinoma: A postpartum cause of "stroke". *Obstetrics and Gynecology,* **45,** 583–588.

Inglis, E. M., and Bruce, A. (1901) Case of cerebral haemorrhage resulting from deciduoma malignum. *Transactions of the Edinburgh Obstetrical Society,* **26,** 119–144.

Javaheri, G., and Sall, S. (1975) Cerebral manifestations of metastatic trophoblastic disease. *American Journal of Obstetrics and Gynecology,* **122,** 989–991.

Novak, E., and Seah, C. S. (1954) Choriocarcinoma of the uterus. *American Journal of Obstetrics and Gynecology,* **67,** 933–961.

Patterson, W. B. (1956) Normal pregnancy after recovery from metastatic choriocarcinoma. *American Journal of Obstetrics and Gynecology,* **72,** 183–187.

Russell, D. J., Jones, H. E., and Auerbach, S. H. (1961) Choriocarcinoma: Report of a case showing unusual metastatic behavior. *Obstetrics and Gynecology,* **17,** 84–88.

Seal, R. M. E., and Millard, A. H. (1955) A case of chorionepithelioma presenting with subarachnoid haemorrhage. *Journal of Obstetrics and Gynaecology of the British Empire,* **62,** 932–934.

Shuangshoti, S., Panyathanya, R., and Wichienkur, P. (1974) Intracranial metastases from unsuspected choriocarcinoma. *Neurology,* **24,** 649–654.

Stilip, T. J., Bucy, P. C., and Brewer, J. I. (1972) Cure of metastatic choriocarcinoma of the brain. *Journal of the American Medical Association,* **221,** 276–279.

Tupasi, T. E., deVeyra, E. A., Perez, M. C., et al. (1968) Neurologic manifestations in metastatic choriocarcinoma. *Proceedings of the Australian Association of Neurologists,* **5,** 435–441.

Van der Werf, A. J. M., Broeders, G. H. B., Vooys, G. P., et al. (1970) Metastatic choriocarcinoma as a complication of pregnancy. *Obstetrics and Gynecology,* **35,** 78–88.

Vaughn, H. G., and Howard, R. G. (1962) Intracranial hemorrhage due to metastatic chorionepithelioma. *Neurology,* **12,** 771–777.

Choriocarcinoma

CSF Chorionic Gonadotrophin

Delfs, E. (1957) Quantitative chorionic gonadotrophin: Prognostic value in hydatidiform mole and chorionepithelioma. *Obstetrics and Gynecology,* **9,** 1–24.

McCormick, J. B. (1954) Gonadotrophin in urine and spinal fluid: Quantitative studies for chorionic moles and choriocarcinomas. *Obstetrics and Gynecology,* **3,** 58–65.

Pastorfide, G. B., Goldstein, D. P., and Kosasa, T. S., (1974) The use of a radioimmunoassay specific for human chorionic gonadotrophin in patients with molar pregnancy and gestational trophoblastic disease. *American Journal of Obstetrics and Gynecology,* **120,** 1025–1028.

Vesell, M., and Goldman, S. (1941) Friedman test on spinal fluid in cases of hydatidiform mole and pregnancy. *American Journal of Obstetrics and Gynecology,* **42,** 272–275.

Zondek, B. (1937) Gonadotropic hormone in the diagnosis of chorionepithelioma. *Journal of the American Medical Association,* **108,** 607–611.

Neonatal Choriocarcinoma

Buckell, E. W. C., and Owen, T. K. (1954) Chorionephithelioma in mother and infant. *Journal of Obstetrics and Gynecology of the British Empire,* **61,** 329, 330.

Daamen, C. B. F., Bloem, G. W. D., and Westerbeek, A. J. (1961) Chorionepithelioma in mother and child. *Journal of Obstetrics and Gynaecology of the British Empire,* **68,** 144–149.

Kelly, D. L., Kushner, J., and McLean, W. T. (1971) Neonatal intracranial choriocarcinoma. *Journal of Neurosurgery,* **35,** 465–471.

Mercer, R. D., Lammert, A. C., Anderson, R., et al. (1958) Choriocarcinoma in mother and infant. *Journal of the American Medical Association,* **166,** 482, 483.

Witzleben, C. L., and Bruninga, G. (1968) Infantile choriocarcinoma: A characteristic syndrome. *Journal of Pediatrics,* **73,** 374–378.

Spinal Cord Disease

TUMORS

Bailey, P., and Bucy, P. C. (1930) Tumors of the spinal canal. Case II. *Surgical Clinics of North America,* **10,** 233–242.

Glaser, G. (1885) Ein Fall von centralem Angiosarkom des Rückenmarks. *Archiv für Psychiatrie und Nervenkrankheiten,* **16,** 87–100.

Mealey, J., and Carter, J. E. (1968) Spinal cord tumor during pregnancy. *Obstetrics and Gynecology,* **32,** 204–209.

O'Connell, J. E. A. (1962) Neurosurgical problems in pregnancy. *Proceedings of the Royal Society of Medicine,* **55,** 577–582.

Rath, S., Mathal, K. V., and Chandy, J. (1967) Multiple meningiomas of the spinal canal: Case report. *Journal of Neurosurgery,* **26,** 639, 640.

Rogers, L. (1955) Tumours involving the spinal cord and its roots. *Annals of the Royal College of Surgeons of England,* **16,** 1–29.

Slooff, J., Kernohan, J. W., and McCarty, C. S. (1964) *Primary Intramedullary Tumors of the Spinal Cord and Filum Terminale,* pp. 165, 166. Philadelphia: W. B. Saunders Co.

Smolik, E. A., Nash, F. P., and Clawson, J. W. (1957) Neurological and neurosurgical complications associated with pregnancy and the puerperium. *Southern Medical Journal,* **50,** 561–572.

Taylor, E. W. (1906) Spinal cord tumor simulating acute myelitis, associated with optic neuritis and painless labor. *Journal of Nervous and Mental Disease,* **33,** 583–585.

VON RECKLINGHAUSEN'S NEUROFIBROMATOSIS

Messina, A. M., and Strauss, R. G. (1976) Pelvic neurofibromatosis. *Obstetrics and Gynecology,* (Suppl.) **47,** 63S–66S.

Sharpe, J. C., and Young, R. H. (1937) Recklinghausen's neurofibromatosis: Clinical manifestations in 31 cases. *Archives of Internal Medicine,* **59,** 299–328.

Swapp, G. H., and Main, R. A. (1973) Neurofibromatosis in pregnancy. *British Journal of Dermatology,* **80,** 431–435.

VERTEBRAL VASCULAR MALFORMATIONS

Aminoff, M. J., and Logue, V. (1974a) Clinical features of spinal vascular malformations. *Brain,* **97,** 197–210.

Aminoff, M. J., and Logue, V. (1974b) The prognosis of patients with spinal vascular malformations. *Brain,* **97,** 211–218.

Askenasy, H., and Behmoaram, A. (1957) Neurological manifestations in haemangioma of the vertebrae. *Journal of Neurology, Neurosurgery and Psychiatry,* **20,** 276–284.

Balado, M., and Morea, R. (1928) Hemangioma extramedular produciendo paraplejias durante el embarazo. *Archivos Argentinos de Neurologia,* **1,** 345–351.

Delmas-Marsalet, P. (1941) Poussées évolutives gravidiques et image lipiodolée caractéristiques des hémangiomes médullaires. *Presse médicale,* **49,** 964–965.

Fields, W. S., and Jones, J. R. (1957) Spinal epidural in hemangioma in pregnancy. *Neurology,* **7,** 825–828.

Hoffmann, W., and Rohr, H. (1959) Wirbel-Angiom und Schwangerschaft. *Nervenarzt,* **30,** 353–357.

Lam, R. L., Roulhac, G. E., and Erwin, H. J. (1951) Hemangioma of the spinal canal and pregnancy. *Journal of Neurosurgery,* **8,** 668–671.

McAllister, V. L., Kendall, B. E., and Bull, J. W. D. (1975) Symptomatic vertebral haemangiomas. *Brain,* **98,** 71–80.

Nelson, D. A. (1964) Spinal cord compression due to vertebral angiomas during pregnancy. *Archives of Neurology,* **11,** 408–413.

Newquist, R. E., and Mayfield, F. H. (1960) Spinal angioma presenting during pregnancy. *Journal of Neurosurgery,* **17,** 541–545.

SPINAL CORD ARTERIOVENOUS MALFORMATIONS

Antoni, N. (1962) Spinal vascular malformations (angiomas) and myelomalacia. *Neurology,* **12,** 795–804.

Bean, W. B., Cogswell, R., Dexter, M., et al. (1949) Vascular changes of the skin in pregnancy: Vascular spiders and palmar erythema. *Surgery, Gynecology and Obstetrics,* **88,** 739–752.

Brion, S., Netsky, M. G., and Zimmerman, H. M. (1952) Vascular malformations of the spinal cord. *Archives of Neurology and Psychiatry,* **68,** 339–361.

Doppman, J. L., Wirth, F. P., DiChiro, G., et al. (1969) Value of cutaneous angiomas in the arteriographic localization of spinal-cord arteriovenous malformations. *New England Journal of Medicine,* **281,** 1440–1444.

Epstein, J. A., Beller, A. J., and Cohen, I. (1949) Arterial anomalies of the spinal cord. *Journal of Neurosurgery,* **6,** 45–56.

Kulowski, J. (1962) Unusual causes of low back pain and sciatica during pregnancy. *American Journal of Obstetrics and Gynecology,* **84,** 627–630.

Newman, M. J. D. (1958) Spinal angioma with symptoms in pregnancy. *Journal of Neurology, Neurosurgery and Psychiatry,* **21,** 38–41.

Newman, M. J. D. (1959) Racemose angioma of the spinal cord. *Quarterly Journal of Medicine,* **28,** 97–108.

Tobin, W. D., and Layton, D. D. (1976) The diagnosis and natural history of spinal cord arteriovenous malformations. *Mayo Clinic Proceedings,* **51,** 637–646.

Other Conditions

Bidzinski, J. (1966) Spontaneous spinal epidural hematoma during pregnancy: Case report. *Journal of Neurosurgery,* **24,** 1017.

Fujimoto, A., Ebbin, A. J., Wilson, M. G., et al. (1973) Successful pregnancy in a woman with meningomyelocele. *Lancet,* **1,** 104.

Male, C. G., and Martin, R. (1973) Puerperal spinal epidural abscess. *Lancet,* **1,** 608, 609.

O'Connell, J. E. A. (1962) Neurosurgical problems in pregnancy. *Proceedings of the Royal Society of Medicine,* **55,** 577–582.

Opitz, J. M. (1973) Pregnancy in woman with meningomyelocele. *Lancet,* **1,** 368, 369.

Silvis, R., Riddle, L. R., and Clark, G. G. (1956) Anterior sacral meningocoele. *American Surgeon* **22,** 554–566.

Yonekawa, Y., Medhorn, H. M., and Nishikawa, M. (1975) Spontaneous spinal epidural hematoma during pregnancy. *Surgical Neurology,* **3,** 327–328.

Benign Intracranial Hypertension

Arbenz, J. P., and Wormser, P. (1965) Pseudotumor cerebri durch Sexualhormone. *Schweizer Medizinische Wochenschrift,* **95,** 1654–1656.

Arseni, C., and Maretsis, M. (1967) Tumors of the lower spinal cord associated with increased intracranial pressure and papilledema. *Journal of Neurosurgery,* **27,** 105–110.

Bickerstaff, E. R. (1975) *Neurological Complications of Oral Contraceptives.* Oxford: Clarendon Press.

Boddie, H. G., Banna, M., and Bradley, W. G. (1974) "Benign" intracranial hypertension: A survey of the clinical and radiological features, and long term prognosis. *Brain,* **97**(2), 313–326.

Elian, M., Ben-Tovim, N., Bechar, M., et al. (1968) Recurrent benign intracranial hypertension (pseudotumor cerebri) during pregnancy. *Obstetrics and Gynecology,* **31,** 685–688.

Foley, J. (1955) Benign forms of intracranial hypertension: "Toxic" and "otitic" hydrocephalus. *Brain,* **78,** 1–41.

Foley, K. M., and Posner, J. B. (1975) Does pseudotumor cerebri cause the empty sella syndrome? *Neurology,* **25,** 565–569.

Gardner, W. J., Spittler, D. X., and Whitten C. (1954) Increased intracranial pressure caused by increased protein content in the cerebrospinal fluid. *New England Journal of Medicine,* **250,** 932.

Greer, M. (1963) Benign intracranial hypertension: III. Pregnancy. *Neurology,* **13,** 670–672.

Greer, M. (1964a) Benign intracranial hypertension: IV. Menarche. *Neurology,* **14,** 569–573.

Greer, M. (1964b) Benign intracranial hypertension: V. Menstrual dysfunction. *Neurology,* **14,** 668–673.

Greer, M. (1965) Benign intracranial hypertension: VI. Obesity. *Neurology,* **15,** 382–388.

Johnston, I., and Paterson, A. (1974a) Benign intracranial hypertension: I. Diagnosis and prognosis. *Brain,* **97,** 289–300.
Johnston, I. and Paterson, A. (1974b) Benign intracranial hypertension: II. CSF pressure and circulation. *Brain,* **97,** 301–312.
Mani, K. S., and Townsend, H. R. A. (1964) The EEG in benign intracranial hypertension. *Electroencephalography and Clinical Neurophysiology,* **14,** 604–610.
Mathew, N. T., Meyer, J. S., and Ott, E. O. (1975) Increased cerebral blood volume in benign intracranial hypertension. *Neurology,* **25,** 646–649.
McCullagh, E. P. (1941) Menstrual edema with intracranial hypertension (pseudotumor cerebri). *Cleveland Clinical Quarterly,* **8,** 202–212.
Mumenthaler, M., Grandjean, P., and Huber, P. (1970) Neurologische Pathologie der hormonalen Antikonzeption. *Schweizer Medizinische Wochenschrift,* **100,** 1585–1594.
Newborg, B. (1974) Pseudotumor cerebri treated by rice/reduction diet. *Archives of Internal Medicine,* **133,** 802–807.
Oldstone, M. B. A. (1966) Disturbance of pituitary-adrenal interrelationships in benign intracranial hypertension (pseudotumor cerebri). *Journal of Clinical Endocrinology,* **26,** 1366–1369.
Paterson, R., DePasquale, N., and Mann, S. (1961) Pseudotumor cerebri. *Medicine,* **40,** 85–99.
Powell, J. L. (1972) Pseudotumor cerebri and pregnancy. *Obstetrics and Gynecology,* **40,** 713–718.
Raynor, R. B. (1969) Papilledema associated with tumors of the spinal cord. *Neurology,* **19,** 700–704.
Thomas, W. A. (1933) Generalized edema occurring only at the menstrual period. *Journal of the American Medical Association,* **101,** 1126–1127.
Walsh, F. B., Clark, D. B., Thompson, R. S., et al. (1965) Oral contraceptives and neuro-ophthalmologic interest. *Archives of Ophthalmology,* **74,** 628–640.
Weisberg, L. A. (1975a) Benign intracranial hypertension. *Medicine,* **54,** 197–207.
Weisberg, L. A. (1975b) The syndrome of increased intracranial pressure without localizing signs: A reappraisal. *Neurology,* **25,** 85–88.

Extraglandular Estrogen Production

Grodin, J. M., Siiteri, P. K., and MacDonald, P. C. (1973) Source of estrogen production in postmenopausal women. *Journal of Clinical Endocrinology,* **36,** 207–214.
Longcope, C. (1971a) Metabolic clearance and blood production rates of estrogens in postmenopausal women. *American Journal of Obstetrics and Gynecology,* **111,** 778–781.
Longcope, C., and Tait, J. F. (1971) Validity of metabolic clearance and interconversion rates of estrone and 17 beta-estradiol in normal adults. *Journal of Clinical Endocrinology,* **32,** 481–490.
MacDonald, P. C., Rombaut, R. P., and Siiteri, P. K. (1967) Plasma precursors of estrogen: I. Extent of conversion of plasma Δ^4-androstenedione to estrone in normal males and nonpregnant normal, castrate and adrenalectomized females. *Journal of Clinical Endocrinology,* **27,** 1103–1111.
McEwan, B. S. (1976) Interactions between hormones and nerve tissue. *Scientific American,* **235,** 48–58.
Siiteri, P. K., and MacDonald, P. C. (1966) Placental estrogen biosynthesis during human pregnancy. *Journal of Clinical Endocrinology,* **26,** 751–761.
Siiteri, P. K. (1973) Role of extraglandular estrogen in human endocrinology. In *Handbook of Physiology,* Section 7: Endocrinology; Vol. II. Female reproductive system, Part 1, Chap. 28, pp. 615–629. Washington, D.C.: American Physiological Society.

CHAPTER NINE

Headache

Headache is the most common neurologic symptom and one of the most distressing. Proper classification is essential before it can be effectively treated. Unfortunately, no one classification of headache is universally accepted by neurologists, physicians in general, and patients. All severe headache is migraine. Many series reported in the literature cannot be compared.

MUSCLE CONTRACTION/TENSION HEADACHE

The most common headache is the muscle contraction/tension headache. This headache consists of dull, persistent pain over the whole head or sometimes localized to the vertex; it typically occurs in the late afternoon or early evening. The head may feel as if it would explode or as if there were a band around it. When severe this type of headache can be incapacitating. The neck muscles are sore and tight.

Muscle contraction headache is part of the premenstrual syndrome. The same headache can happen at any time during pregnancy.

Treatment consists of aspirin or other analgesics, rest in a quiet room, neck and shoulder massage, soaking in a warm bath, and either hot or cold packs on the neck. The benzodiazepine minor tranquilizers (meprobamate, chlordiazepoxide, and especially diazepam) often alleviate an acute muscle contraction/tension headache, but long-term use of these drugs for chronic headaches of this type is not beneficial. I rely instead upon environmental changes, tricyclic antidepressants, and psychiatric counselling.

The regular use of benzodiazepine tranquilizers cannot be recommended for pregnant women or lactating mothers. First, there is a suspicion that the risk of orofacial clefts increases if these drugs are taken during the first trimester of gestation (Milkovich and van der Berg, 1974; Saxen, 1975; Safra and Oakley, 1975), but conflicting evidence has also been reported (Belafsky et al., 1969; Hartz et al., 1975). The definitive study has yet to be done.

Second, benzodiazepine drugs are poorly metabolized by the fetus and neonate. Diazepam quickly crosses the placenta. Twelve minutes after a maternal intravenous injection, concentrations of diazepam in the umbilical cord and maternal plasma are equal. If diazepam has been chronically ingested during gestation, it and its *N*-dimethyl metabolite accumulate in fetal lungs, heart, brain, and liver (Mandelli et al., 1975). Infants whose mothers took 10 to 15 mg diazepam daily for 1 to 3 weeks before delivery had pharmacologically potent plasma diazepam levels 10 days after birth (Kanto et al., 1974).

There are wide individual variations in the clearance of diazepam by newborns. In full-term babies diazepam has an average half-life of 31 hours (Mandelli et al., 1975). This is faster than the half-life usually observed in premature babies but slower than that in older infants (Morselli et al., 1973).

Thirdly, variable but significant amounts of diazepam and its active metabolite are excreted in breast milk (Cole and Hailey, 1975). Chronic use of diazepam is not recommended for lactating mothers (Stirrat, 1976).

VASCULAR HEADACHE

Vascular headaches are attributed to cerebral vasodilation. This category includes migraine, cluster headaches, and toxic vascular headaches. Cluster headaches will not be discussed here, as they afflict men almost exclusively. Toxic vascular headaches are caused by fever, carbon dioxide retention, and nitrites.

Migraine

Classic migraine is a severe, throbbing, often unilateral, headache associated with nausea and vomiting; it follows a prodromal stage of scintillating scotomas. The initial phase is attributed to intense cerebral vasoconstriction. Ophthalmoplegia, hemiplegia, aphasia, and paresthesias can occur instead of the more common visual changes. If the vertebral-basilar system is involved, bilateral blindness occurs, associated with vertigo, dysarthria, incoordination, transient memory loss, or even quadriparesis and loss of consciousness. The aura lasts 20 to 30 minutes.

Ergotamine tartrate taken during this period will usually abort the subsequent vasodilation, headache, photophobia, and nausea, which can last several days. If headache develops, rest in a quiet room plus various combinations of analgesics, sedatives, and antiemetics will give symptomatic relief.

Classic migraine is mainly a disease of women of childbearing age. It often begins about the time of menarche. The frequency of the attacks can decrease with age, but some women experience a flare at menopause. A history of motion sickness in childhood is not unusual. Patients with migraine tend to have an obsessive-compulsive personality. Attacks can be precipitated by tyramine in fermented cheese (Hannington, 1967; Ryan, 1974) or by β-phenylethylamine in chocolate, cheese, and red wine (Sandler et al., 1974).

Menstrual Migraine

Menstruation is another provocative stimulus for a sizeable group of women (Fig. 9.1). Ovulation may be also. Brian Somerville (1972a, b; 1975) has shown this to be an estradiol-withdrawal phenomenon. Almost daily plasma estradiol and progesterone levels were measured in a group of women with classic migraine which recurred every month about the time of menstruation. Progesterone injections beginning 3 to 6 days before the expected onset of bleeding did delay menorrhagia but not migraine, which occurred at the usual time, corresponding to dropping estradiol levels. Later withdrawal bleeding was unaccompanied by migraine. Injections of estradiol in oil did postpone the headache until after menstrual bleeding, when plasma estradiol levels had declined.

The duration of exposure to high estradiol concentrations, or the concurrent exposure to elevated progesterone levels may be a factor. This is suggested by the clinical observation that ovulatory migraine is rare, but menstrual migraine is common. Migraine can occur when estradiol concentrations have declined to low levels after being elevated by estradiol-in-oil injections for 7 to 10 days in the preluteal menstrual cycle when progesterone levels were low (Somerville, 1975).

Migraine and the Pill

The Pill increases the frequency or severity or both of migraine for most women (Whitty et al., 1966; Desrosiers, 1973). Attacks usually occur between courses of the Pill. Migraine which develops *de novo* while a woman is taking the Pill does not always abate after the Pill is stopped. There is no relationship between a history of migraine during pregnancy and the effect of the Pill (Whitty et al., 1966). Statistically

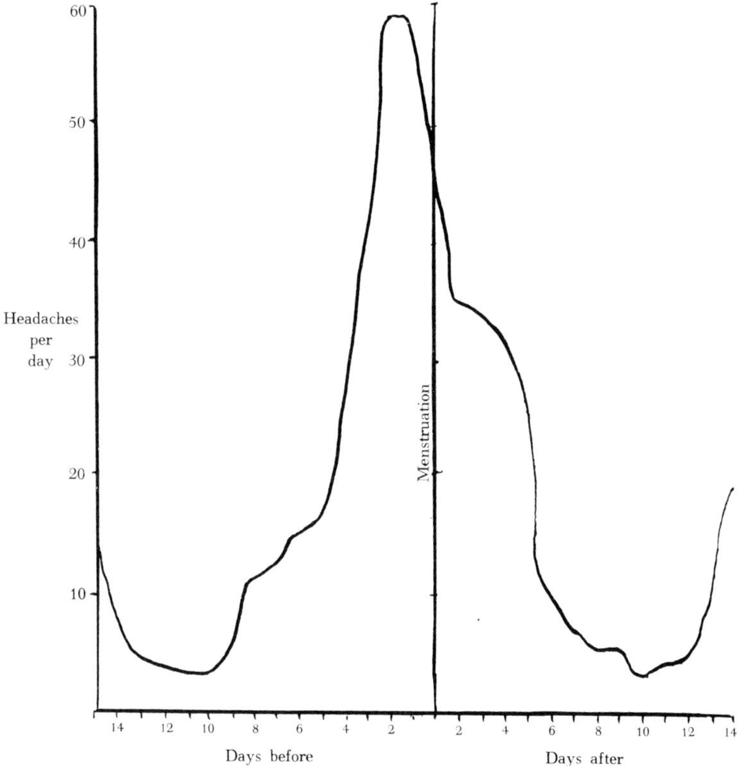

Figure 9.1. Distribution of 512 headaches during the menstrual cycle. From Dalton, K. (1973) Progesterone suppositories and pessaries in the treatment of menstrual migraine. *Headache*, **12**, 152.

significant prospective studies of the effect of strongly progestrogenic Pills versus strongly estrogenic Pills on women with pre-existing migraine have not been done. A change in the type of Pill may result in decreased attacks of migraine. Most women stop taking the Pill.

Migraine and Pregnancy

The improvement of classic migraine during pregnancy is such a common observation of neurologists that few have statistically studied the phenomenon. Somerville (1972c) found that, of the 77 per cent who improved during pregnancy, 30 per cent were completely free of migraine for that period. However, 23 per cent either failed to improve or worsened. Migraine can begin during pregnancy, usually in the first trimester (Callaghan, 1968; Somerville, 1972c). Migraine probably does

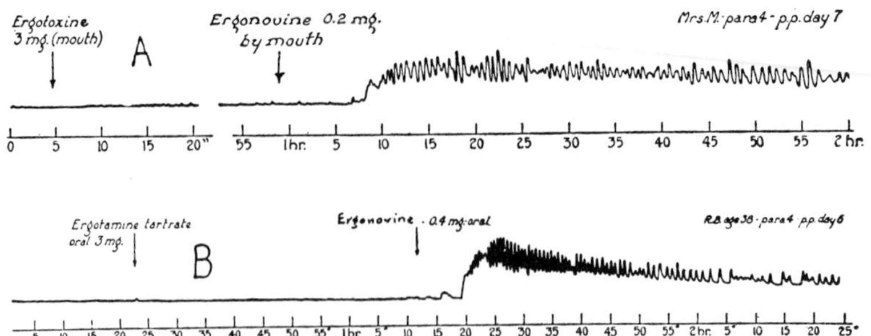

Figure 9.2. Kymographic tracings of uterine motility in postpartum women in response to oral ergotoxine, ergotamine tartrate, and ergonovine. From Davis, M. E., Adair, F. L., and Pearl, S. (1936) The present status of oxytocics in obstetrics. *Journal of the American Medical Association,* **107**, 262. Copyright 1936, American Medical Association.

not increase the risk of toxemia, although one retrospective study found this to be true (Rotton et al. 1959).

Treatment for Migraine

Early administration of ergot alkaloids is the traditional treatment of acute migraine. These compounds should be avoided during pregnancy owing to their oxytocic effect. However, oral ergotamine tartrate lacks an oxytocic action (Fig. 9.2). Parenteral ergotamine tartrate does have a delayed effect upon the uterus (Davis et al. 1936). Although ergonovine maleate has been used to treat migraine, ergotamine tartrate is preferred. Ergonovine is a water-soluble ergot alkaloid which has a prompt, brisk oxytocic effect after oral or parenteral administration.

Nomenclature adds to the confusion. Ergonovine maleate has two other generic names outside the United States—ergometrine and ergobasine. In the United States ergonovine is marketed under the trade name Ergotrate, which can easily be confused with ergotamine tartrate.

All the foregoing information to the contrary, it takes a brave physician to give oral ergotamine tartrate to a pregnant woman. The headache is self-limited. Treatment of acute migraine of pregnancy consists of analgesics, sedatives, and the avoidance of known precipitating factors (Table 9.1).

Ergot alkaloids are not recommended for use by lactating mothers (Stirrat, 1976). Ergotamine excreted in breast milk may cause vomiting, diarrhea, and unstable blood pressure (Fomina, 1934).

Propranolol, 40 to 160 mg daily in four divided doses, has been used as a prophylactic agent for patients with frequent migraines (Weber and Reinmoth, 1972; Wideroe and Vigander, 1974). Propranolol should be used with caution for this purpose during pregnancy. Propranolol can

Table 9.2. Dietary therapy of migraine during pregnancy

Avoid alcohol, especially red wines and champagne
Avoid strong or aged cheeses
Avoid chicken livers, pickled herring, canned figs, and pods of broad beans
Use monosodium glutamate sparingly
Avoid cured meats (hot dogs, bacon, salami) if they cause headache
Eat three regular meals per day. Avoid fasts

Adapted from Dalessio, D. J. (1975) Neurologic complications. In *Medical Complications During Pregnancy,* Chap. 16, pp. 642–688. ed. Burrow, G. N., and Ferris, T. F. Philadelphia: W. B. Saunders Company.

cross the human placenta (Barnes, 1970). In animal experiments propranolol has been found to impair fetal response to anoxia. Infants born of mothers taking large amounts of propranolol (180 to 240 mg daily) were depressed at birth and had postnatal hypoglycemia and bradycardia (Gladstone et al. 1975).

REFERENCES

Menstrual Headache

Dalton, K. (1973) Progesterone suppositories and pessaries in the treatment of menstrual migraine. *Headache,* **12,** 151–159.

Grant, E. C. G. (1975) The influence of hormones on headache and mood in women. *Hemicrania,* **6,** 2–10.

Kashiwagi, T., McClure, J. N., and Wetzel, R. D. (1972) The menstrual cycle and headache type. *Headache,* **12,** 103, 104.

Selby, G., and Lance, J. W. (1960) Observations on 500 cases of migraine and allied vascular headache. *Journal of Neurology, Neurosurgery, and Psychiatry,* **23,** 23–32.

Sommerville, B. W. (1972a) The role of estradiol withdrawal in the etiology of menstrual migraine. *Neurology,* **22,** 355–365.

Sommerville, B. W. (1972b) The influence of progesterone and estradiol upon migraine. *Headache,* **12,** 93–102.

Sommerville, B. W. (1975) Estrogen-withdrawal migraine: I. Duration of exposure required and attempted prophylaxis by premenstrual estrogen administration. *Neurology,* **25,** 239–244.

Waters, W. E., and O'Connor, P. J. (1971) Epidemiology of headache and migraine in women. *Journal of Neurology, Neurosurgery, and Psychiatry,* **34,** 148–153.

Headache on the Pill

Bickerstaff, E. R. (1975) *Neurological Complications of Oral Contraceptives.* Oxford: Clarendon Press.

British Medical Journal (1968) Headache on the Pill. *British Medical Journal,* **3,** 388, 389.

Desrosiers, J. J. J. (1973) Headaches related to contraceptive therapy and their control. *Headache,* **13,** 117–124.

Diddle, A. W., Gardner, W. H., and Williamson, P. J. (1969) Oral contraceptive medications and headache. *American Journal of Obstetrics and Gynecology,* **104,** 507–511.

Grant, E. C. G. (1968) Relation between headaches from oral contraceptives and development of endometrial arterioles. *British Medical Journal,* **3,** 402–405.

Larsson-Cohn, U., and Lundberg, P. C. (1970) Headache and treatment with oral contraceptives. *Acta Neurologica Scandinavica,* **46,** 267–278.

Mears, E., and Grant, E. C. G. (1962) "Anovlar" as an oral contraceptive. *British Medical Journal,* **2,** 75–79.

Phillips, B. M. (1968) Oral contraceptive drugs and migraine. *British Medical Journal,* **2,** 99.

Whitty, C. W. M., Hockaday, J. M., and Whitty, M. M. (1966) The effect of oral contraceptives on migraine. *Lancet,* **1,** 856–859.

Headache During Pregnancy

Callaghan, N. (1968) The migraine syndrome in pregnancy. *Neurology,* **18,** 197–201.

Dalessio, D. J. (1975) Neurologic complications. In *Medical Complications During Pregnancy,* Chap. 16, pp. 642–688. ed. Burrow, G. N., and Ferris, T. F. Philadelphia: W. B. Saunders Company.

Dooling, E. C., and Sweeney, V. P. (1974) Migrainous hemiplegia during breast-feeding. *American Journal of Obstetrics and Gynecology,* **118,** 568–570.

Rotton, W. N., Sachtleben, M. R., and Friedman, E. A. (1959) Migraine and eclampsia. *Obstetrics and Gynecology,* **14,** 322–329.

Somerville, B. W. (1972c) A study of migraine in pregnancy. *Neurology,* **22,** 824–828.

Treatment

Barnes, A. B. (1970) Chronic propranolol administration during pregnancy. *Journal of Reproductive Medicine,* **5,** 179–180.

Davis, M. E., Adair, F. L., and Pearl, S. (1936) The present status of oxytocics in obstetrics. *Journal of the American Medical Association,* **107,** 261–267.

Davis, M. E., Adair, F. L., Rogers, G., et al. (1935) A new active principle in ergot and its effects on uterine motility. *American Journal of Obstetrics and Gynecology,* **29,** 155–167.

Fomina, P. I. (1934) Untersuchungen über den Übergang des aktiven Agens des Mutterkorns in die Milchstillender Mütter. *Archiv fur Gynaekologie,* **157,** 275.

Friedman, A. P. (1971) Metabolic abnormalities in migraine. *Annals of Internal Medicine,* **75,** 801, 802.

Gladstone, G. R., Hordof, A., and Gersony, W. M. (1975) Propranolol administration during pregnancy: Effects on the fetus. *Journal of Pediatrics,* **86,** 962–964.

Hanington, E. (1967) Preliminary report on tyramine headache. *British Medical Journal,* **2,** 550, 551.

Moir, J. C. (1974) Ergot: From "St. Anthony's fire" to the isolation of its active principle, ergometrine (ergonovine). *American Journal of Obstetrics and Gynecology,* **120,** 291–296.

Ryan, R. E. (1974) A clinical study of tyramine as an etiological factor in migraine. *Headache,* **14,** 43–48.

Sandler, M., Youdim, M. B. H., and Hanington, E. (1974) A phenylethylamine oxidising defect in migraine. *Nature,* **250,** 335–337.

Stirrat, G. M. (1976) Prescribing problems in the second half of pregnancy and during lactation. *Obstetric and Gynecologic Survey,* **31,** 1–7.

Weber, R. B., and Reinmuth, O. M. (1972) The treatment of migraine with propranolol. *Neurology,* **22,** 366–369.

Wideroe, T., and Vigander, T. (1974) Propranolol in the treatment of migraine. *British Medical Journal,* **2,** 699–701.

Perinatal Benzodiazepine Metabolism

Belafsky, H. A., Breslow, S., Hirsch, L. M., et al. (1969) Meprobamate during pregnancy. *Obstetrics and Gynecology,* **34,** 378–386.

Cavanagh, D., and Condo, C. S. (1964) Diazepam: A pilot study of drug concentrations in maternal blood, amniotic fluid and cord blood. *Current Therapeutic Research,* **6,** 122–126.

Cole, A. P., and Hailey, D. M. (1975) Diazepam and active metabolite in breast milk and their transfer to the neonate. *Archives of Diseases of Childhood,* **50,** 741, 742.

deSilva, J. A. F., D'Arconte, L., and Kaplan, J. (1964) The determination of blood levels and the placental transfer of diazepam in humans. *Current Therapeutic Research,* **6,** 115–121.

Hartz, S. C., Heinonen, O. P. Shapiro, S., et al. (1975) Antenatal exposure to meprobamate and chlordiazepoxide in relation to malformations, mental development, and childhood mortality. *New England Journal of Medicine,* **292,** 726–728.

Idänpään-Heikkilä, J. E., Jouppila, P. I., Puolakka, J. O., et al. (1971) Placental transfer and fetal metabolism of diazepam in early human pregnancy. *American Journal of Obstetrics and Gynecology,* **109,** 1011–1016.

Kanto, J., Erkkola, R., and Sellman, R. (1974) Perinatal metabolism of diazepam. *British Medical Journal,* **1,** 641–642.

Mandelli, M., Morselli, P. L., Nordio, S., et al. (1975) Placental transfer of diazepam and its disposition in the newborn. *Clinical Pharmacology and Therapeutics,* **17,** 564–572.

McCarty, G. T., O'Connell, B., and Robinson, A. E. (1973) Blood levels of diazepam in infants of two mothers given large doses of diazepam during labour. *Journal of Obstetrics and Gynaecology of the British Commonwealth,* **80,** 349–352.

Milkovich, L., and van den Berg, B. J. (1974) Effects of prenatal meprobamate and chlordiazepoxide hydrochloride on human embryonic and fetal development. *New England Journal of Medicine,* **291,** 1268–1271.

Morselli, P. L., Principi, N., Tognoni, G., et al. (1973) Diazepam elimination in premature and full term infants and children. *Journal of Perinatal Medicine,* **1,** 133–141.

Safra, M. J., and Oakley, G. P. (1975) Association between cleft lip with or without cleft palate and prenatal exposure to diazepam. *Lancet,* **2,** 278–480.

Saxen, I. (1975) Associations between oral clefts and drugs taken during pregnancy. *International Journal of Epidemiology,* **4,** 37–44.

Stirrat, G. M. (1976) Prescribing problems in the second half of pregnancy and during lactation. *Obstetric and Gynecologic Survey,* **31,** 1–7.

CHAPTER TEN

Epilepsy

Epilepsy is the most common serious neurologic problem encountered by an obstetrician. It involves 0.3 to 0.5 per cent of all pregnancies (Janz, 1975). Parents with epilepsy wonder what effect it may have upon their progeny, and obstetricians wonder what advice to give and how to manage the disorder.

The natural history of epilepsy shows fluctuations—with the seasons, with the age of the patient, with emotional stress, and with compliance to a drug schedule. Fluctuations are especially common at times of hormonal change—puberty, menses, pregnancy, and menopause. Puberty is a common time for a seizure disorder to develop, to be exacerbated, or, as in the case of centrencephalic epilepsy, to improve. This is true of both sexes.

SEXUAL REFLEX EPILEPSY

Specific factors can provoke fits in susceptible patients. Sleep, hyperventilation (alkalemia), and flashing lights are three stimuli which have been incorporated into standard EEG tests. Reflex epilepsy is the term given to convulsions which typically follow a specific signal—for example, reading, hearing music, or smelling a particular odor. Sexual intercourse can be the sensory stimulus necessary to trigger convulsions (Hoenig and Hamilton, 1960). Synchronous spike-wave activity in the amygdala and septal regions of the limbic system has been recorded from depth electrodes during coitus and sexual climax in humans (Health, 1972).

SEXUAL TEMPORAL LOBE SEIZURES

The stimulus for reflex epilepsy is not to be confused with the aura of temporal lobe epilepsy, which is experienced only by the patient. During temporal lobe epilepsy patients can perform complex stereotyped acts and may appropriately interact with others and their surroundings. Some patients know they have had another seizure when they find themselves in a strange room or cooking breakfast at 2 A.M. A few rare cases of temporal lobe sexual seizures have been reported (Erickson, 1945; Blumer and Walker, 1967). In the following case there was a right temporal lobe focus (Freemon and Nevis, 1969).

The patient was a 36-year-old, right-handed housewife who complained of a 3- to 4-year history of unusual spells characterized by an aura of itching in the perineum and a feeling "like a red hot poker" was being inserted into her vagina and a hot sun was descending onto her face. The patient would spread her legs apart, beat with both hands on her chest, verbalize her sexual needs, often in vulgarities, and place her hand over her perineum. Although the patient had no memory for any of these motor movements she sometimes could converse with her husband during the automatisms with enough meaning to indicate that she understood him. An example is her question, "Are you ready for me?" His "no" was immediately followed by, "Well, you had better get ready."

The patient usually came to her senses immediately without postictal drowsiness, but about one time in five the spell would proceed to urinary incontinence, tonic extension of neck and legs, and tonic flexion of both arms. Falling to the ground, the patient would become cyanotic and develop tonic-clonic jerking movements symmetrically in all four extremities.

Though most of these episodes occurred in the home, others occurred in social situations that caused the patient a good deal of embarrassment. The frequency of these seizures was three to four in a period of 2 to 3 days each month.

NARCOLEPSY

Narcolepsy is in no way related to epilepsy. I mention it in this context only because gynecologists need to be aware that sudden unconsciousness during coitus is not always caused by a seizure or a subarachnoid hemorrhage. A quite embarrassed woman may tell only her gynecologist of the sudden onset of sleep during coitus, a typical trait of narcolepsy (Zarcone, 1973).

CATAMENIAL EPILEPSY

Sir William Gowers (1881) and no doubt others before him observed that for some women the frequency of seizures is related to the menstrual cycle. Alfred Gordon (1909) collected the first series—23 women who were seizure free between menses but who regularly had convulsions precisely a day before or during the first days of menstrual bleeding.

Although this association was commonly observed and tacitly accepted, it was not proved until John Laidlaw (1956) analyzed the meticulous records of St. Faith's Hospital for epileptics in Brentwood, Essex. The staff had faithfully recorded 41,870 major fits and 12,913 menstrual cycles in 50 chronically institutionalized epileptics over a 25 year period! Twenty-eight per cent of these women did not have a clear exacerbation of seizures at the time of menses. Seizures were exacerbated in the remainder whether their menses were regular or irregular. The data for the entire series are summarized in Figure 10.1. There is a definite reduction in frequency of seizure during the luteal phase and a definite increase during and just before menstruation. A small increase is noted at the expected time of ovulation.

Menstrual Cycle EEG Changes

Serial electroencephalograms of normal women throughout their menstrual cycles have been analyzed with ever increasing sophistication, but the basic observation remains unchanged. The mean frequency of the alpha rhythm increases slightly, about 0.3 Hz, during the luteal phase (deBarenne and Gibbs, 1942; Lamb et al., 1953; Creutzfeld et al., 1976) (Fig. 10.2). The EEG of women subject to catamenial epilepsy showed more abnormalities during menses (Logothetis et al., 1959).

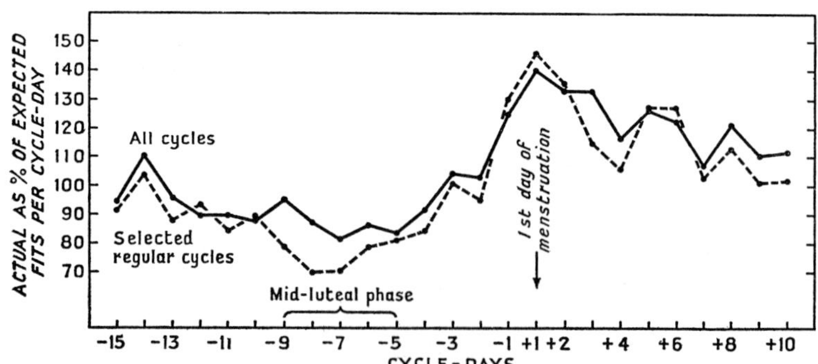

Figure 10.1. The catamenial exacerbation of epilepsy. The distribution of 41,870 major fits according to day of the menstrual cycle in 50 chronically institutionalized women over 25 years. The distribution is identical for women with either regular or irregular cycles. From Laidlaw, J. (1956) Catamenial epilepsy. *Lancet,* **2,** 1236.

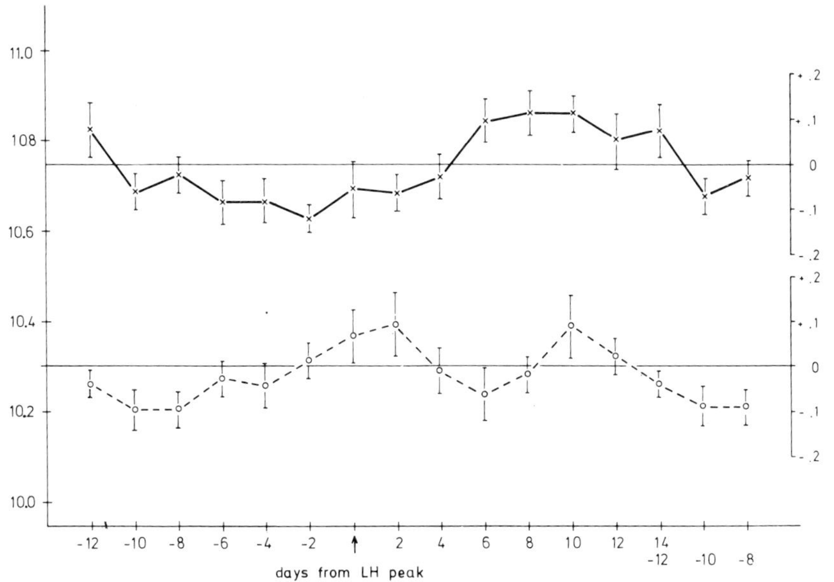

Figure 10.2. Fluctuation of the weighted mean alpha frequency (Hz) during monthly cycles. (x – x) indicates normal menstrual cycles, (o - - - o) indicates the ovulation-controlled cycles of women taking the Pill. Arrow denotes the peak of LH secretion for normal cycles or the midcycle day for women taking the Pill. From Creutzfeldt, O. D., Arnold, P. M., Backer, D., et al. (1976) EEG changes during spontaneous and controlled menstrual cycles and their correlation with psychological performance. *Electroencephalography and Clinical Neurophysiology,* **40**, 123.

Treatment

Catamenial epilepsy often responds to the administration of acetazolamide 250 mg or 500 mg daily from 5 to 7 days before the expected onset of menses until the cessation of bleeding (Ansell and Clarke, 1956a, b; Poser, 1974).

EFFECT OF THE PILL

The Pill can be used by most epileptics. Those women, usually severe epileptics, whose condition is aggravated throughout the cycle should obviously discontinue the Pill (Bickerstaff, 1975). If seizures occur only during withdrawal bleeding, they may be alleviated by taking acetazolamide during the 1 week hiatus in Pill cycles.

The mean frequency of the alpha rhythm of women taking the Pill does not fluctuate during a cycle. It is 0.5 Hz lower than the average alpha frequency of ovulating women (Creutzfeld et al. 1976) (Fig. 10.2).

EFFECT OF PREGNANCY

The effect of pregnancy upon epilepsy is unpredictable for the individual patient and difficult to study in any group. Only a few large representative series exist (Suter and Klingman, 1957; Knight and Rhind, 1975). Often only poorly controlled cases are referred to neurologists. Neither the thoroughness of diagnosis nor the philosophy of management is uniform. Pregnant patients may take their medicine more conscientiously. Or, concerned by potential teratogenic risk, they may omit anticonvulsants without telling their obstetricians. Morning nausea may dictate a change in the routine drug schedule. Then too, seizure frequency naturally fluctuates.

A review of five series accumulated since hydantoin anticonvulsants became available shows that epilepsy during pregnancy became worse in 50 per cent of patients, remained unchanged in 42 per cent, and improved in 8 per cent. Deterioration of epilepsy usually started in the first half of pregnancy (Sabin and Oxorn, 1956). Maternal age and age at onset of epilepsy were not relevant factors (Knight and Rhinds, 1975). About half of the patients could expect the same response in subsequent pregnancies; the other half were inconsistent in response (Knight and Rhind, 1975).

Risk Factors

The chances of an increased frequency of seizures during pregnancy are correlated with the frequency before pregnancy (Fig. 10.3). Almost all epileptics who have more than one fit per month can expect their condition to become worse during pregnancy. Only 25 per cent of those with more than 9 months between seizures can expect an increase in seizure frequency (Knight and Rhind, 1975). Women who regularly experience catamenial seizures probably do have more fits while pregnant, but this has not been statistically proved (Burnett, 1946; Knight and Rhind, 1975).

Alteration in phenytoin pharmacokinetics results in lower blood levels and an increased frequency of seizures (Mygind et al., 1976). Excessive weight gain and fluid accumulation have been associated with poor seizure control (Suter and Klingman, 1957).

EFFECT OF EPILEPSY UPON PREGNANCY

The course of pregnancy is unaffected by idiopathic epilepsy for most women (Baptisti, 1938; McClure, 1955). However, the national statistics of Norway clearly show that epileptic women and their offspring are

Table 10.1. Effect of pregnancy upon seizure frequency in epilepsy

Study	Pregnancies	Seizure frequency (%) *Increased*	*No change*	*Decreased*
Burnett (1946)	19	42	52	6
McClure (1955)	20	55	25	20
Sabin (1956)	55	33	52	15
Sutor (1957)	120	61	33	6
Knight (1975)	84	45	50	5
Total pregnancies	298			
Weighted averages		50	42	8

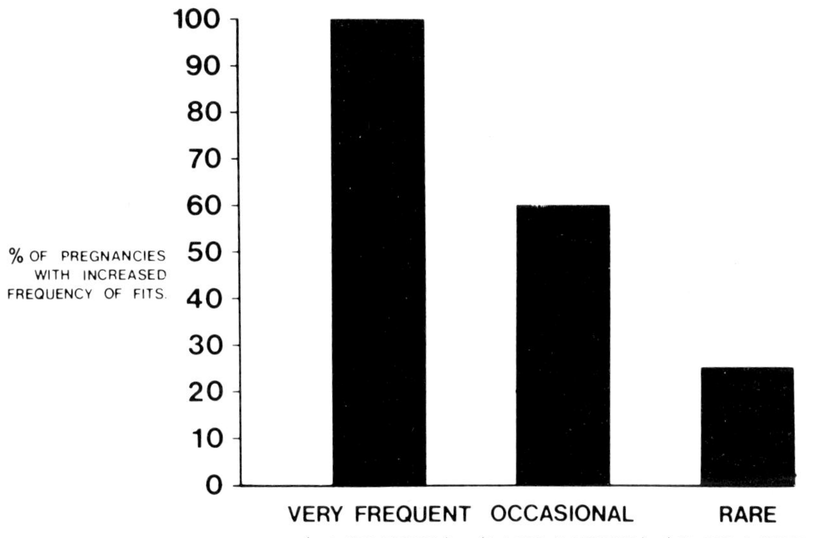

Figure 10.3. Relationship between pregestational seizure frequency and the effect of pregnancy upon seizure frequency in 60 pregnancies. From Knight, A. H., and Rhind, E. G. (1975) Epilepsy and pregnancy: A study of 153 pregnancies in 59 patients. *Epilepsia*, **16,** 104.

at higher risk (Table 10.2). Spontaneous abortion was not considered in the Norwegian study.

Status epilepticus is a serious threat to mother and fetus but is not an indication for abortion. Healthy infants have been delivered even though the mother had experienced status epilepticus (Knight and Rhind, 1975).

Lactation and Epilepsy

The ability to lactate is unimpaired. The use of bromides and chronic use of diazepam should be avoided by lactating mothers because their milk could contain enough of these drugs to cause neonatal depression (Stirrat, 1976).

Seizure activity will rarely increase only for the duration of lactation (Turner, 1907).

ISOLATED GESTATIONAL SEIZURES

The seizure of any woman who convulses for the first time while pregnant should be considered symptomatic. If the "seizure" is not hysterical, a work-up should be started to rule out infections, metabolic/hy-

Table 10.2. Frequency of maternal complications and the fate of pregnancy in Norway

	Epilepsy	No epilepsy	Significance
Total pregnancies	371	125,423	
Hyperemesis gravidarum	1.3%	0.8%	
Vaginal hemorrhage	5.1%	2.2%	$p < 0.001$
Toxemia	7.5%	4.7%	$p < 0.01$
Birth by			
Cesarean section	3.2%	1.1%	$p < 0.001$
Forceps/vacuum extractor	6.3%	2.4%	$p < 0.001$
Gestation < 37 weeks	8.9%	5.0%	$p < 0.01$
Birth weight < 2500 g	7.4%	3.7%	$p < 0.001$
Hypoxia at birth	1.9%	0.7%	
Any congenital malformation	4.5%	2.2%	
Cleft palate or lip	1.1%	0.6%	
Infant mortality rates (per 1000 births)			
Stillbirth	5.3	7.8	
Perinatal death	31.8	14.6	$p < 0.005$
Neonatal death	29.3	8.0	$p < 0.001$
Postneonatal death	5.3	3.4	

From Bjerkedal, T., and Bahna, S. L. (1973). The course and outcome of pregnancy in women with epilepsy. *Acta Obstetrica et Gynecologica Scandinavica*, **52**, 245, 247.

poxic/toxic factors, neoplasms, arteriovenous malformations, arterial emboli, cerebral venous thrombosis, and eclampsia. The differential diagnosis and investigative scheme are discussed later in Chapter 11.

If no cause is found for an isolated convulsion, anticonvulsants are withheld by many neurologists. The second fit is always treated. Idiopathic epilepsy can begin at any age; by chance alone it may begin during a pregnancy.

COUNSELLING

Genetic Factors

The genetic factors of epilepsy are difficult to assess since we are unable to classify etiologically all recurrent seizure disorders. Indeed, we confess our ignorance by labelling about 70 per cent idiopathic. The inheritance of those inborn errors of metabolism that cause seizures has been well delineated. Few of these patients reach adulthood.

Petit mal is a clinical description of a momentary absence without major motor movements but often with eye-blinking. This type of seizure can occur as a primary event from the deep central gray matter or as a secondary phenomenon from a cortical focus, usually in a temporal lobe. The distinction can be made by the EEG. Wilder Penfield proposed the term centrencephalic epilepsy to denote the primary disorder which is characterized electroencephalographically by paroxysmal, bilaterally synchronous, 3-per-second spike-and-wave patterns. Typically, this condition begins in childhood and fades away during adolescence. Ethosuximide is the effective drug of choice. Metrakos and Metrakos (1961) found that centrencephalic epilepsy, strictly defined, was inherited, probably as an autosomal dominant trait with age-dependent penetrance. Other investigators agree that it is inherited by disagree about the manner (Doose et al., 1973). Since this disorder is rare in adults, only young prospective mothers will require counselling for it.

Grand Mal Epilepsy

The existence of hereditary factors in epilepsy is apparent from studies of twins (Lennox, 1951). Monozygotic twins without evidence of perinatal brain damage have a high—84 per cent—concordance for epilepsy. Dizygotic twins have a much lower but still significant concordance—10 per cent.

Many retrospective studies have found that families of epileptics have a higher frequency of seizures than relatives of a control group. The younger the age of the proband at the onset of epilepsy, the stronger the family history of convulsions. This is also true of electroencephalographic abnormalities in relatives whether or not they have ever had a seizure (Lennox, 1940). Patients whose seizures started between the ages of 6 and 15 usually have one parent and at least one sibling with an EEG abnormality (Rodin and Gonzalez, 1966). Seizure disorders which begin at an older age are more likely to have a post-traumatic cause.

Retrospective studies show that hereditary factors exist in epilepsy. They do not answer the question that most epileptic fathers and mothers ask or want to ask: "What are the chances that my child will have epilepsy?" If the cause of the parent's epilepsy is known, the answer is reasonably easy, as post-traumatic or postencephalitic epilepsy carries no increase in risk to offspring. But most epilepsy is idiopathic. A large, prospective, long-term, well-controlled study at the Mayo Clinic provides the best answer to the question of probability (Annegers et al., 1976) (Fig. 10.4). Approximately 0.7 per cent of children of parents without a history of seizures have at some time a seizure of some type—febrile, symptomatic, or idiopathic. About 0.5 per cent of children of such parents develop idiopathic epilepsy. Seizures occur four times more frequently among children of epileptic mothers. This is true of all types of maternal seizure disorders and regardless of seizure control during pregnancy.

The Mayo Clinic study did not find a higher incidence of the disorder in the offspring if the father was an epileptic. Other studies (Echeveria,

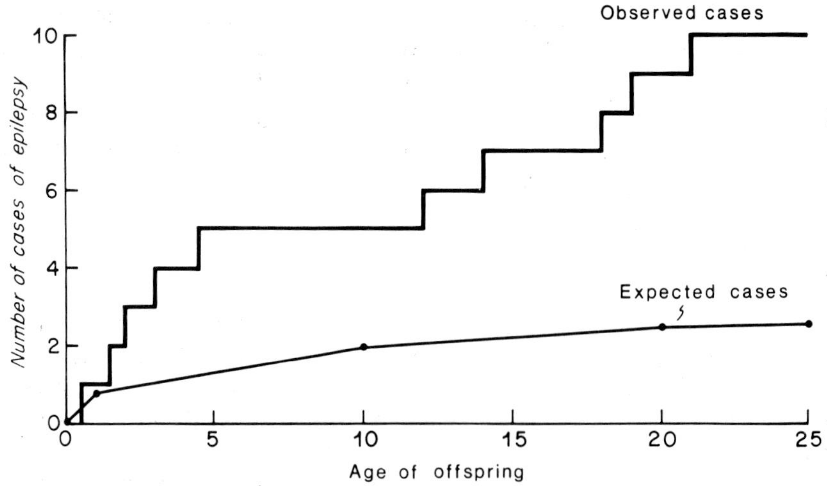

Figure 10.4. Incidence of epilepsy in offspring of mothers with epilepsy. From Annegers, J. F., Hauser, W. A., Elochack, L. R., et al. (1976) Seizure disorders in offspring of parents with a history of seizures—A maternal-paternal difference? *Epilepsia,* **17**, 6.

1880; Thom and Walker, 1922) agreed that children of epileptic mothers are more likely to develop epilepsy than are children of affected fathers, but the risk was higher in both categories than in children of unaffected parents.

Teratogenic Effect of Anticonvulsants

The possible teratogenic effect of anticonvulsants was not a concern until the thalidomide catastrophe, even though phenobarbital and phenytoin had been in use since 1912 and 1938, respectively. After Meadows (1968) noted several cases of cleft lip among the children of epileptic mothers, almost every journal has published similar studies of the various aspects of this subject.

Congenital malformations are more frequent among infants of epileptic mothers whether the mothers have been treated or not, but the highest frequency occurs in the treated group. The difference may be due to the severity of maternal disease or to an anticonvulsant effect. For children of treated epileptic mothers, the overall irsk of congenital malformations doubles. It is not known whether children of mothers who convulse during pregnancy are at greater risk of malformation than those whose mothers are free of seizures. Fetal hypoxia in the first trimester could cause malformations.

The most common malformations are orofacial clefts and congenital heart lesions (Table 10.3). Among populations of European ancestry, the incidence of orofacial clefts is 0.2 to 0.6 per cent of births (Janz, 1975; Bjerkedal and Bahna, 1973). Among Orientals this incidence is much higher. Thus, the incidence of orofacial clefts among children of treated epileptic mothers is from two to four times the expected rate.

Congenital heart disease is two to four times more common than ex-

Table 10.3. Frequency of congenital malformations in 1,726 children of epileptic mothers treated during pregnancy

Malformation	Incidence
Orofacial clefts	1.8%
Congenital heart disease	1.5%
Skeletal abnormalities	1.0%
Anencephaly	0.3%
Microcephaly	0.3%
Hydrocephaly	0.1%
Neural tube defects	0.3%
Hypospadias	0.5%
Intestinal atresia	0.3%

From Janz, D. (1975). The teratogenic risk of antiepileptic drugs. *Epilepsia*, **16**, 162.

pected (Janz, 1975). All types of lesions have been reported, but septal defects are the most common. The coincidence of cleft lip and cardiac septal defects does not exceed the 3 to 5 per cent that is to be expected.

Incomplete development of distal phalanges and rudimentary nails have been attributed to anticonvulsants (Loughnan et al., 1973; Aase, 1974; Hanson and Smith, 1975).

Dysmorphic children have followed maternal ingestion of all types of anticonvulsants in all sorts of combinations. There has been no attempt to correlate maternal plasma anticonvulsant concentrations with subsequent congenital malformations in humans. Other factors—maternal age, maternal diabetes, a family history of congenital abnormality—are rarely considered.

Phenytoin (diphenylhydantoin) has been the drug most impugned. It caused orofacial clefts and other malformations in rodents (Mercer-Parot and Tuchman-Duplessis, 1974). However, phenytoin did not induce congenital defects in a limited study in rhesus monkeys (Wilson, 1973). Nor do hydantoin anticonvulsants need to be part of the mother's drug regimen for her child to develop cleft lip or congenital heart disease (Janz, 1974) (Table 10.4).

Data from the Finnish Register of Congenital Malformations suggest that maternal epilepsy, regardless of drug regimen, is the decisive risk factor (Table 10.5). One study that used a relatively small sample did find that there were twice as many malformed infants among those children whose epileptic mothers used phenytoin daily during the first 4 lunar months of gestation as among children of epileptic mothers whose anticonvulsant intake, if any, did not include phenytoin (Monson et al., 1973). However, the same investigators, when collaborating with Finnish health officials, could not confirm this (Shapiro et al., 1976). The malformation rate was almost identical no matter what anticonvulsant was used. It is clear that phenobarbital cannot be considered a teratogen. The malformation rate among nonepileptic women taking phenobarbital during gestation did not increase (Shapiro et al., 1976).

Table 10.4. Drug regimen in pregnancy followed by birth of children with selected malformations

Regimen	Orofacial clefts	Heart lesion
Barbiturates	29, alone in 5	21, alone in 6
Hydantoins	22, alone in 4	14, alone in 1
Diones	7, alone in 2	6, alone in 2
Carbamazepine	–	1, alone in 1
Ethosuximide	2, alone –	
Benzodiazepines	1, alone –	1, alone –

From Janz, D. (1975). The teratogenic risk of antiepileptic drugs. *Epilepsia,* **16,** 165.

Table 10.5. Congenital malformation rate among children of epileptic women according to anticonvulsant regimen

	Number of mother/child pairs	Total malformation rate (per cent)
No convulsive disorder	49,977	6.4
Phenobarbital daily in first trimester	95	5.3
Phenobarbital at other times	7,741	6.6
Convulsive disorder	305	10.5
Phenobarbital daily in first trimester	75	9.3
Phenobarbital after first trimester	124	11.3
No phenobarbital	106	10.4
Phenytoin daily in first trimester	102	11.8
Phenytoin after first trimester	78	9.0
No phenytoin	97	11.3

Data from Shapiro, S., Slone, D., Hartz, S. C., et al. (1976) Anticonvulsants and parental epilepsy in the development of birth defects. *Lancet*, **1**, 272–275.

It should be stressed that although congenital malformations are relatively more common among the offspring of epileptic mothers, the absolute frequency is low. An epileptic woman should not be discouraged from bearing children for this reason. However, if she is over 35 years of age and has diabetes and a strong family history of cleft lip, she need not be encouraged.

MANAGEMENT OF EPILEPSY DURING PREGNANCY

Epilepsy should be treated with the fewest number of drugs in the smallest possible amounts to control convulsions. Therapeutic blood levels should be attained with one major anticonvulsant before a second is added. A non-neurologist should use the well-established, well-studied drugs for which blood tests are obtainable. These drugs are also the least expensive.

The two most reliable questions for determining the efficacy of seizure control are: (1) What has been the longest time between seizures? and (2) How many fits have you had in one day?

During pregnancy additional factors must be considered. Weight gain should be restricted and fluid retention prevented, since these factors may increase the frequency of seizures during pregnancy (Suter and Klingman, 1957). Also, anticonvulsants have hematologic complications of importance during pregnancy.

Chronic administration of phenobarbital, phenytoin, and primidone can cause a macrocytic anemia due to an abnormality of folic acid metabolism (Malpas et al., 1966). Such anemia has been observed during the third trimester of pregnancy when it could be dangerous (Gatenby, 1960). Folic acid deficiency has been correlated with third trimester hemorrhage (Streiff and Little, 1967).

A coagulation defect similar to that caused by a vitamin K deficiency was found in half of the babies of unselected epileptic mothers taking anticonvulsants (Mountain et al., 1970). Neonatal hemorrhage is less frequent but can be fatal (Bleyer and Skinner, 1976). Infants at risk should be given 1 mg of phytonadione intramuscularly soon after birth. If hemorrhage occurs, fresh plasma transfusions will be needed, since there is a lag of several hours before vitamin K is effective.

Anticonvulsants

Bromide

The use of sodium bromide was a significant advance in the treatment of epilepsy when it was introduced by Sir Charles Locock in 1857. It is included here as a matter of historic interest. Bromide replaces chloride throughout the body. A therapeutic blood level is 15 mEq/1 (about 90 mg/dl). Bromide crosses the placenta. It is excreted in human milk (Kwit, 1935). Neonatal bromism from maternal antepartum ingestion of bromides is rare but is still encountered (Mangurten and Ban, 1974; Pleasure and Blackburn, 1975). Symptoms include hypotonia, hyporeflexia, lethargy, and irritability. Rashes and lethargy have been attributed to bromide from breast milk (van der Bogart, 1921).

Phenobarbital

Phenobarbital was introduced as an anticonvulsant by Alfred Hauptman in 1912. It can be administered orally, intramuscularly, or intravenously. Phenobarbital can be derived from the metabolic transformation of primidone and mephobarbital. The customary adult dose is 1 to 2 mg/kg/day; usually a total of 90 to 120 mg is given daily. Therapeutic phenobarbital blood levels range from 15 to 40 μg/ml (1.5 to 4.0 mg/dl), although drowsiness may be encountered in the upper part of that range.

Phenobarbital and other barbiturates readily cross the placenta. Maternal and fetal serum concentrations may reach equilibrium within 30 minutes (Plowman and Persson, 1957). Cord serum phenobarbital levels are linearly dependent upon maternal levels (Melchoir et al., 1967) (Fig. 10.5). The cord blood to maternal blood phenobarbital concentration ratio is 0.95.

Unlike shorter acting barbiturates, phenobarbital is primarily ex-

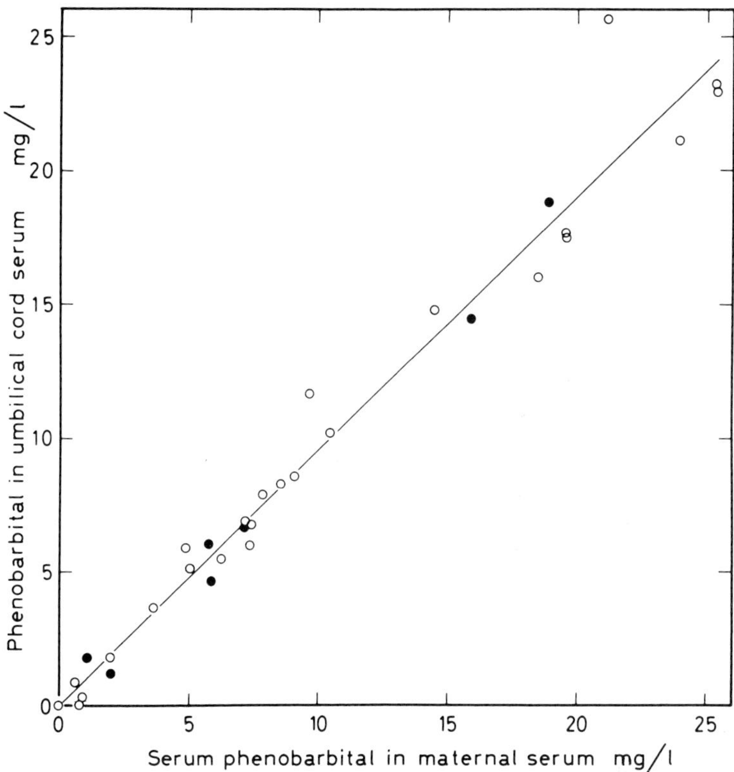

Figure 10.5. Phenobarbital concentrations in umbilical cord and maternal serum at delivery. ○ indicates patients who received phenobarbital; ● indicates patients who received primidone. From Melchior, J. C., Svensinark, O., and Trolle, D. (1967) Placental transfer of phenobarbitone in epileptic women, and elimination in newborns. *Lancet,* **2,** 860. Courtesy of J. C. Melchior.

creted by the kidney. An alkaline urine increases the rate of excretion. The half-life in adults is 4 to 5 days (i.e., the blood level of the drug drops 10 to 20 per cent daily). Phenobarbital clearance apparently increases during gestation (Mygind et al., 1976; Lander et al., 1977) (Fig. 10.6). Toxicity can develop during the first postpartum month unless the woman is closely watched. The rate of phenobarbital elimination by neonates varies from 1 per cent daily to the adult range (10 to 20 per cent) (Melchoir et al., 1967). This rate could not be correlated with neonatal maturity. Urinary pH was not considered.

Phenobarbital is excreted in breast milk (Tyson et al, 1938). The phenobarbital concentration of human milk is 10 to 30 per cent of that of maternal serum (Westerink and Glerum, 1965) Neonatal lethargy has not been attributed to the small amount so ingested.

Infants born of barbiturate addicts and epileptic mothers who took

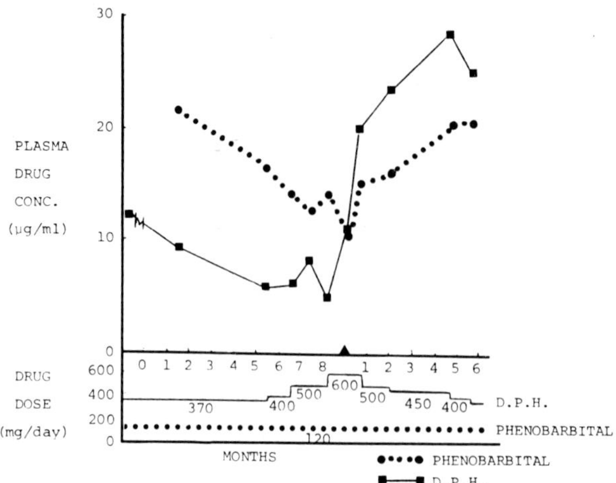

Figure 10.6. Plasma concentrations of phenytoin (diphenylhydantoin) and phenobarbital during pregnancy and the puerperium. Childbirth is indicated by the solid triangle. Drug doses are shown. From Lander, C. M., Edwards, V. E., Eadie, M. J., et al. (1977) Plasma anticonvulsant concentrations during pregnancy. *Neurology,* **27**, 129. © 1977 by Harcourt Brace Jovanovich, Inc.

barbiturates throughout pregnancy may exhibit withdrawal symptoms (Desmond et al., 1972). Hyperexcitability, tremor, high-pitched cry, and feeding problems (although the child always seems hungry) usually begin 1 week after birth. Normally, the child has left the hospital. Apgar scores at birth are typically normal. Hyperexcitability can last 2 to 4 months.

Phenytoin

Phenytoin (diphenylhydantoin) was introduced as an anticonvulsant by Merritt and Putnam in 1938. Usually phenytoin is readily absorbed from the gastrointestinal tract. Intramuscular injections are painful and irregularly absorbed. Since phenytoin is soluble only in alkaline solutions, and dextrose solutions are acidic, intravenous doses must be given in plain saline solutions. The maximum safe adult intravenous infusion rate is 50 mg/minute. The usual daily dose for adults is 4 to 5 mg/kg, or a total of 300 to 400 mg daily. The intravenous or oral loading dose is 1 gram. Effective plasma levels range between 10 and 20 μg/ml (i.e., 1 to 2 mg/dl).

It is suspected that phenytoin pharmacokinetics is altered by pregnancy, since pregnant women taking 300 to 400 mg/day have been found to have plasma concentrations that average only 3.6 μg/ml (Mirkin 1971b). Using the ratio between daily dosage and plasma level as a measure, the clearance of phenytoin from plasma more than doubles during gestation (Mygind et al. 1976; Lander et al., 1977) (Fig. 10.6). Some pregnant women have required as much as 1200 mg of phenytoin daily to achieve a therapeutic blood level (Strauss and Bernstein, 1974). Pre-pregnant clearance rates return to normal within the first postpartum month (Lander et al., 1977). Close observation is needed to prevent toxicity.

The apparent clearance calculation assumes normal gut absorption and protein binding (Fig. 10.7). In one case gut absorption of phenytoin was low during pregnancy (Ramsay et al., 1976). The percentage of protein-bound phenytoin (about 90 per cent) does not change during pregnancy (Hooper et al., 1974). Increased metabolism of phenytoin during gestation may be expected but has not been definitively studied in humans. In rats just the opposite occurred (Gutová et al., 1976).

Phenytoin quickly and freely penetrates the placental barrier in both rodents and humans (Mirkin, 1971a,b). Maternal venous plasma and umbilical cord plasma phenytoin concentrations are almost identical if the mother consistently receives phenytoin throughout pregnancy. The distribution of phenytoin in both human and rat fetuses after a single maternal intravenous dose parallels the maternal distribution pattern.

The half-life of transplacentally transferred phenytoin averages about 1 day (Rane et al., 1974). Similarly, after a single dose, the plasma halftime of phenytoin in healthy adults is 22 ± 9 hours (Arnold, 1970). The range in infants is quite broad—from 6 hours (Rane et al., 1974) to 60 hours (Mirkin, 1971b). Mirkin (1971b) observed a slow excretion phase in the first 2 days of life which was succeeded by a fast phase.

The pharmacokinetics of phenytoin excretion in human milk has not been thoroughly investigated. Phenytoin concentrations in human milk

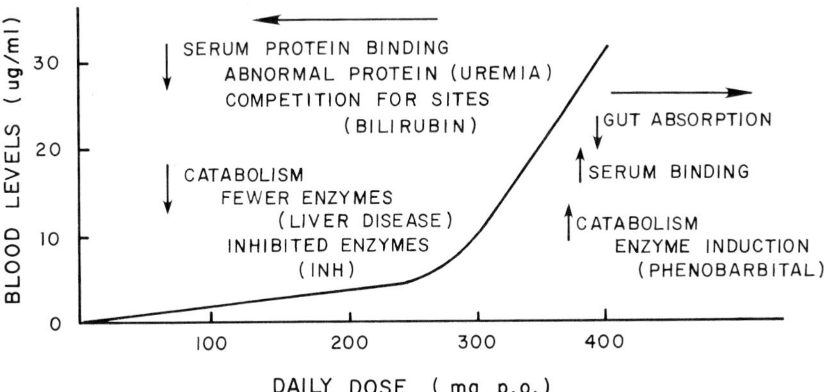

Figure 10.7. Factors which can alter the phenytoin (diphenylhydantoin) serum concentration response to an oral dose of phenytoin.

ranged from 1.5 to 2.6 μg/ml, with maternal plasma levels ranging from 5.5 to 8.4 μg/ml (Mirkin, 1971b). The small amount so ingested (1 or 2 mg/day) does not interfere with the rapid clearance of phenytoin from babies of mothers chronically treated with phenytoin (Rane, 1974). No adverse effect has been attributed to phenytoin in human milk (Mirkin, 1971a).

Diazepam

Diazepam is an ineffective oral anticonvulsant. It is extremely effective for short periods of time if given intravenously to control status epilepticus or eclampsia (p. 223). Regular ingestion of diazepam during gestation or while lactating is not recommended. Diazepam is readily transferred to the fetus, where it accumulates without any significant fetal or neonatal metabolism (p. 183).

Other Anticonvulsants

Other anticonvulsant drugs have been poorly studied with regard to alteration of pharmacokinetics during pregnancy, placental transfer, changes in fetal and neonatal metabolism, and excretion in breast milk. Congenital malformations have been ascribed to certain drugs despite lack of documentation that they actually cross the placenta. It is hoped that the availability of data on therapeutic blood levels of these anticonvulsant drugs will alter this situation.

Primidone. Primidone readily crosses the human placenta and can be found in the infant's urine at least 2 days after birth (Martinez and Snyder, 1973). Primidone is transformed to phenobarbital.

Ethosuximide. Ethosuximide is the drug of choice for centrencephalic epilepsy. Transplacental transfer of this agent has been demonstrated in rats (Chang et al., 1972). Ethosuximide concentrations in maternal and fetal rat tissue were approximately equal.

Carbamazepine. Carbamazepine is often effective against focal temporal lobe epilepsy. In one case, its metabolism was relatively unchanged during gestation (Lander et al., 1977).

REFERENCES

Sexual Epilepsy

Blumer, D., and Walker, A. E. (1967) Sexual behavior in temporal lobe epilepsy. *Archives of Neurology*, **16**, 37–43.

Erickson, T. C. (1945) Erotomania (nymphomania) as an expression of cortical epileptiform discharge. *Archives of Neurology and Psychiatry*, **53**, 226–231.

Freemon, F. R., and Nevis, A. H. (1969) Temporal lobe sexual seizures. *Neurology*, **19**, 87–90.

Heath, R. G. (1972) Pleasure and brain activity in man. *Journal of Nervous and Mental Disease,* **154,** 3–18.
Hoenig, J., and Hamilton, C. M. (1960) Epilepsy and sexual orgasm. *Acta Psychiatrica et Neurologica Scandinavica,* **35,** 448–456.
Zarcone, V. (1973) Narcolepsy. *New England Journal of Medicine,* **288,** 1156–1166.

Catamenial Epilepsy

Ansell, B., and Clarke, E. (1956a) Acetazolamide in treatment of epilepsy. *British Medical Journal,* **1,** 650–654.
Ansell, B., and Clarke, E. (1956b) Epilepsy and menstruation: The role of water retention. *Lancet,* **2,** 1232–1235.
Creutzfedlt, O. D., Arnold, P. M., Backer, D., et al. (1976) EEG changes during spontaneous and controlled menstrual cycles and their correlation with psychological performance. *Electroencephalography and Clinical Neurophysiology,* **40,** 113–131.
de Barenne, D., and Gibbs, F. A. (1942) Variations in the electroencephalogram during the menstrual cycle. *American Journal of Obstetrics and Gynecology,* **44,** 687–690.
Dickerson, W. W. (1941) The effect of menstruation on seizure incidence. *Journal of Nervous and Mental Diseases,* **94,** 160–169.
Gordon, A. (1909–1910) Epilepsy in its relation to menstrual periods. A study of twenty-three cases. *Pennsylvania Medical Journal,* **13,** 347–354.
Gowers, W. R. (1881) *Epilepsy and Other Convulsive Diseases, Their Causes, Symptoms, and Treatment.* London:
Laidlaw, J. (1956) Catamenial epilepsy. *Lancet,* **2,** 1235–1237.
Lamb, W. M., Ulett, G. A., Masters, W. H., et al. (1953) Premenstrual tension: EEG, hormonal, and psychiatric evaluation. *American Journal of Psychiatry,* **109,** 840–848.
Logothetis, J., Harner, R., and Morrell, F. (1959) The role of estrogens in catamenial epilepsy. *Neurology,* 352–360.
Poser, C. M. (1974) Modification of therapy for exacerbation of seizures during menstruation. *Journal of Pediatrics,* **84,** 779.

Pregnancy

Baptisti, A. (1938) Epilepsy and pregnancy: A review of the literature and a study of thirty-seven cases. *American Journal of Obstetrics and Gynecology,* **35,** 818–824.
Bjerkedal, T., and Bahna, S. L. (1973) The course and outcome of pregnancy in women with epilepsy. *Acta Obstetrica et Gynecologica Scandinavica,* **52,** 245–248.
Burnett, C. W. F. (1946) A survey of the relation between epilepsy and pregnancy. *Journal of Obstetrics and Gynaecology of the British Empire,* **53,** 539–556.
Dimsdale, H. (1959) The epileptic in relation to pregnancy. *British Medical Journal,* **2,** 1147–1150.
Knight, A. H., and Rhind, E. G. (1975) Epilepsy and pregnancy: A study of 153 pregnancies in 59 patients. *Epilepsia,* **16,** 99–110.
Lennox, W. G., and Lennox, M. A. (1960) *Epilepsy and Related Disorders.* Boston: Little, Brown and Co.
McClure, J. H. (1955) Idiopathic epilepsy in pregnancy. *American Journal of Obstetrics and Gynecology,* **70,** 296–301.
Sabin, M., and Ozorn, H. (1956) Epilepsy and pregnancy. *Obstetrics and Gynecology,* **7,** 175–179.
Stirrat, G. M. (1976) Prescribing problems in the second half of pregnancy and during lactation. *Obstetric and Gynecologic Survey,* **31,** 1–7.
Suter, C., and Klingman, W. O. (1957) Seizure states and pregnancy. *Neurology,* **7,** 105–118.
Turner, W. A. (1907) *Epilepsy, A Study of the Idiopathic Disease.* London: Macmillan.

Genetics

Annegers, J. F., Hauser, W. A., Elveback, L. R., et al. (1976) Seizure disorders in offspring of parents with a history of seizures—A maternal-paternal difference? *Epilepsia,* **17,** 1–9.

Brain, W. R. (1926) The inheritance of epilepsy. *Quarterly Journal of Medicine,* **19,** 299–309.

Bray, P. F., and Wiser, W. C. (1965) Hereditary characteristics of familial temporal-central focal epilepsy. *Pediatrics,* **36,** 207–211.

Doose, H., Gerken, H., Horstmann, T., et al. (1973) Genetic factors in Spike-wave absences. *Epilepsia,* **14,** 57–75.

Esheverria, M. G. (1880) Marriage and hereditariness of epileptics. *Journal of Mental Science,* **26**, 346–369.

Lennox, W. G., Gibbs, E. L., and Gibbs, F. A. (1940) Inheritance of cerebral dysrhythmia and epilepsy. *Archives of Neurology and Psychiatry,* **44,** 1155–1183.

Lennox, W. G. (1951) The heredity of epilepsy as told by relatives and twins. *Journal of the American Medical Association,* **146,** 529–536.

Metrakos, J. D., and Metrakos, K. (1960) Genetics of convulsive disorders: I. Introduction, problems, methods and base lines. *Neurology,* **10,** 228–240.

Metrakos, K., and Metrakos, J. D. (1960) Genetics of convulsive disorders: II. Genetic and electroencephalographic studies in centrencephalic epilepsy. *Neurology,* **11,** 474–483.

Rodin, E., and Gonzalez, S. (1966) Hereditary components in epileptic patients. *Journal of the American Medical Association,* **198,** 221–225.

Thom, D. A., and Walker, G. S. (1922) Epilepsy in the offspring of epileptics. *American Journal of Psychiatry,* **78,** 613–627.

Anticonvulsants

Teratogenic Effects

Aase, J. M. (1974) Anticonvulsant drugs and congenital abnormalities. *American Journal of Diseases of Children,* **127,** 758.

Fedrick, J. (1973) Epilepsy and pregnancy: A report from the Oxford Record Linkage Study. *British Medical Journal,* **2**, 442–447.

German, J., Ehlers, K. H., Kowal, A., et al. (1970) Possible teratogenicity of trimethadione and paramethadione. *Lancet,* **2,** 261, 262.

Hanson, J. W., and Smith, D. W. (1975) The fetal hydantoin syndrome. *Journal of Pediatrics,* **87**, 285–290.

Hill, R. M., Verniaud, W. M., Horning, M. G., et al. (1974) Infants exposed in utero to antiepileptic drugs. *American Journal of Diseases of Children,* **127,** 645–653.

Janz, D. (1975) The teratogenic risk of antiepileptic drugs. *Epilepsia,* **16**, 159–169.

Loughnan, P. M., Gold, H., and Vance, J. C. (1973) Phenytoin teratogenicity in man. *Lancet,* **1,** 70–72.

Meadow, S. R. (1968) Anticonvulsant drugs and congenital abnormalities. *Lancet,* **2,** 1296.

Mercier-Parot, E., and Tuchmann-Duplessis, H. (1974) The dysmorphic potential of phenytoin: Experimental observations. *Drugs,* **8,** 340–353.

Meyer, J. G. (1973) The teratological effects of anticonvulsants and the effects on pregnancy and birth. *European Neurology,* **10,** 179–190.

Monson, R. R., Rosenberg, L., Hartz, S. C., et al. (1973) Diphenylhydantoin and selected congenital malformations. *New England Journal of Medicine,* **289,** 1049–1052.

Shapiro, S., Slone, D., Hartz, S. C., et al. (1976) Anticonvulsants and parental epilepsy in the development of birth defects. *Lancet,* **1,** 272–275.

Spiedel, B. D., and Meadow, S. R. (1972) Maternal epilepsy and abnormalities of the fetus and newborn. *Lancet,* **2,** 839–843.

Spiedel, B. D., and Meadow, S. R.: (1974) Epilepsy, anticonvulsants and congenital malformations. *Drugs,* **8,** 354–365.

Wilson, J. G. (1973) Present status of drugs as teratogens in man. *Teratology,* **7,** 3–16.

Zackai, E. H., Mellman, W. J., Neiderer, B., et al. (1975) The fetal trimethadione syndrome. *Journal of Pediatrics,* **87,** 280–284.

Hematologic Side Effects

Bleyer, W. A., and Skinner, A. L. (1976) Fatal neonatal hemorrhage after maternal anticonvulsant therapy. *Journal of the American Medical Association,* **235**, 626, 627.

Finch, E., and Lorber, J. (1954) Methaemoglobinaemia in the newborn, probably due to phenytoin excreted in human milk. *Journal of Obstetrics and Gynaecology of the British Empire,* **61,** 833, 834.

Gatenby, P. B. B. (1960) Anticonvulsants as a factor in megaloblastic anaemia in pregnancy. *Lancet,* **2,** 1004, 1005.

Malpas, J. S., Spray, G. H., and Witts, L. J. (1966) Serum folic-acid and vitamin-B_{12} levels in anticonvulsant therapy. *British Medical Journal,* **1,** 955–957.

Mountain, K. R., Hirsh, J., and Gallus, A. S. (1970) Neonatal coagulation defect due to anticonvulsant drug treatment in pregnancy. *Lancet,* **1,** 265–268.

Strauss, R. G., and Bernstein, R. (1974) Folic acid and Dilantin antagonism in pregnancy. *Obstetrics and Gynecology,* **44,** 345–347.

Streiff, R. R., and Little, B. (1967) Folic acid deficiency in pregnancy. *New England Journal of Medicine,* **276,** 776–779.

BROMIDE

Kwit, N. T., and Hatcher, R. A. (1935) Excretion of drugs in milk. *American Journal of Diseases of Children,* **49,** 900–904.

Mangurten, H. H., and Ban, R. (1974) Neonatal hypotonia secondary to transplacental bromism. *Journal of Pediatrics,* **85,** 426–428.

Pleasure, J. R., and Blackburn, M. G. (1975) Neonatal bromide intoxication: Prenatal ingestion of a large quantity of bromides with transplacental accumulation in the fetus. *Pediatrics,* **55,** 503–506.

van der Bogert, F. (1921) Bromin poisoning through mother's milk. *American Journal of Diseases of Children,* **21,** 167–169.

PHENOBARBITAL

Desmond, M. M., Schwanecke, R. P., Wilson, G. S., et al. (1972) Maternal barbiturate utilization and neonatal withdrawal symptomatology. *Journal of Pediatrics,* **80,** 190–197.

Finster, M., Mark, L. C., Morishima, H. O., et al. (1966) Plasma thiopental concentrations in the newborn following delivery under thiopental-nitrous oxide anesthesia. *American Journal of Obstetrics and Gynecology,* **95,** 621–629.

Flowers, C. E. (1957) Placental transmission of sodium barbital. *Obstetrics and Gynecology,* **9,** 332–335.

Flowers, C. E. (1959) The placental transmission of barbiturates and thiobarbiturates and their pharmacological action on the mother and the infant. *American Journal of Obstetrics and Gynecology,* **78,** 730–742.

Lander, C. M., Edwards, V. E., Eadie, M. J., et al. (1977) Plasma anticonvulsant concentrations during pregnancy. *Neurology,* **27,** 128–131.

Mayo, C. W. (1942) Appearance of a barbiturate in human milk. *Proceedings of the Mayo Clinic,* **17,** 87, 88.

Melchior, J. C., Svensmark, O., and Trolle, D. (1967) Placental transfer of phenobarbitone in epileptic women, and elimination in newborns. *Lancet,* **2,** 860, 861.

Mygind, K., Dam, M., and Christiansen, J. (1976) Phenytoin and phenobarbitone plasma clearance during pregnancy. *Acta Neurologica Scandinavica,* **54,** 160–166.

Plowman, L., and Persson, B. H. (1957) On the transfer of barbiturates to the human foetus and their accumulation in some of its vital organs. *Journal of Obstetrics and Gynaecology of the British Empire,* **64,** 706–711.

Tyson, R. M., Shrader, E. A., and Perlman, H. H. (1938) Drugs transmitted through breast milk: II. Barbiturates. *Journal of Pediatrics,* **13,** 86–90.

Westerink, D., and Glerum, J. H. (1965) Scheiding en microbepaling van Fenobarbital en Fenytoine in Moedermelk. *Pharmaceutisch Weekblad,* **100,** 577–583.

PHENYTOIN

Baughman, F. A., and Randinitis, E. J. (1970) Passage of diphenylhydantoin across the placenta. *Journal of the American Medical Association,* **213,** 466.

Gutová, M., Borga, O., and Rane, A. (1976) Kinetics of phenytoin in pregnant rats and non-pregnant rats. *Acta Pharmacologica et Toxicologica,* **38,** 254–259.

Hooper, W. D., Bochner, F., Eadie, M. J., et al. (1974) Plasma protein binding of diphenylhydantoin: Effects of sex hormones, renal and hepatic disease. *Clinical Pharmacology and Therapeutics,* **15,** 276–282.

Lander, C. M., Edwards, V. E., Eadie, M. J., et al. (1977) Plasma anticonvulsant concentrations during pregnancy. *Neurology,* **27,** 128–131.

Mirkin, B. L. (1971a) Placental transfer and neonatal elimination of diphenylhydantoin. *American Journal of Obstetrics and Gynecology,* **109**, 930–933.

Mirkin, B. L. (1971b) Diphenylhydantoin: Placental transport, fetal localization, neonatal metabolism, and possible teratogenic effects. *Journal of Pediatrics,* **78**, 329–337.

Mirkin, B. L. (1973) Drug distribution in pregnancy. In *Fetal Pharmacology,* Boreus, L. ed. New York: Raven Press.

Mygind, K. I., Dam, M., and Christiansen, J. (1976) Phenytoin and phenobarbitone plasma clearance during pregnancy. *Acta Neurologica Scandinavica,* **54,** 160–166.

Ramsey, R. E., Wilder, B. J., Strauss, R., et al. (1976) Status epilepticus during pregnancy: Effects of gastrointestinal malabsorption on phenytoin kinetics and seizure control. *Neurology,* **26**, 344.

Rane, A., Garle, M., Borga, O., et al. (1974) Plasma disappearance of transplacentally transferred diphenylhydantoin in the newborn studied by mass fragmentography. *Clinical Pharmacology and Therapeutics,* **15,** 39–45.

Spellacy, W. N., Cohn, J. E., Buhi, W. C., et al. (1975) Effects of Diuril and Dilantin on blood glucose and insulin levels in late pregnancy. *Obstetrics and Gynecology,* **45**, 159–162.

Strauss, R. G., and Bernstein, R. (1974) Folic acid and Dilantin antagonism in pregnancy. *Obstetrics and Gynecology,* **44**, 345–347.

Watson, J. D., and Spellacy, W. N. (1971) Neonatal effects of maternal treatment with the anticonvulsant drug diphenylhydantoin. *Obstetrics and Gynecology,* **37**, 881–885.

Westerink, D., and Glerum, J. H. (1965) Scheidung en microbepaling van Fenobarbital en Fenytoine in Moedermelk. *Pharmaceutisch Weekblad,* **100,** 577–583.

Other Anticonvulsants

Chang, T., Dill, W. A., Glazko, A. J. (1972) Ethosuximide: Absorption, distribution, and excretion. In *Antiepileptic Drugs,* ed. Woodbury, D. M., Penry, J. K., and Schmidt, R. P., pp. 417–423. New York: Raven Press.

Martinez, G., and Snyder, R. D. (1973) Transplacental passage of primidone. *Neurology,* **23,** 381–383.

CHAPTER ELEVEN

Eclampsia and Other Causes of Peripartum Convulsions

ECLAMPSIA

Clinical Presentation

Eclampsia is a hypertensive disease of women in the second half of pregnancy characterized by proteinuria, edema, hyperreflexia, convulsions, and coma. The term toxemia of pregnancy includes the entire spectrum of acute or subacute hypertension during gestation. If a previously normotensive woman develops hypertension above 140/90 mm Hg with significant proteinuria or persistent edema of the hands, face, and legs, the condition is classified as mild pre-eclampsia. If any of the criteria listed in Table 11.1 exist, the stage is called severe pre-eclampsia. These diagnostic criteria are too strict. Eclampsia may evolve in less than 6 hours. Women may have convulsions at blood pressures of 140/90 mm Hg. Whatever the label, treatment must be intensified, and the termination of pregnancy should be considered. Hyperreflexia and headache are important features of severe pre-eclampsia but are not included as specific diagnostic criteria. When convulsions or coma ensues, the condition is called eclampsia. The progression of events is significant (Fig. 11.1).

Toxemia usually is a disease of poorly nourished young primigravidas. It is more common in multiple or advanced extrauterine pregnancies. Eclampsia can occur before the twentieth week of gestation, but it is extremely rare (Lindheimer et al., 1974). True eclamptic convulsions may occur on the first postpartum day. "Late postpartum eclampsia" usually proves to be postpartum cerebral vein thrombosis

Table 11.1. One strict set of diagnostic criteria for severe pre-eclampsia

Blood pressure over 160/110 mm Hg on two occasions, 6 hours apart
Proteinuria over 5 g/24 hrs or 4+ on "dip stick"
Oliguria (daily urine flow of less than 400 ml)
Pulmonary edema or cyanosis
Visual symptoms
(Hyperreflexia, headache)

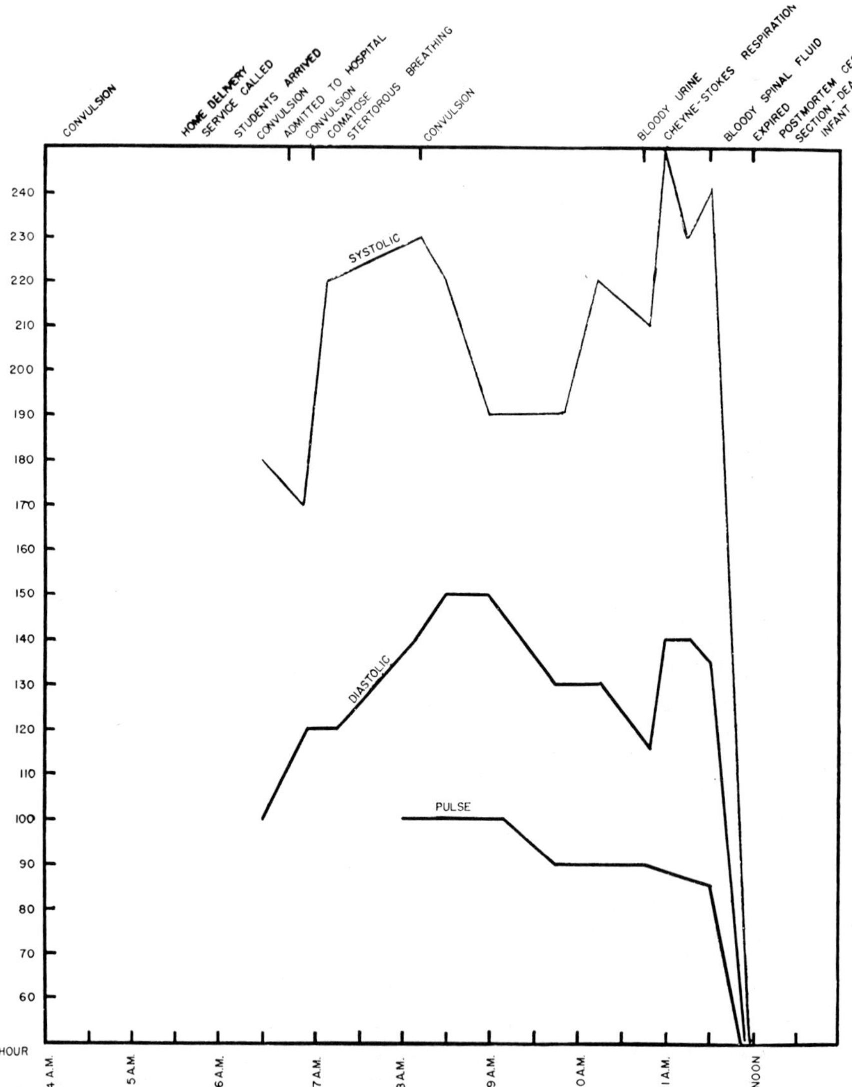

Figure 11.1. The progression of events in eclampsia. Death from a large intracerebral hematoma. From Parks, J., and Pearson, J. W. (1943) Cerebral complications occurring in the toxemias of pregnancy. *American Journal of Obstetrics and Gynecology,* **45,** 778.

(Sheehan and Lynch, 1973). A few rare cases of verified late postpartum eclampsia are associated with retained placental fragments (Chapman and Karimi, 1973). Recurrent eclampsia is unusual.

The cause of toxemia is unknown. So many hypotheses have been advanced that toxemia has been called a disease of theories. The literature is immense, but definitive studies are sparse. Neither the source of hypertension nor the manifestations of the disease in other organ systems will be discussed here. I shall limit myself to an attempt to make sense of the cerebral manifestations and to describe a rational mode of treatment.

The cerebral manifestations of eclampsia can be explained as sequelae of hypertension. Like any hypertensive patient, an eclamptic woman may have a large hemorrhage in the basal ganglia, pons, cerebellum, thalamus, or cerebral lobe (Fig. 11.2). These hemorrhages are often fatal, especially if the hematoma ruptures into the ventricles. If the patient remains conscious, vomiting is common. Coma without seizures can occur. Large intracerebral hematomas do not cause the progressive sequence of cerebral signs and symptoms that are usually associated with the term eclampsia.

Hyptertensive Encephalopathy

Hypertensive encephalopathy describes the common cerebral syndrome of eclampsia, upon which the symptoms of a large deep intracerebral hematoma may be superimposed. The term hypertensive encepha-

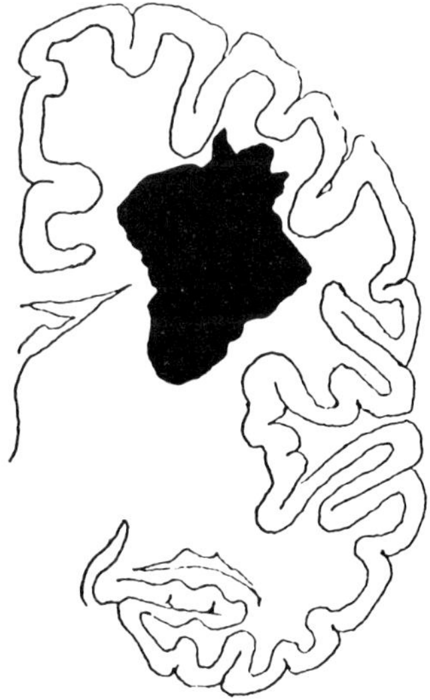

Figure 11.2. A large deep hematoma may cause coma and death without convulsions. From Sheehan, H. L., and Lynch, J. B. (1973) *Pathology of Toxaemia of Pregnancy*. Edinburgh: Churchill Livingstone. Courtesy of Prof. H. L. Sheehan.

lopathy should be restricted to a largely reversible acute or subacute cerebral disorder associated with accelerating severe hypertension, but it is often incorrectly applied to any cerebrovascular disease co-existent with hypertension (Ziegler et al., 1965). The symptoms are headache and confusion, progressing to cortical blindness, convulsions, and coma. The generalized or occipital headache is increased by cough or the Valsalva maneuver.

Pathology

In hypertensive encephalopathy the brain is swollen with multiple microinfarctions (Fig. 11.3) and punctate hemorrhages dotting the cortical gray matter and, to a lesser extent, white matter. All areas of the cortex are involved, but the occipital and parietal areas are more extensively affected than other areas. Some small hemorrhages can be found at the juxtaposition of the gray and white zones. These cortical and subcortical lesions cause the characteristic confusion and seizures and contribute to coma (Fig. 11.4).

Cerebral edema in eclampsia was consistently observed by nineteenth century German pathologists as well as by more modern authors. Sheehan and Lynch (1973) dispute these observations on the basis of average brain weights. I think that most neuropathologists would dis-

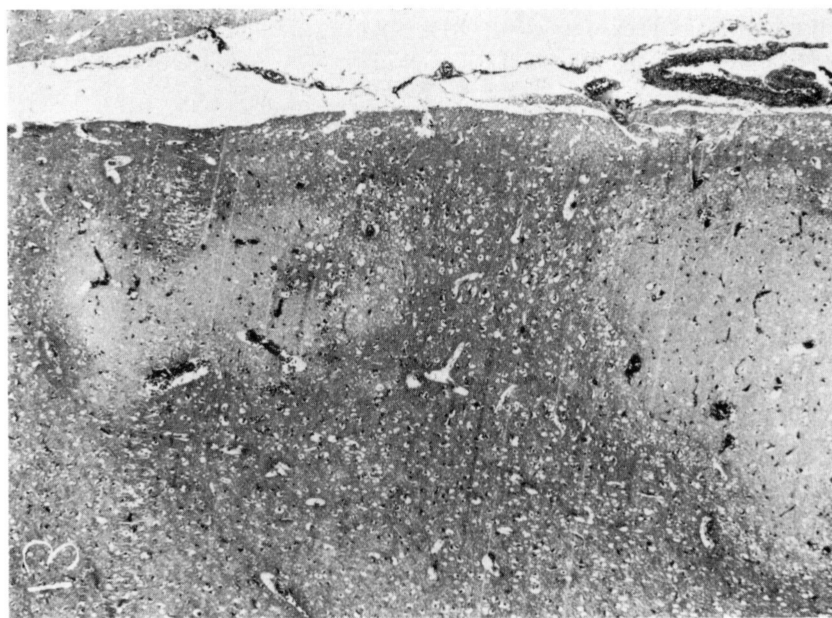

Figure 11.3. Multiple small areas of necrosis in the cerebral cortex of a woman who died from eclampsia 19 hours after her first convulsion. From Sheehan, H. L., and Lynch, J. B. (1973) *Pathology of Toxaemia of Pregnancy*. Edinburgh: Churchill Livingstone. Courtesy of Prof. H. L. Sheehan.

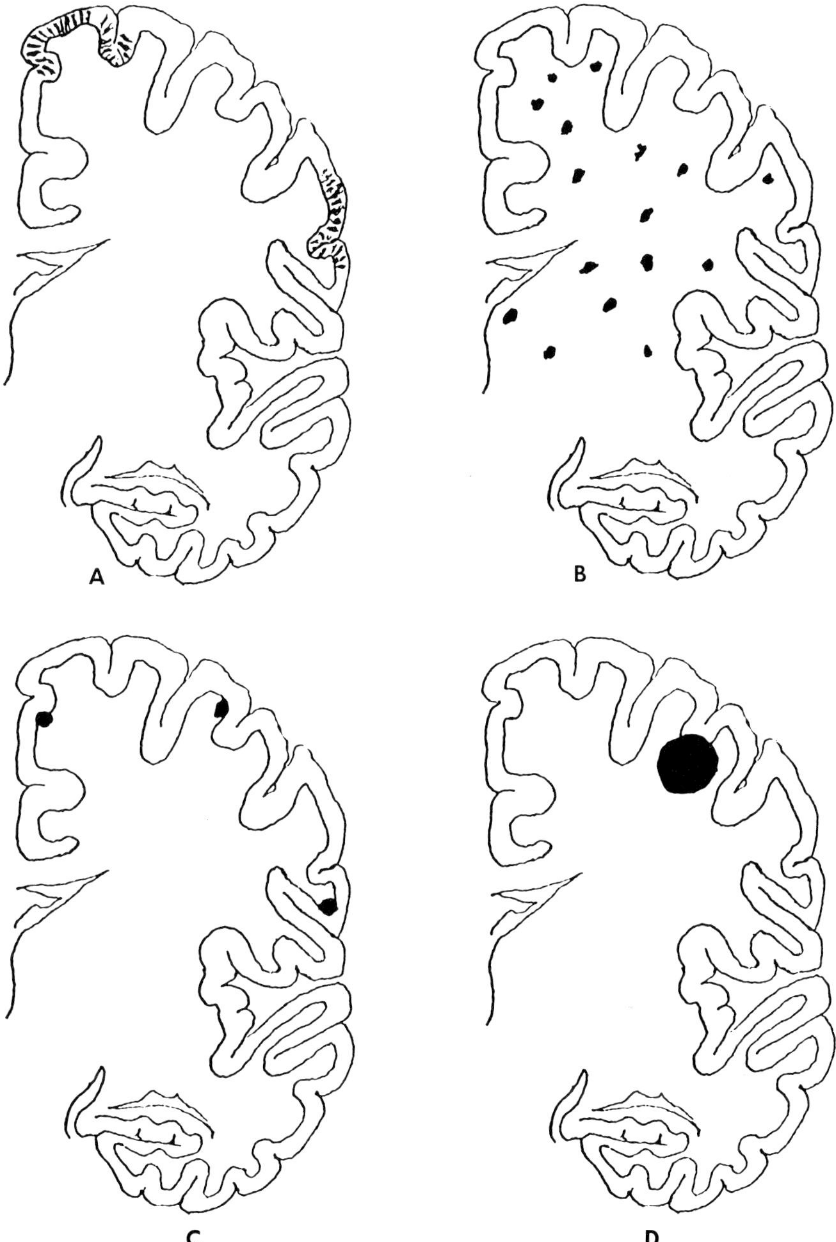

Figure 11.4. Diagrammatic illustrations of the four most common pathological changes in the hypertensive encephalopathy of eclampsia. A, Cortical petechiae. B, Multiple white matter softenings of petechiae. C, Subcortical hemorrhages. D, Medium-sized subcortical hematomas. From Sheehan, H. L., and Lynch, J. B. (1973) *Pathology of Toxaemia of Pregnancy*. Edinburgh: Churchill Livingstone. Courtesy of Prof. H. L. Sheehan.

agree with their theory and would prefer to rely upon the appearance of the brain with swollen gyri and the grooving of uncal, cerebellar, and falcian herniations. As Sheehan states, the method of proving cerebral edema consists of determining the water content of gray and white matter almost immediately after death. In their study, this was not done. Sheehan and Lynch base their conclusion upon the fact that 30 "normal" brains weighed an average of 1200 grams—the same weight as five eclamptic brains. However, the normal brains ranged in weight from 900 to 1400 grams, whereas the eclamptic brains weighed 1100 to 1340 grams. Within the enclosed space of the cranium, the sudden addition of small volumes can drastically increase intracranial pressure; such an increase is of great clinical importance. Cerebral edema was dramatically described by Zangemeister (1911), who attempted to treat three eclamptic women by trephining the skull. When the dura was opened, brain exuded. Eclamptogenic cerebral edema may continue to form and may cause death after hypertension has been corrected (Jewett, 1973).

Cerebral Perfusion Autoregulation

The pathogenesis of hypertensive encephalopathy deals with cerebral blood flow (CBF) autoregulation. In a normotensive individual, pregnant or not, cerebral perfusion is maintained at a constant level, about 55 ml/min/100 g tissue, and can vary with pCO_2 and other factors (Olesen, 1974; McHenry et al., 1974). Hypercapnia increases cerebral perfusion, and hypocapnia decreases cerebral perfusion. Thus, forced

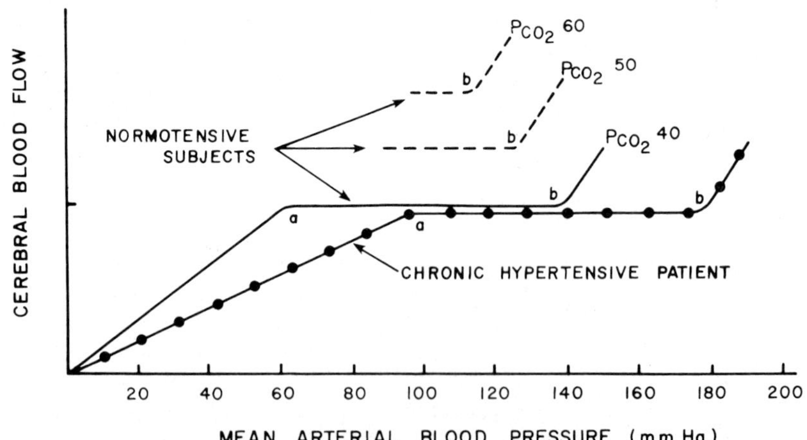

Figure 11.5. Ranges of cerebral blood flow autoregulation in normotensive and chronically hypertensive patients. Points marked *a* and *b* are the lower and upper limits of autoregulation, respectively. Hypercarbic limits are postulated but are supported by animal experiments.

hyperventilation can effectively decrease cerebral blood flow and cerebral edema.

Cerebral perfusion remains constant over a broad range of systemic blood pressures (Olesen, 1974). In normotensive individuals the range extends from about 60 to about 140 mm Hg mean arterial blood pressure (MABP) (Fig. 11.5). Mean arterial blood pressure can be approximated by adding one-third of the pulse pressure to the diastolic blood pressure. The zone of constant cerebral blood flow shifts to a higher range if the patient's customary MABP is elevated—i.e., in chronic hypertension (Strangaard, 1973, 1976).

Below the range of autoregulation, cerebral blood flow is directly proportional to systemic blood pressure. Thus, a mean arterial pressure of 70 mm Hg may be well within the zone of autoregulation of a normotensive patient but in the shock range of a chronic hypertensive patient.

Hypertensive encephalopathy results if the mean arterial blood pressure exceeds the upper limit of autoregulation. As the blood pressure rises, an arteriolar spasm limits cerebral perfusion. This effect was initially noted by Bayliss (1902). Subsequent workers (Forbes, 1928; Fog, 1938, 1939; Byrom, 1954; Meyer et al., 1960) have developed more elegant methods of defining the phenomenon. The constriction

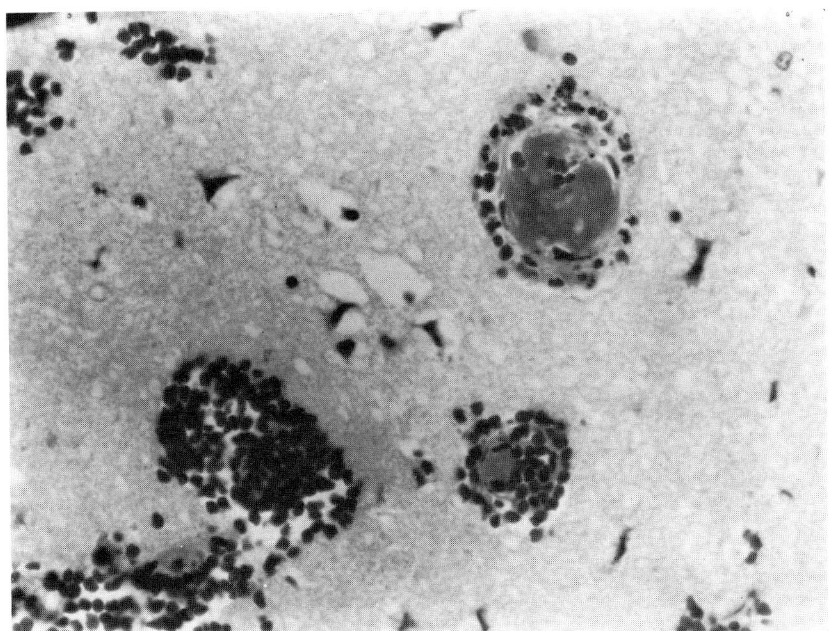

Figure 11.6. Cortical petechia in eclampsia at 24 hours after first convulsion. Note a thrombosis in a precapillary. From Sheehan, H. L., and Lynch, J. B. (1973) *Pathology of Toxaemia of Pregnancy*. Edinburgh: Churchill Livingstone. Courtesy of Prof. H. L. Sheehan.

may be severe enough to cause ischemia or infarction in a few areas, but overall cerebral blood flow is maintained at a constant rate. At some point the ability of the arterial spasm to limit cerebral perfusion is exceeded. The pathologic damage is perivascular (Fig. 11.6). Cerebral fibrinoid arteriolonecrosis has been demonstrated in acutely hypertensive monkeys (Rodda and Denny-Brown, 1966), in which trypan blue dye was used to stain some of these spastic arterioles. Proteins seep through the now porous blood-brain capillary barrier. Haeggendal and Johansson (1972) have postulated that the sudden increase in intracapillary pressure, occurring when the upper limit of autoregulation is exceeded, disrupts the tight junctions of the capillary endothelial cells and allows extravasation of protein and fluid (Fig. 11.7). They demonstrated the exudation of Evans blue dye in experiments on cats. Peroxidase, used as a tracer protein, can penetrate these formerly tight junctions in another model (Giacomelli et al., 1970).

The upper limit of cerebral blood flow autoregulation is directly proportional to the premorbid mean arterial blood pressure and inversely proportional to pCO_2. In healthy young normotensive patients, a sudden

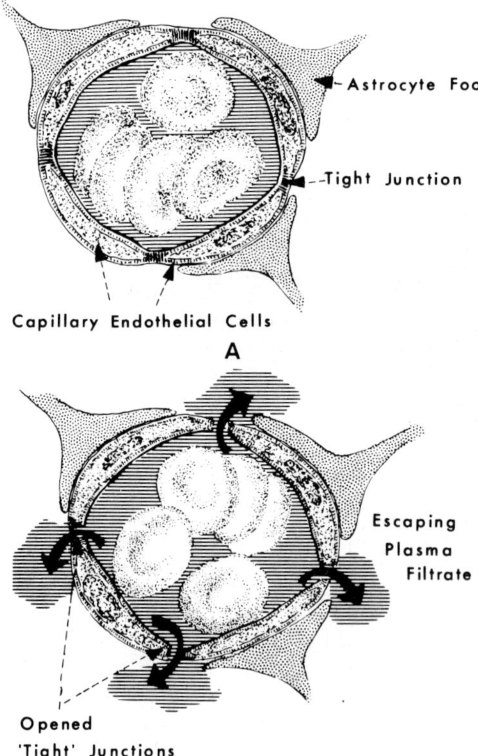

Figure 11.7. A, A normal capillary wall with tight junctions. B, The increased permeability of endothelial cells and "tight" junction of the capillary wall in vasogenic edema. From Fishman, R. A. (1975) Brain Edema. *New England Journal of Medicine,* **293,** 708.

sustained rise in blood pressure to 180/110 mm Hg *or less* can cause hypertensive encephalopathy. In chronic hypertensives, the upper limit varies between 150 and 200 mm Hg MABP. The higher a patient's customary mean arterial pressure, the higher the upper and lower limits of autoregulation (Strandgaard, 1973, 1976; Strandgaard et al., 1975, 1976). One series of experiments in dogs demonstrated the importance of pCO_2 upon the upper limit of cerebral blood flow autoregulation (Ekstrom-Jodal et al., 1972). During normocapnia, cerebral blood flow remained stable at least to 200 mm Hg. In hypercapnia the upper limit of autoregulation dropped to 125 to 150 mm Hg. This observation has therapeutic implications that are still unproved. Certainly drugs that depress respiration to the point of retaining carbon dioxide should be avoided. Whether or not hypocapnia induced by forced hyperventilation can readjust the brain's tolerance of elevated pressures once the arterioles have been damaged is unknown. Without doubt hypocapnia can decrease cerebral blood flow.

Visual Manifestations

Serial funduscopic observations are of clinical importance, since ocular manifestations parallel cerebral events. Thirty to fifty per cent of eclamptic women complain of visual symptoms, often with great alarm (Dieckman, 1952) (Table 11.2). In fact, Professor Skinner (1970) believes that the French pathologist Francis de la Croix de Sauvages introduced the term eclampsia, derived from the Greek verb εκλαμπειγ, *to shine forth,* because "flashes of light [are] seen before the eyes."

The initial change is arteriolar narrowing without arteriovenous crossing compression (Fig. 11.8). Angiospasm may be severe enough to cause central retinal arterial occlusion (Carpenter, 1953). Reversal of this acute focal or generalized arteriolar spasm has been commonly observed in eclampsia. Byrom (1963) found the same phenomenon in acutely hypertensive rats. Reversal will not occur if the hypertension is chronic. Similar but clinically impractical changes in the bulbar conjunctival vascular bed have been documented (Landesman et al., 1954).

Retinal edema, not papilledema, is the next change. Retinal edema, as indicated by an inability to focus clearly upon the retina, begins in the periphery and may not be seen until the posterior pole is involved. By that time retinal hemorrhages and exudates are common. Detachment of an edematous retina was detected in 2 per cent of one large series of pre-eclamptic and eclamptic women (Hallum, 1936). This change is often missed, since the lesion is peripheral (Fig. 11.9). Vision usually improves rapidly as the edema abates after delivery. Reattachment within 10 days is common (Hallum, 1936; Clapp, 1919).

Cortical blindness in hypertensive encephalopathy is caused by multiple microinfarctions and microhemorrhages with edema in the

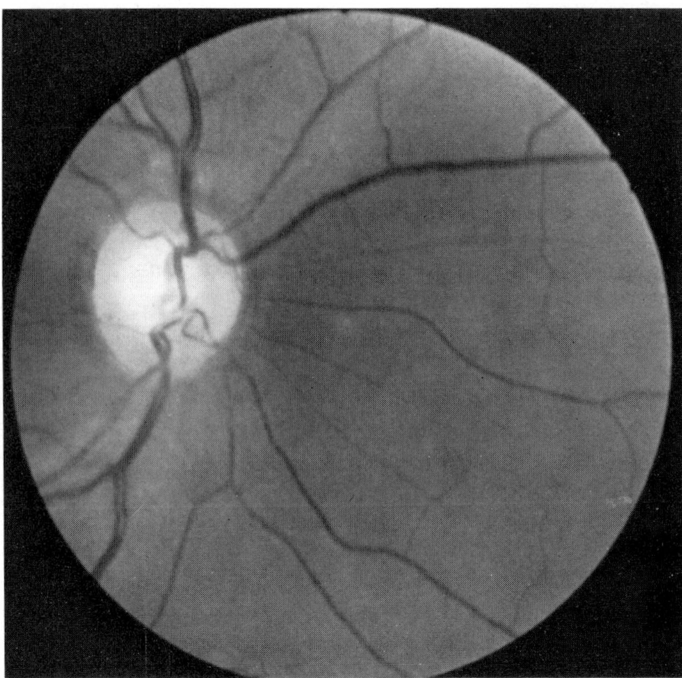

Figure 11.8. Retinal photograph in toxemia demonstrating arteriolar narrowing. From Burrow, G. N., and Ferris, T. F. (1975) *Medical Complications During Pregnancy*. Philadelphia: W. B. Saunders Company. Courtesy of F. Finnerty.

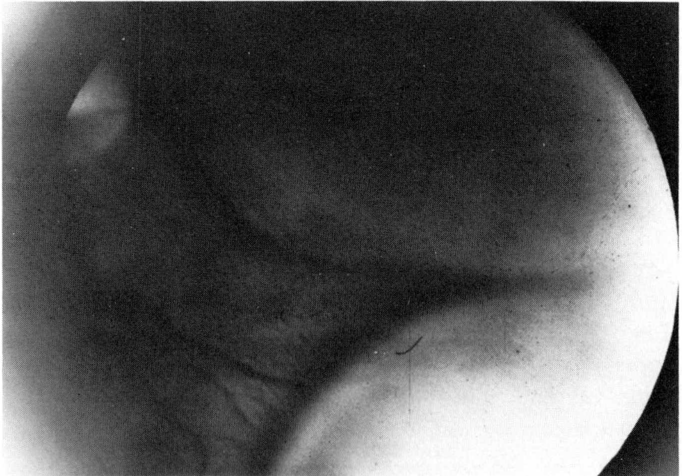

Figure 11.9. The buckled retina of an exudative retinal detachment caused by eclampsia. From Galin, M. A., Harris, L. S., Baras, I., et al. (1974) Ophthalmic surgery in pregnancy. In *Surgical Disease in Pregnancy*. ed. Barber, H. R. K., and Graber, E. A. Philadelphia: W. B. Saunders Company.

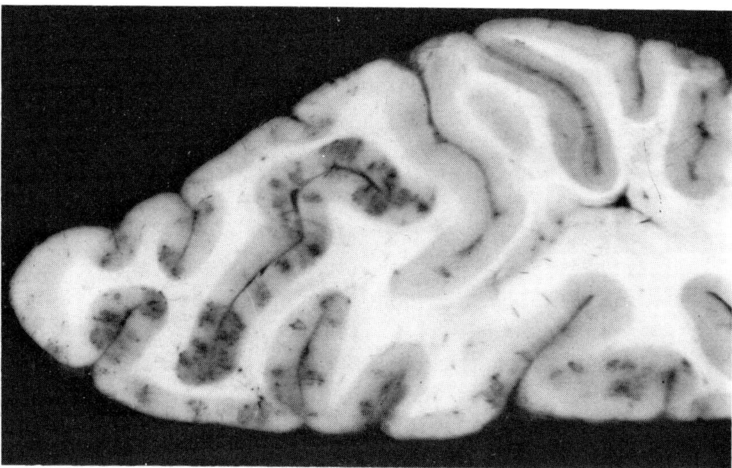

Figure 11.10. Cortical petechiae in the occipital pole of a woman who died of eclampsia 14 hours after her first seizure. These multiple lesions of the occipital (visual) cortex produce cortical blindness. From Sheehan, H. L., and Lynch, J. B. (1973) *Pathology of Toxaemia of Pregnancy*. Edinburgh: Churchill Livingstone. Courtesy of Prof. H. L. Sheehan.

occipital gray matter (Fig. 11.10) Cortical blindness has the same clinical importance as a seizure. The toxemic woman with cortical blindness should be classified as eclamptic. The syndrome need not be complete in that light may be perceived (Jellinek et al., 1964). The pupils continue to react to light (a midbrain reflex), but the ability to blink in response to a threat is lost. If the lesion is complete, optokinetic nystagmus is absent, and the patient is indifferent to his blindness (Anton's syndrome).

Papilledema in eclampsia signifies cerebral edema. The woman may be cortically blind. It should be stressed that arteriolar narrowing and retinal edema are the first funduscopic signs of hypertensive encephalopathy. If the hypertension is corrected after significant cerebral damage, papilledema may develop after the retinal arterioles have regained their normal caliber.

Table 11.2. Visual manifestations of hypertensive encephalopathy

Primary ocular changes
Arteriolar spasm
Central retinal artery occlusion
Retinal edema, hemorrhages
Retinal detachment
Secondary to cerebral disease
Cortical blindness
Papilledema

Differential Diagnosis

Not every woman near term who has convulsions has eclampsia. The evolution of signs and symptoms may leave little doubt that the diagnosis is eclampsia. Atypical eclampsia is a suspect diagnosis.

First, was the fit real? A good rule is to observe the first seizure critically while protecting the patient from injury. In generalized convulsions, pupillary light reflexes and corneal reflexes are lost. Eyes roll upward in their sockets or, in "aversive" seizures, are driven conjugately away from the cerebral hemisphere containing the seizure focus. Following eye movements are lost. The ability to blink in response to a threat is also lost. Clonic movements may start in one limb first (i.e., a Jacksonian seizure), but bilateral clonic movements are synchronous. Neither running movements nor thrashing of the head from side to side constitutes seizure activity. Babinski responses can be present during a seizure or for awhile afterward.

Hyperventilation can trigger a true seizure in a susceptible patient. Psychogenic hyperventilation can cause a spell that resembles a seizure, but the sequence is reversed—first clonic movements occur and then a tonic phase. During the clonic phase of the hyperventilation syndrome, pupillary light reflexes are present, and the patient often can respond to requests. The diagnosis can be verified by arterial blood gas values, which will show an acute respiratory alkalosis.

If the seizure is real, it should be considered a symptom of some condition—whether pre-existing epilepsy, meningitis, hypoxia, a metabolic disorder, or some form of cerebrovascular disease. The list could be endless. In the context of a woman in labor, the differential diagnosis must include diseases demanding prompt treatment (Table 11.3). A few rare conditions often initially misdiagnosed as eclampsia are reviewed at the end of this chapter.

Hypertension is a key differential sign. It does not occur in water intoxication, hypoglycemia, or cerebral venous thrombosis. It is a feature of toxemia, pheochromocytoma, spontaneous subarachnoid hemorrhage, and sometimes thrombotic thrombocytopenic purpura. Toxemia early in pregnancy may indicate a hydatidiform mole or a pheochromocytoma. Pheochromocytoma should be considered if labile hypertension exists with orthostatic hypotension. The hypertension of subarachnoid hemorrhage can be extremely high with wide fluctuations. The abrupt onset of severe headache, vomiting, and nuchal rigidity can herald either a subarachnoid hemorrhage or a hypertensive intracerebral hemorrhage. Coma without convulsions may develop in either state. However, the peripheral edema and massive proteinuria characteristic of toxemic hypertension are not typical of a spontaneous subarachnoid hemorrhage. Late postpartum eclampsia is usually caused by cerebral phlebothrombosis.

Table 11.3. Differential diagnosis of seizures at time of childbirth

	Blood pressure	Proteinuria	Fits	Timing	CSF	Other features
Eclampsia	+++	+++	+++	Third trimester	Early: RBC 0–1,000; Protein 50 to 150 mg/dl; Late: grossly bloody	Platelets normal or ↓; RBC normal
Epilepsy	Normal	Normal to +	+++	Any trimester	Normal	Low anticonvulsant levels
Subarachnoid hemorrhage	+ to +++ (labile)	0 to +	+	Any trimester	Grossly bloody	
Thrombotic thrombocytopenic purpura	Normal to +++	++	++	Third trimester	RBC 0 to 100	Platelets ↓ ↓; RBC fragmented
Amniotic fluid embolus	Shock	–	+	Intrapartum	Normal	Hypoxia, cyanosis; Platelets ↓ ↓; RBC normal
Cerebral vein thrombosis	+	–	++	Postpartum	Normal (early)	Headache; Occasional pelvic phlebitis
Water intoxication	Normal	–	++	Intrapartum	Normal	Oxytocin infusion rate > 45 mU/min; Serum Na < 124 mEq/l
Pheochromocytoma	+++ (labile)	+	+	Any trimester	Normal	Neurofibromatosis
Autonomic stress syndrome of high paraplegics	+++ (with labor pains)	–	–	Intrapartum	Normal	Cardiac arrhythmia
Toxicity of local anesthetics	Variable	–	++	Intrapartum	Normal	

Table 11.4. Initial diagnostic studies of seizures by a pregnant woman at term

Hemogram with platelet count
Blood sugar
BUN
Serum sodium
Save serum and/or plasma for later use
Lumbar puncture

Diagnostic Evaluation

A sufficient work-up can be accomplished in short order. A diagnostic lumbar puncture is indicated in a woman with eclampsia to rule out infection and gross subarachnoid hemorrhage as causes of seizures and coma (Table 11.4). The procedure should not be delayed by any fears of herniation. At one time the removal of 20 to 30 ml of cerebrospinal fluid was tried as a therapy for eclampsia (Spillman, 1922). Once 101 ml were removed without apparent mishap. This therapy was discontinued when it became apparent that it did not alter the number of seizures.

Cerebrospinal fluid protein is normal in pre-eclampsia and is moderately elevated (60 to 100 mg/dl) in most cases of eclampsia (Morrison, 1971). A value of 200 mg/dl has been recorded in hypertensive encephalopathy (Adams, 1953). In this context, cerebrospinal fluid protein reflects the increased permeability of the blood-brain barrier.

Cerebrospinal fluid is not bloody in pre-eclampsia or early in the course of eclampsia. As red cells are leached into the cerebrospinal fluid from the cortical petechiae, the fluid becomes blood-tinged. Red blood cell counts of below 5000 cells per cubic millimeter are common (Fish, 1972). Cerebrospinal fluid which is grossly bloody after the first convulsion usually indicates a cause other than eclampsia. Grossly bloody cerebrospinal fluid associated with other features of eclampsia often denotes an intracerebral hemorrhage. It is a bad omen.

Electroencephalography has not been fully utilized in this disorder. The EEG pattern during eclampsia is predictable—diffusely slow, sometimes with focal features and intermittent seizure activity (Jost, 1948; Whitacre et al., 1947). One woman had a normal EEG 38 hours before her first eclamptic convulsion (Kolstad, 1961). No systematic follow-up study has been reported. The EEG may be normal within 6 months, but some minor abnormality may persist.

Other studies should include a serum sodium test to exclude water intoxication, a blood urea nitrogen study to rule out uremia, and a hemogram with platelet count to detect TTP. If local anesthetic agents have been injected, draw and save a sample of plasma or serum as soon after the fit begins as possible. Blood levels of both lidocaine and procaine groups can be determined. A knowledge of the clinical features of seizures and hypertension during pregnancy is almost sufficient to exclude rare causes in the differential diagnosis.

Treatment

The ultimate treatment of any disease is removal of its cause. If eclampsia exists, the pregnancy should be terminated. If the cerebrospinal fluid is grossly bloody, the woman should be delivered promptly without attempting to lower blood pressure. Grossly bloody cerebrospinal fluid in a woman at term from either a spontaneous subarachnoid hemorrhage or hypertensive intracerebral hematoma indicates a poor maternal prognosis and, unless the fetus is delivered promptly by cesarean section, a poor fetal prognosis. In eclampsia with a clear or only microscopically bloody cerebrospinal fluid, the pregnancy should be terminated with deliberate speed but not in haste. There is time to secure the diagnosis and to begin treatment which will lower the risk to mother and fetus during delivery.

The treatment of eclamptic hypertensive encephalopathy must be designed to (1) lower systemic blood pressure, (2) stop convulsions, and (3) decrease cerebral edema if symptomatic (Table 11.5). Concurrently, uterine blood flow must be maintained and diuresis of edema must be started. Only drugs which neither cause fetal depression nor alter fetal metabolism and hemodynamics should be used.

Treatment with Antihypertensives

The ideal antihypertensive drug for eclampsia swiftly lowers the systemic blood pressure to normal without causing absolute hypotension. Uterine and placental perfusion must be maintained. Lower systemic blood pressure allows relaxation of cerebral angiospasm. Arteries

Table 11.5. Treatment of eclampsia before termination of pregnancy

Hypertension
Diazoxide: 300 mg IV push or hydralazine IV drip
Furosemide: 20 or 40 mg IV
Convulsions
Prevent injury and hypoxia
Observe patient for focal features and progression of events
Dextrose: 50 ml of a 50 per cent solution IV
For one seizure—
Phenytoin: 0.5 to 1.0 g IV in 100 ml normal saline at 50 mg/min
For status epilepticus—
Diazepam: 5 mg IV each 5 minutes until convulsions cease (usually $\leq$ 20 mg)
Phenytoin: 1.0 g IV as above
Phenobarbital: 200 mg IV initially
Cerebral edema
Hyperventilation
Hypothermia after delivery if needed

to the brain are physiologically and pharmacologically different from arteries to the muscles and other organs. If an agent, such as carbon dioxide, interferes with the maintenance of cerebral arteriolar spasm without substantially reducing systemic hypertension, hypertensive encephalopathy can be worsened. The cerebral capillary beds would no longer be protected from high pressure flow.

In eclampsia obstetricians need drugs that actively dilate the systemic arteries but not the arteries to the brain. Unless the mechanism of cerebral perfusion autoregulation has been pathologically or pharmacologically impaired, cerebral angiospasm will smoothly relax on a reflex basis as the systemic blood pressure falls. Diazoxide and hydralazine are the drugs that best fit the obstetrician's requirements. Finnerty (1963, 1974) and Cameron (1976) have had excellent results using diazoxide as the treatment of choice in hypertensive encephalopathy, including eclampsia. Diazoxide works within minutes, but the extent of the drop in blood pressure cannot be regulated. Significantly decreased uterine perfusion is a potential hazard which has not been encountered by the proponents of diazoxide. Absolute hypotension has not occurred either. Some physicians prefer intravenous hydralazine because the end point can be titrated. Intramuscular hydralazine acts too slowly for use in eclampsia but has been used in slowly evolving pre-eclampsia. Either drug can be used intravenously in eclampsia. Since diazoxide is a new drug and has an effect upon the myometrium, its pharmacology will be reviewed here. The use and pharmacology of hydralazine is familiar to most physicians and is described fully in standard pharmacology texts.

DIAZOXIDE

Pharmacology. Diazoxide is a benzothiadiazine derivative which directly relaxes arteriolar smooth muscle. Like hydralazine, it affects the cardiovascular autonomic reflexes which increase the heart rate and cardiac output. The same factor prevents absolute hypotension unless plasma and intracellular volumes have been depleted, which is usually not the case in edematous eclamptic women. Diazoxide-induced sodium retention and plasma volume expansion can be counterbalanced by concurrent use of diuretics (Table 11.6). Finnerty (1974) recommends routine use of furosemide.

Diazoxide is unique among antihypertensive drugs in that it acts within minutes and its effect lasts for several hours, often long enough for the pregnancy to be terminated (Fig. 11.11). The standard intravenous dose is 5 mg/kg body weight. A 300 mg ampoule is used unless the patient weighs more than 200 pounds. Rapid injection, using a push, is essential for maximal effect and the highest concentration of free, active diazoxide. Slow infusion permits more diazoxide to be bound to al-

Table 11.6 Effects of combined diazoxide and furosemide treatment

	Diazoxide	Furosemide	Diazoxide and furosemide
Blood pressure	↓ ↓	↓	↓ ↓ ↓
Cardiac output	↑ ↑	↓ ↑	↑ ↑
Sodium balance	++	−−	−
Urinary output	↓ ↓	↑ ↑	↑

From Finnerty, F. A. (1974) Hypertensive emergencies. In *Hypertension Manual,* ed. Laragh, J. H. New York: Yorke Medical Books, p. 808.

bumin and thus unavailable to vasodilator receptors. The patient should remain recumbent and have her blood pressure checked every 5 minutes for the first 30 minutes. Maximal effect usually occurs within 5 minutes. If the initial injection is not completely effective, an identical dose can be repeated 30 minutes later. Diazoxide remains effective for 3 to 4 hours.

Precautions and Side Effects. Extravascular injection of diazoxide is irritating for 1 to 2 hours because the solution is alkaline. Nausea is minimized by an empty stomach. Diazoxide produces hyperglycemia

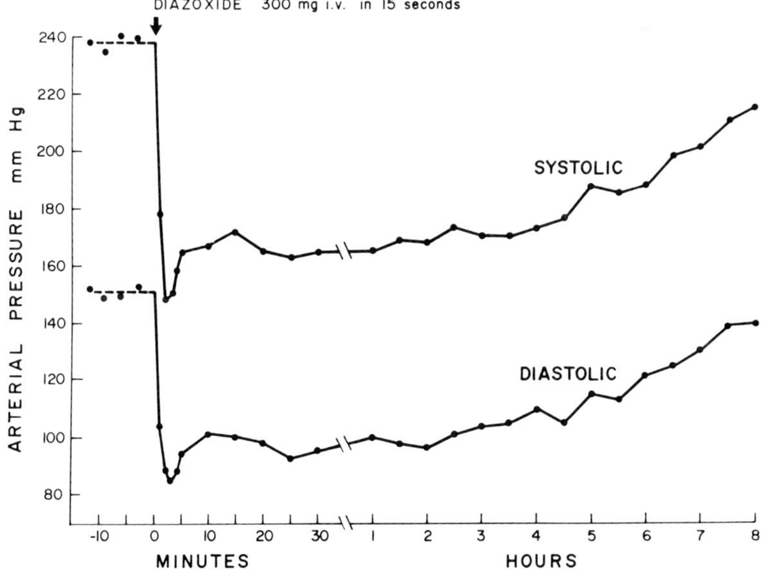

Figure 11.11. Time course of antihypertensive action of diazoxide in a patient with accelerated primary hypertension. From Koch-Weser, J. (1976) Drug therapy: Diazoxide. *New England Journal of Medicine,* **294,** 1272. Courtesy of J. Koch-Weser.

principally by reducing insulin secretion. Hyperglycemia is often mild and is reversible by discontinuing the medication. Severe hyperglycemia has been provoked by regular use of diazoxide for several days without daily blood sugar determinations.

Long-term use of oral diazoxide for treatment of hyperinsulinism has altered phenytoin metabolism (Roe et al., 1975). Low blood levels of phenytoin were attributed to rapid inactivation by para-hydroxylation. An in vitro study demonstrated that diazoxide competitively displaced phenytoin from its albumin binding sites (Roe et al., 1975). The amount of nonprotein-bound phenytoin increased by 40 per cent or more. Similarly, diazoxide displaces warfarin anticoagulants from albumin (Sellers, 1970).

Uterine Effects. Obstetricians must be aware that diazoxide induces uterine inertia. This has not been a clinical problem, since oxytocin promptly reestablishes active labor (Finnerty, 1974). Diazoxide powerfully relaxes gravid and nongravid human myometrium (Landesman and Wilson, 1968; Landesman et al., 1968) (Fig. 11.12).

All currently available antihypertensive drugs decrease uteroplacental perfusion (Ladner et al., 1970 a and b). Diazoxide administered to normotensive pregnant ewes at 10 mg/kg (twice the standard human

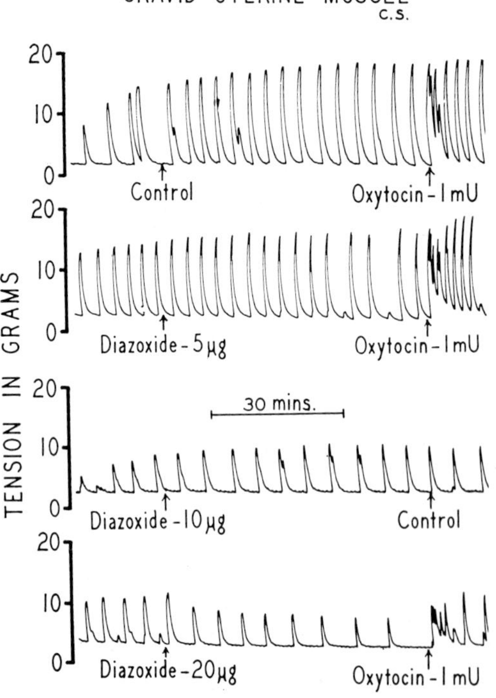

Figure 11.12. The effect of diazoxide upon gravid human myometrium. No significant relaxant effect is observed until the dose of diazoxide in the muscle bath reaches 20 μg/ml. The relaxant effect continues until it is reversed by oxytocin. From Landesman, R., and Wilson, K. H. (1968) The relaxant effect of diazoxide on isolated gravid and nongravid human myometrium. *American Journal of Obstetrics and Gynecology,* **101,** 122.

dose) diminished uterine blood flow by 40 per cent 30 minutes after injection (Nuwayhid et al., 1975). Despite these changes, fetal hemodynamics were unaltered as measured by fetal blood pressure, heart rate, pO_2, and pH. Uterine perfusion in hypertensive gravid subjects before and after administration of diazoxide has not been measured.

Fetal Effects. Diazoxide quickly crossed the ovine placenta (Boulos et al., 1971). Diazoxide injected directly into the sheep fetus is quickly lost to the maternal circulation (Nuwayhid et al., 1975). As previously mentioned, fetal hemodynamics and oxygenation are unaltered.

Fetal hyperglycemia has been demonstrated in sheep after periodic injections over 5 days (Boulos et al., 1971). The validity of these measurements has been questioned, since (1) fetal blood sugar concentrations were twice maternal levels even before diazoxide was given, and (2) both maternal and fetal blood levels were higher than expected (Nuwayhid et al., 1975). Nevertheless, a 10 to 20 per cent increase in the concentration of ovine fetal blood sugar within 30 to 120 minutes after injection has been observed consistently, although statistical limits of confidence can overlap with the normal range. A thorough study of human fetal effects and metabolism has not been reported.

Treatment with Anticonvulsants

The best anticonvulsant for hypertensive encephalopathy is the best antihypertensive drug. Although seizures may originate from recent foci of infarction, hemorrhage, and edema, convulsions in this circumstance probably signify additional cerebral lesions. Obviously this statement can be neither proved nor disproved, but it is supported by the frequency of seizures before and after effective antihypertensive medication (Finnerty, 1974).

If seizures persist after the hypertension is controlled, there are several well-established anticonvulsants (e.g., diazepam, phenytoin, barbiturates) available. Magnesium sulfate is not an anticonvulsant, although it is believed to be one by many physicians in some countries. Since the metabolism and effects of magnesium are controversial, they will be discussed first.

MAGNESIUM

Pharmacology. Magnesium is a chiefly intracellular divalent cation (Mg^{++}) essential for a myriad of enzymatic reactions. The serum level is normally between 1.6 and 2.1 mEq/1. One-third is protein bound. Analogous to another predominantly intracellular cation potassium, serum

Mg^{++} levels need not reflect intracellular stores. Almost all Mg^{++} is excreted by the kidneys (Wacker and Parisi, 1968; Fishman, 1965).

Hypermagnesemia blocks neuromuscular transmission by decreasing the amount of acetylcholine released in response to a nerve action potential (del Castillo and Engback, 1954). An excess of calcium antagonizes this effect by increasing the amount of acetylcholine liberated (del Castillo and Stark, 1952). Stretch reflexes are diminished if serum Mg^{++} concentrations exceed 4 mEq/1 and are lost at 10 mEq/1. Above 5 mEq/1 cardiac conduction is prolonged, as measured by the PR interval and the QRS duration. Complete heart block may occur below 10 mEq/1. Respiratory paralysis occurs between 10 and 15 mEq/1 (Wacker and Parisi, 1968).

Edmond Lazard (1925) popularized the parenteral use of magnesium sulfate to control eclamptic convulsions. Numerous proponents have devised intramuscular and intravenous dosage schedules of varying complexity. All have been designed to maintain serum levels of between 3 and 6 mEq/1 (about 3 to 7 mg/dl). All authorities recommend that before more magnesium is administered (1) reflexes should be present, (2) respiratory rate should be at least 16/minute, (3) adequate volumes of urine are being excreted, and (4) calcium gluconate should be at hand in case of cardiac arrhythmia or respiratory depression. More recent schedules include the use of antihypertensive agents.

The rationale for the use of magnesium sulfate to control eclamptic convulsions has long been debated. First, the risks of respiratory depression and arrhythmias have deterred some physicians. Second, magnesium is not an antihypertensive agent, although an intravenous infusion may cause a transient reduction in blood pressure. Third, prolonged use will depress neonatal respiration. Fourth, hypermagnesemia has never been shown to stop cerebral seizure activity. Its neuromuscular blockade prevents tonic-clonic limb movements.

Even magnesium sulfate's staunchest proponents admit that seizures can occur in spite of "therapeutic" magnesium levels. For instance, one primigravida had six convulsions in spite of a serum magnesium concentration of 6.3 mEq/1. Convulsions ceased after 200 mg of phenobarbital was given intravenously (Chesley and Tepper, 1957). Only rarely has an EEG been recorded during a run of eclamptic convulsions, and none has been reported during magnesium therapy. But it is unlikely that magnesium even reaches the brain. The concentration of magnesium in the cerebrospinal fluid is remarkably independent of the serum concentration.

The cerebrospinal fluid magnesium concentration, 2.4 mEq/1, is significantly higher than the unbound serum level. The calcium-magnesium ratio in the cerebrospinal fluid is closely regulated in normal subjects (Harris and Sonnenblick, 1955). Hypermagnesemia in the range considered therapeutic for eclampsia does elevate Mg^{++} in cerebrospinal fluid *but very slowly*. Plasma magnesium maintained in the 3 to 8 mEq/l range in ten patients for 3 to 48 hours increased magnesium in the cerebrospinal fluid only marginally from 2.35 mEq/l to 2.65 mEq/l. A plasma magnesium level that was kept between 6.3 and 11 mEq/l for 1 week resulted in a cerebrospinal fluid magnesium level of 3.5 mEq/l (Pritchard, 1955). Similar results were found in dogs (Oppelt et al., (1963) (Fig. 11.13).

The intrathecal injection of magnesium sulfate causes spinal anesthesia. Five milliliters of a 25 per cent magnesium sulfate solution paralyzes the legs and bladder for 12 to 24 hours. A larger amount causes respiratory paralysis. Intrathecal magnesium sulfate has been used to control eclamptic convulsions, but in several instances it stopped clonic movements only in the legs (Alton and Lincoln, 1925).

The best evidence that acute hypermagnesemia has no appreciable effect upon the central nervous system is a study performed by two investigators with themselves as subjects. In spite of serum magnesium levels of 15.3 and 14.6 mEq/l respectively, these two normal subjects were aware of their surroundings and keenly perceived pain (Somjen et

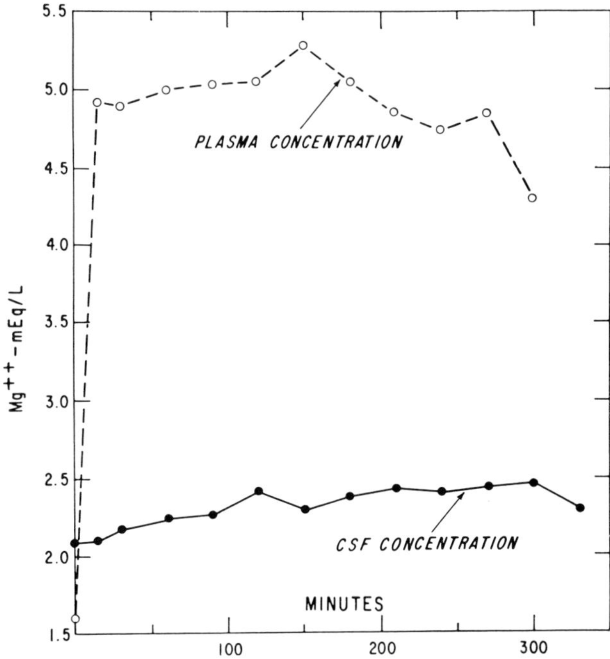

Figure 11.13. CSF and plasma magnesium concentrations during intravenous magnesium infusions in dogs. From Oppelt, W. W., MacIntyre, I., and Rall, D. P. (1963) Magnesium exchange between blood and cerebrospinal fluid. *American Journal of Physiology,* **205,** 960.

al., 1966). Memory, vision, hearing, and conjugate eye movements remained intact, although there was profound paralysis of all skeletal muscles. The EEG did not show any changes characteristic of anesthesia. The alpha rhythm diminished in amplitude and persistence but quickly reappeared with verbal stimulation (i.e., the normal response of a slightly drowsy individual).

Chronic hypermagnesemia can occur in patients with chronic renal failure who are unable to excrete magnesium ingested as an antacid or laxative (Randall et al., 1964). Whether central nervous system depression attributable to hypermagnesemia occurs in this complex situation has not been established.

Magnesium sulfate has been called a "peripherally acting anticonvulsant," which is almost by definition a bad medicine. Unless status epilepticus has produced major complications by muscle exertion (i.e., myoglobinuria, hyperthermia, or hypoxia with severe lactic acidosis), muscle paralysis is not indicated. If complete paralysis is desired, far safer and more effective agents than $MgSO_4$ are available. EEG monitoring is essential as a guide to anticonvulsant therapy while the patient is paralyzed.

Neonatal Hypermagnesemia. In normal pregnancy, concentrations of magnesium in maternal and cord blood serum are identical (Lipsitz, 1971). After parenteral administration of $MgSO_4$ to normal and toxemic pregnant women, there is a delayed increase in the concentration of fetal magnesium (Pritchard, 1955). The fetal level reaches 90 per cent of the maternal concentration in 3 hours (Chesley and Tepper, 1957).

Neonatal hypermagnesemia is manifest by a weak or absent cry, flaccidity, hyporeflexia, and respiratory distress. Symptomatic neonatal magnesium toxicity occurs if administration of maternal magnesium sulfate has continued for more than 24 hours (Lipsitz, 1971). It is not statistically correlated with maternal or fetal magnesium levels or total magnesium dose.

Usually conservative treatment (ventilation and fluids) leads to marked clinical improvement within 24 to 36 hours (Lipsitz, 1971). Normal serum levels of magnesium can be expected within 3 days. Calcium can temporarily improve hypotonia, but exchange transfusions will rapidly reverse severe magnesium toxicity (Brady and Williams, 1967).

ANTICONVULSANTS IN PREGNANCY

Many effective anticonvulsants exist. The three best drugs for the obstetrician are probably phenytoin (the new generic name for diphenylhydantoin), phenobarbital, and diazepam. These drugs are familiar, effective, and available at minimal cost. Although more questions remain to be answered, the effects of these drugs on fetal metabolism have been studied enough to allow them to be used with relative safety.

Basic care of the convulsing patient should not be overlooked. Injury must be avoided. Sustained hypoxia must be prevented by nasotracheal intubation if the seizure is prolonged or cannot be broken. A bolus of concentrated dextrose is never amiss and is often forgotten. Critical observation of the seizure itself is of diagnostic significance—its onset, progression, and focal features, if any. Serial convulsions do not necessarily indicate status epilepticus. The term status epilepticus is applied to two or more fits which follow each other without recovery of consciousness between attacks.

Diazepam. Diazepam is an excellent drug to break status epilepticus long enough for the physician to collect his wits, insert an oral airway, start a dependable intravenous line, and administer longer acting drugs such as phenytoin and phenobarbital. Oral diazepam is not an effective anticonvulsant. Diazepam given intravenously stops seizures quickly, but its effect may last only 20 minutes. Convulsions in adults usually stop after one or two 5 mg injections, but 20 mg or more may be needed.

Obstetric Use and Safety. In obstetrics diazepam has been used to relieve anxiety and reduce analgesic needs during normal labor. The amounts administered intravenously have ranged from 5 to 10 mg (Yeh et al., 1974) to 20 mg (Niswander, 1969) and even 40 mg (Kawathekar et al., 1973). In uncomplicated labor a total dose of 5 or 10 mg calms the mother adequately without producing an adverse effect upon maternal, fetal, or neonatal pH, pO_2, or pCO_2. Maternal and fetal heart rates rise transiently (Yeh et al., 1974). Neonatal hypotonia and respiratory depression, as judged by Apgar scores, was not more frequent in infants who had received up to 20 mg of diazepam intravenously than in those whose mothers had not received any (Flowers et al., 1969; Niswander, 1969). Large total doses of diazepam (i.e., 100 to 250 mg IV) in addition to other respiratory depressants can cause neonatal depression and maternal stupor (McCarthy et al., 1973; Kawathekar et al., 1973). Rarely will such large amounts be needed to control seizures. Perinatal diazepam metabolism is reviewed elsewhere (cf p. 183).

Phenytoin. Phenytoin can be infused whether or not the patient is in status epilepticus. A full 1.0 g loading dose of phenytoin can be administered at once or in two 500 mg increments. Phenytoin can be infused at a rate of 50 mg per minute without significant risk of cardiac arrhythmia. Phenytoin must be diluted in a simple isotonic saline solution, since it will crystallize in acidic dextrose solutions. Phenytoin should not be injected intramuscularly because absorption is variable.

The effects of this drug on the fetus have been discussed in Chapter 10. Fetal respiratory depression is not a problem.

Phenobarbital. Phenobarbital is a basic drug in the treatment of the actively convulsing patient. After an isolated seizure, 100 mg of phenobarbital given parenterally is recommended. In status epilepticus, a previously untreated patient needs 200 mg initially, followed by 100 mg every 6 hours for the first day.

Phenobarbital quickly crosses the placenta in significant amounts. Neonatal respiratory depression can occur.

Cerebral Edema

Eclampsia produces generalized swelling of the entire cortex by increasing capillary permeability. This condition is called diffuse vasogenic cerebral edema (Fishman, 1975), and therapeutic measures must be selected carefully; for instance, mannitol would not be appropriate. Mannitol is effective if a gradient of osmotic pressure is established between the vascular space and its surrounding tissue. The blood-brain capillary barrier must be intact. If it is damaged, mannitol and its sphere of hydration escape into tissue, and a gradient does not develop. In fact, swelling increases. If the lesion is isolated, additional swelling is more than offset at least temporarily by shrinkage of normal brain. However, if the entire cortex has a leaky blood-brain barrier, as in eclampsia, mannitol would not only fail to improve the situation but actually worsen it.

Hyperventilation and hypothermia affect the whole brain. Hyperventilation decreases cerebral perfusion and may help reestablish the autoregulation of cerebral blood flow, as previously discussed. Intubation and forced hyperventilation can begin before delivery if necessary. Short term hyperventilation has no significant fetal effect (Miller, 1974). Hypothermia decreases cerebral oxygen and metabolic needs. Hypothermia has been safely used in brain operations during gestation. In an eclamptic woman whose pregnancy must be terminated, hypothermia can await a prompt delivery.

PHEOCHROMOCYTOMA

Pheochromocytomas that present during pregnancy are regularly confused with pre-eclampsia (Table 11.7). Only one quarter of such tumors in cases reported in English have been detected before childbirth. Fully one third of these tumors were detected at autopsy (Schenker and Chowers, 1971). The fetal prognosis is poor whether or not the diagnosis is established antepartum unless delivery is by cesarean section. Overall fetal wastage amounts to 60 per cent. Maternal mortality decreases from 55 per cent to 25 per cent or less if the diagnosis is known (Schenker and Chowers, 1971) because vaginal delivery

Table 11.7. Initial clinical diagnoses in 67 cases of pheochromocytoma associated with pregnancy

Acute toxemia		43%
Pre-eclampsia	37%	
Eclampsia	6%	
Essential hypertension		16%
Neurosis		6%
Obstetric complication		6%
Nephritis		6%
Neurologic conditions (migraine, epilepsy, brain tumor)		7%
Hyperthyroidism		1%
Other		9%

Data from Schenker, J. G., and Chowers, I. (1971) Pheochromocytoma and pregnancy: Review of 89 cases. *Obstetric and Gynecologic Survey*, **26**, 740. © 1971, The Williams & Wilkins Co., Baltimore.

precipitates a massive release of catecholamines owing to the uterus pressing upon the tumor. Life is threatened by the ensuing hypertensive crisis and cardiac arrhythmias.

Effect of Pregnancy

The effect of pregnancy upon the growth of a pheochromocytoma is undetermined. Some patients who have had hypertension only during pregnancy proved to harbor pheochromocytomas (Gemmell, 1955; Hendee et al., 1959).

Clinical Presentation

Pheochromocytomas must be suspected if paroxysmal hypertension is associated with palpations, pounding headaches, nasal congestion, and sweating (Table 11.8). However, sustained hypertension is more common than the classic presentation. Sustained hypertension beginning in the first half of pregnancy cannot by definition be toxemia. Orthostatic hypotension, a regular feature of pheochromocytomas, does not occur in eclampsia. Seizures occurred in 10 per cent of cases of pheochromocytoma associated with pregnancy—a higher frequency than expected. These seizures may imitate eclampsia (Davies and Short, 1955).

A careful history may find that headaches occur whenever the woman assumes a certain position. She may have developed the habit of sleeping in a chair or in another specific position to avoid inducing the symptoms that are caused by the enlarged uterus pressing upon the tumor.

Table 11.8. Incidence of signs and symptoms in 89 cases of pheochromocytoma associated with pregnancy

Hypertension (sustained or paroxysmal)	82%
Headaches	66%
Palpitations	36%
Sweating	33%
Blurred vision	17%
Anxiety	15%
Convulsions	10%
Dyspnea	10%

From Schenker, J. G. and Chowers, I. (1971) Pheochromocytoma and pregnancy: Review of 89 cases. *Obstetric and Gynecologic Survey,* **26,** 740. © 1971, The Williams & Wilkins Co., Baltimore.

Pheochromocytomas are associated with von Recklinghausen's neurofibromatosis, medullary thyroid carcinoma, and parathyroid hyperplasia. A search should be conducted for obvious signs of neurofibromatosis—cutaneous or mucosal neurofibromas, numerous café-au-lait spots, and axillary freckles.

Diagnostic Studies

The presence of a pheochromocytoma is confirmed by the presence of elevated urinary excretion of catecholamine metabolites—metanephrines or vanillylmandelic acid (VMA) (Crout et al., 1961). Excretion of vanillylmandelic acid continues to be normal in the third trimester in uncomplicated pregnancies and in those complicated by chronic hypertension and severe pre-eclampsia (Table 11.9). Urinary epinephrine and norepinephrine excretion is transiently increased by the stress of normal delivery (Zuspan, 1970) and eclampsia (Zuspan, 1972). A concomitant rise in serum dopamine β-hydroxylase confirms that these catecholamines are released by the sympathetic nervous system (Hashimoto et al., 1974).

Urinary epinephrine and norepinephrine levels can be of value in determining the site of the tumor (Crout, 1964). Only the adrenals and the organ of Zuckerkandl possess the O-methyl transferase that is necessary for producing epinephrine (Axelrod, 1962). Thus, pheochromocytomas confined to those locations secrete epinephrine and norepinephrine. If only norepinephrine is secreted, the tumor can be almost anywhere, but the majority are located in the adrenal. Approximately 10 per cent of pheochromocytomas are extra-adrenal. Another 10 per cent are multiple.

Table 11.9. Urinary excretion of catecholamines and their metabolites

Upper limit of normal[a]	
Total catecholamines	0.1 mg/day
Total metanephrines	1.3 mg/day
Vanillylmandelic acid	6.0 mg/day
Third trimester pregnancy VMA excretion[b]	
Uncomplicated	4.1 mg/day
Severe pre-eclampsia	4.3 mg/day
Chronic hypertension	4.8 mg/day

[a]Data from Crout, J. R., Pisano, J. J., and Sjoerdsma, A. (1961) Urinary excretion of catecholamines and their metabolites in pheochromocytonia. *American Heart Journal,* **61,** 375–381.

[b]Data from Pekkarinen, A., and Castren, O. (1968) Excretion of vanillylmandelic acid (VMA) in the third trimester of normal and toxaemic pregnancy and other clinical conditions. *Annales Chirurgiae et Gynaecologiae Fenniae,* **57,** 373–381.

The next most valuable test is an intravenous pyelogram with tomograms. Although abdominal radiography is usually best avoided during pregnancy, the need to demonstrate an adrenal mass in this potentially lethal disease is paramount. Computerized tomography may become more valuable in these circumstances.

Perirenal carbon dioxide injections and selective arteriography can be dangerous whether the patient is pregnant or not. These procedures and pharmacological tests—the phentolamine test and the histamine and tyramine provocative tests—are usually avoided in pregnant women owing to the high fetal risk and low yield. Maternal and fetal deaths have occurred during a phentolamine test (Roland, 1959).

Treatment

The timing of surgery depends upon the duration of gestation and the viability of the fetus. In the first two trimesters, most surgeons proceed with the operation. Considering the natural history of pheochromocytomas during pregnancy, the risk of inducing an abortion must be taken. In the third trimester, the gravid uterus prevents adequate operative exposure of the tumor. If the fetus has a reasonable chance for survival, a cesarean section can be immediately followed by excision of the tumor. This minimizes risk from an anesthetic, which is considerable in this condition.

If the fetus lacks a few weeks of in utero growth needed for survival, this time can be bought by using α- and β-adrenergic blocking agents, phenoxybenzamine and propranolol, respectively, to control the hypertension and arrhythmias (Griffith et al., 1974). Unresectable invasive pheochromocytomas can be managed in a similar manner (Simawis et al., 1972). Although cesarean section is almost unanimously recommended, vaginal delivery may be possible with use of these blocking agents (Awitti-Sunga and Ursell, 1975).

Excretion of urinary catecholamine metabolites should be measured after surgery to determine whether the tumor was completely excised; thereafter it should be measured at regular intervals to exclude recurrences or metastases.

Placental Transfer of Catecholamines

Maternal catecholamines can cross the placenta to some extent (Morgan et al., 1972). Only trace amounts are found in amniotic fluid (Thiery et al., 1967). Single intravenous injections of norepinephrine in pregnant women produce fetal bradycardia (Beard, 1962). The mechanism has not been proved. One woman with a pheochromocytoma had persistent tachycardia while the fetus maintained a normal fetal heart rate (Thiery et al., 1967). At delivery, cord blood catecholamine levels were within the normal range. The maternal venous norepinephrine level was nine times higher than expected. This difference has been attributed to fetal and placental metabolism of monoamine oxidase and catechol-O-methyl transferase (Morgan et al., 1972).

THROMBOTIC THROMBOCYTOPENIC PURPURA

Thrombotic thrombocytopenic purpura (TTP, thrombotic microangiopathy) is a rare syndrome which is important to obstetricians because it should be considered in the differential diagnosis of eclampsia, gestational seizures without hypertension, and stroke. The condition has been reported in both sexes at all ages, but most cases occur in adolescent and young adult women. Approximately three times more cases have been reported in pregnant and puerperal women than in other women in the same age group. Whether this higher incidence indicates a true association or a statistical aberration in reporting is not known.

The clinical syndrome consists of (1) thrombocytopenic purpura, (2) Coombs' negative hemolytic anemia with fragmented red cells, (3) fever, (4) renal dysfunction, and (5) a variety of neurologic manifestations. Before the florid onset of the full syndrome, indolent prodromal symptoms may be present without known cause. At autopsy, hyaline thrombi fill the arterioles and capillaries of multiple organs.

The presenting complaint is a neurologic one in 60 per cent of cases (Amorosi and Ultmann, 1966). One-third of patients complain of headache. Almost all patients exhibit signs of cerebral cortical dysfunction. Changes in mental status range from confusion and inattention to coma. Seizures occur in half the patients. Weakness and aphasia may be persistent but often dramatically resolve within hours. Seizures and transient ischemic attacks (TIA's) have been observed months before the underlying cause is apparent.

Most pregnant women with TTP are admitted to the hospital during the second half of pregnancy. If not in labor at the time, they soon are. Eclampsia is the usual working diagnosis—not unreasonably, since various combinations of hypertension, proteinuria, edema, retinal hemorrhages, and neurologic signs are present. Unless petechiae, ecchymoses, or purpuric patches are present, there is little reason to suspect a hemorrhagic disorder. Usually a macerated fetus or a stillborn infant is expelled. Rarely is the infant viable. Postpartum hemorrhage is not heavy, as might be anticipated. Some nonpregnant woman with this disorder have presented with menorrhagia (Amorosi and Altmann, 1966). The placenta either is not mentioned in most reports or is said to be grossly normal. One microscopically examined placenta showed multiple infarctions and intervillous thromboses, which would be the logical cause of placental insufficiency and subsequent abortion (Reisfield, 1959). After childbirth the course of the disease is precipitously downhill. Seventy per cent of patients die within 2 weeks. One woman who survived for 2 years after a splenectomy for TTP during her first pregnancy died after a relapse during her second pregnancy (Piver et al., 1968). Onset of TTP began 1 week postpartum in two women (Harrison, 1958; Solomon et al., 1963), both of whom died.

The diagnosis is established by demonstrating hemolytic anemia (negative on Coombs' test), a low platelet count, and erythroid hyperplasia with increased megakaryocytes on bone marrow examination. The most important study is examination of a peripheral blood smear for fragmented, distorted erythrocytes. Gross or microscopic hematuria occurs. Proteinuria, pyuria, and casts are found. Some of these alterations in coagulation factors are also seen in eclampsia (Pritchard et al., 1976).

Neurologic studies are nonspecific for TTP and reflect the clinical status. The EEG may be normal or show focal slowness, but it is frequently diffusely slow due to the widespread involvement of the cerebral microvasculature. Lumbar puncture is usually normal but may show increased tension or a mildly elevated protein concentration. Subarachnoid hemorrhage is unusual except as a preterminal event.

All infants viable at birth were unaffected. Infant platelet counts in TTP were normal in the two instances reported (Solomon et al., 1963; Barrett and Marshall, 1975). TTP is not a contraindication for vaginal delivery, in contrast to idiopathic thrombocytopenic purpura (ITP). The infant's platelet count in ITP is depressed, since the antiplatelet antibodies cross the placenta. This places the fetus in jeopardy of intracranial hemorrhage during vaginal delivery. Because of lack of accumulated experience, it is not known whether cesarean section is indicated in TTP if the fetus has a reasonable chance for survival. It is logical to assume that continuation of pregnancy increases the likelihood of placental disease and in utero fetal death. Thus, induction of labor or cesarean section may be necessary in late pregnancy to salvage the fetus.

There is no consistently effective treatment for TTP. Most patients receive steroids with little effect. Splenectomy may remove the mechanism of clearing distorted red cells, but the basic process remains. Splenectomy can be done during pregnancy (McElin et al., 1950) and has benefitted several women.

WATER INTOXICATION

Water intoxication is a rare and preventable cause of intrapartum convulsions. Although convulsions and hyponatremia secondary to polydipsia in a pregnant schizophrenic have been reported (Goodner et al., 1971), the most common cause has been the misuse of oxytocin. Typically, large amounts of oxytocin (40 to 1300 mU of oxytocin per minute) in large amounts of dextrose and water (3 to 9 liters) are continuously infused for 12 to 24 hours in an attempt to induce termination of a missed midtrimester abortion. During this time the patient becomes confused, stuporous, and convulsed, and lapses into coma. Brisk reflexes are common. The presence of a normal blood pressure and a review of the drug order sheet will differentiate this clinical syndrome from eclampsia.

A serum sodium concentration of below 120 mEq/1 confirms the diagnosis. Cerebral intracellular swelling is present when the EEG shows diffuse slowing with delta waves (< 3 Hz). This slowness quickly abates as hyponatremia is corrected.

Treatment consists of discontinuing the oxytocin infusion. Since a brisk diuresis of dilute urine begins within 30 minutes, it is not usually necessary to administer hypertonic saline solutions. As the free water is cleared, the patient becomes alert but does not remember the episode.

Oxytocin is structurally similar to antidiuretic hormone (vasopressin). Oxytocin has a dose-related antidiuretic effect in humans beginning about 15 minutes after a constant infusion has begun (Abdul-Karim and Assali, 1961). A single injection has no appreciable effect on free water clearance. The antidiuretic effect of vasopressin is equalled by that of oxytocin when oxytocin is infused at a rate greater than 45 mU per minute (Fig. 11.14). An infusion rate of less than 20 mU per minute,

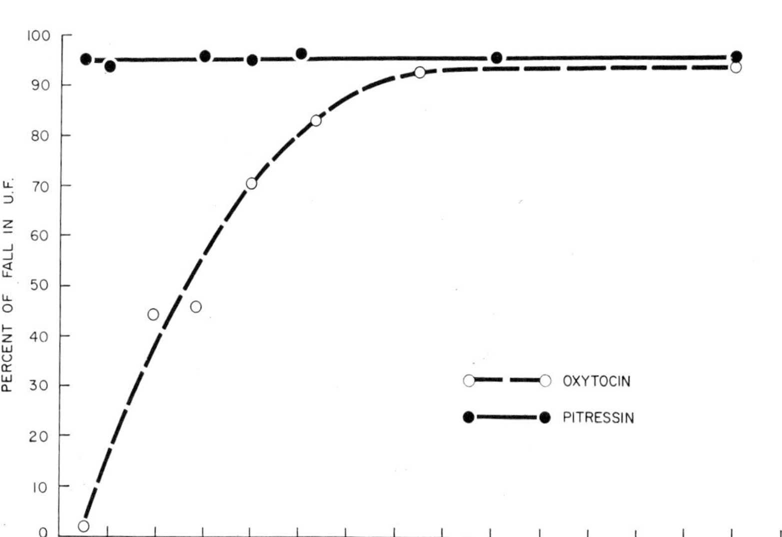

Figure 11.14. The oxytocin and pitressin dose-response relationship as measured by percentage of fall in urine flow (U.F.). Above 45 mU/min the antidiuretic action of oxytocin equals that of pitressin. From Abdul-Karim, R., and Assali, N. S. (1961) Renal function in pregnancy: V. Effects of oxytocin on renal hemodynamics and water and electrolyte excretion. *Journal of Laboratory and Clinical Medicine,* **57**, 529.

as when labor is being induced at term, causes clinically insignificant changes in water metabolism and does not cause hyponatremic seizures.

Water intoxication can be prevented by using concentrated amounts in isotonic saline solution if large amounts of oxytocin are required.

TOXICITY OF LOCAL ANESTHETICS

The incidence of convulsions due to high blood levels of "local" anesthetic agents is 3 to 4 per 10,000 abortions or deliveries in which these agents are used for regional nerve blocks (Smith et al., 1964; Berger et al., 1974). The rate of occurrence is directly proportional to the total amount injected. Confusion, sleepiness, whole body or circumoral numbness, dysarthria, and blurred vision precede seizures. Euphoria, fasciculations, tachycardia, and moderately elevated blood pressure are particularly common with lidocaine and its congeners (Foldes et al., 1960; Foldes et al., 1965). With very high blood levels of these agents, direct depression of the respiratory center and the myocardium causes respiratory and cardiac arrests.

The duration of toxicity depends upon the type of local anesthetic and its total dose. Inactivation of the local amide anesthetic agents (e.g., lidocaine) by the liver takes about twice as long as the hydrolysis of para-aminobenzoic acid ester drugs (e.g., procaine) by plasma cholinesterase. The hydrolysis rate varies within the procaine group (Foldes et al., 1965). Chloroprocaine is rapidly hydrolyzed and has low toxicity (Foldes et al., 1960). Prolonged seizures due to procaine should suggest a plasma cholinesterase deficiency. Procaine and its congeners should not be administered to patients with myasthenia gravis who take cholinesterase inhibitors.

Lidocaine has more CNS toxicity at an equivalent dose per kilogram of body weight than para-aminobenzoic acid ester agents (Foldes et al., 1960). In accordance with the manufacturers' recommendations, not more than 100 mg of epinephrine-free lidocaine should be injected into each paracervical region. The total dose of epinephrine-free lidocaine, not exceeding 3.5 mg/kg, should not be repeated at intervals of less than 90 minutes. Inadvertent intravenous injection may occur in the vascular paracervical region of pregnant women even when aspiration before injection was bloodless (Grimes and Cates, 1976). Symptoms appear within 1 to 5 minutes, although absorption may be slower. Toxic reactions with lidocaine blood levels of 5 to 12 μg/ml have been reported (Grimes and Cates, 1976). Reactions to lidocaine last about 20 minutes, or about twice as long as reactions to procaine drugs (Foldes et al., 1965).

The standard treatment consists of administration of oxygen and the intravenous injection of either 50 to 250 mg of thiopental or 5 to 10 mg of diazepam. Premedication with diazepam may prevent some reactions by raising the seizure threshold (deJong and Heavner, 1972). A bolus of 50 per cent dextrose is always appropriate. If cardiorespiratory arrest occurs, appropriate resuscitative measures and bicarbonate will be needed. A "crash cart" should be accessible in the delivery room.

Prognosis is good if hypoxia is prevented. The electroencephalogram may return to normal within an hour after a toxic seizure if there is no hypoxia (Foldes et al., 1960; Mark et al., 1964).

REFERENCES

Eclampsia

GENERAL REFERENCES

Chapman, K., and Karimi, R. (1973) A case of postpartum eclampsia of late onset confirmed by autopsy. *American Journal of Obstetrics and Gynecology,* **117**, 858–861.

Jewett, J.F. (1973) Fatal intracranial edema from eclampsia. *New England Journal of Medicine,* **289**, 976, 977

Lindheimer, M.D., Spargo, B.H., and Katz, A.I. (1974) Eclampsia during the 16th gestational week. *Journal of the American Medical Association,* **230**, 1006–1008.
Parks, J., and Pearson, J.W. (1943) Cerebral complications occurring in the toxemias of pregnancy. *American Journal of Obstetrics and Gynecology,* **45**. 774–785.
Sheehan, H.L., and Lynch, J.B. (1973) *Pathology of Toxaemia of Pregnancy.* Baltimore: The Williams & Wilkins Co.
Zangemeister, W. (1911) Beitrag zur Auffassung und Behandlung der Eklampsie. *Deutsche Medizinische Wochenschrift,* **37**, 1879–1881.

HYPERTENSIVE ENCEPHALOPATHY—PATHOPHYSIOLOGY

Adams, R.D., and vander Eecken, H.M. (1953) Vascular diseases of the brain. *Annual Review of Medicine,* **4**, 213–252.
Bayliss, W.M. (1902) On the local reactions of the arterial wall to changes of internal pressure. *Journal of Physiology,* **28**, 220–231.
Betz, E. (1972) Cerebral blood flow: Its measurement and regulation. *Physiological Reviews,* **52**, 595–630.
Byrom, F.B. (1954) The pathogenesis of hypertensive encephalopathy and its relation to the malignant phase of hypertension. *Lancet,* **2**, 201–211.
Dimsdale, H.B., Robertson, D.M., Chiang, T.Y., et al. (1972) Hypertensive cerebral microinfarction and cerebrovascular reactivity. *European Neurology,* **6**, 29–33.
Eastman, J.W., and Cohen, S.N. (1975) Hypertensive crisis and death associated with phencyclidine poisoning. *Journal of the American Medical Association,* **231**, 1270, 1271.
Ekström-Jodal, B., Häggendal, E., Linder, L.E., and Nilsson, N.J. (1972) Regulation of cerebral blood flow. *European Neurology,* **6**, 6–10.
Fog, M. (1938) The relationship between the blood pressure and the tonic regulation of the pial arteries. *Journal of Neurology and Psychiatry,* **1**, 187–197.
Fog, M. (1939) Cerebral circulation: II. Reaction of pial arteries to increase in blood pressure. *Archives of Neurology and Psychiatry,* **41**, 260–268.
Forbes, H.S. (1928) The cerebral circulation: I. Observation and measurement of pial vessels. *Archives of Neurology and Psychiatry,* **19**, 751–761.
Giacomelli, F., Wiener, J., and Spiro, D. (1970) The cellular pathology of experimental hypertension: V. Increased permeability of cerebral arterial vessels. *American Journal of Pathology,* **59**, 133–159.
Häggendal, E., and Johansson, B. (1972) Pathophysiological aspects of the blood-brain barrier change in acute arterial hypertension. *European Neurology,* **6,** 24–28.
Lassen, N.A., and Agnoli, A. (1972) The upper limit of autoregulation of cerebral blood flow—On the pathogenesis of hypertensive encephalopathy. *Scandinavian Journal of Clinical Laboratory Investigation,* **30**, 113–116.
McHenry, L.C., West, J.W., Cooper, E.S., et al. (1974) Cerebral autoregulation in man. *Stroke,* **5**, 695–706.
Meyer, J.S., Waltz, A.G., and Gotoh, F. (1960) Pathogenesis of cerebral vasospasm in hypertensive encephalopathy: I. Effects of acute increases in intraluminal blood pressure on pial blood flow; II. The nature of increased irritability of smooth muscle of pial arterioles in renal hypertension. *Neurology,* **10**, 735–744; 859–867.
Olesen, J. (1974) Cerebral blood flow: Methods for measurement, regulation, effects of drugs and changes in disease. *Acta Neurologica Scandinavica,* **50** (Suppl. 57), 1–125.
Rodda, R., and Denny-Brown, D. (1966) The cerebral arterioles in experimental hypertension. II. The development of arterionecrosis. *American Journal of Pathology,* **49**, 365–375.
Skinhøj, E., and Strandgaard, S. (1973) Pathogenesis of hypertensive encephalopathy. *Lancet,* **1**, 461–462.
Strandgaard, S. (1973) The lower and upper limit for autoregulation of cerebral blood flow. *Stroke,* **4,** 323.
Strandgaard, S. (1976) Autoregulation of cerebral blood flow in hypertensive patients: The modifying influence of prolonged antihypertensive treatment on the tolerance to acute, drug-induced hypotension. *Circulation,* **53**, 720–727.
Strandgaard, S., Jones, J.V., MacKenzie, E.T., et al. (1975) Upper limit of cerebral blood

flow autoregulation in experimental renovascular hypertension in the baboon. *Circulation Research,* **37**, 164–167.

Strandgaard, S., MacKenzie, E.T., Jones, J.V., et al. (1976) Studies on the cerebral circulation of the baboon in acutely induced hypertension. *Stroke,* **7**, 287–290.

Strandgaard, S., Olesen, J., Skinhøj, E., et al. (1973) Autoregulation of brain circulation in severe arterial hypertension. *British Medical Journal,* **1**, 507–510.

Ziegler, D.W., Zosa, A., and Zileli, T. (1965) Hypertensive encephalopathy. *Archives of Neurology,* **12**, 472–478.

Visual Changes

Byrom, F.B. (1963) The nature of malignancy in hypertensive disease: Evidence from the retina of the bat. *Lancet,* **1**, 516–520.

Carpenter, F., Kava, H.L., and Plotkin, D. (1953) The development of total blindness as a complication of pregnancy. *American Journal of Obstetrics and Gynecology,* **66**, 641–647.

Chesley, L.C. (1972) The origin of the word "eclampsia." *Obstetrics and Gynecology,* **39**, 802–804.

Clapp, C.A. (1919) Detachment of the retina in eclampsia and toxemia of pregnancy. *American Journal of Ophthalmology,* **2**, 473–485.

Dieckamnn, W.J. (1952) *The Toxemias of Pregnancy,* 2nd ed., pp. 240–249. St. Louis: C. V. Mosby Co.

Hallum, A. V. (1936) Eye changes in hypertensive toxemia of pregnancy. *Journal of the American Medical Association,* **106**, 1649–1651.

Jellinek, E.H., Painter, M., Prineas, J., et al. (1964) Hypertensive encephalopathy with cortical disorders of vision. *Quarterly Journal of Medicine,* **33**, 239–256.

Landau, J., Koren, Z., and Sadovsky, E. (1960) Detachment of retina in eclampsia of pregnancy in a severely anemic patient. *Obstetrics and Gynecology,* **15**, 231–234.

Landesman, R., Douglas, R.G., and Holze, E. (1954) The bulbar conjunctival vascular bed in the toxemias of pregnancy. *American Journal of Obstetrics and Gynecology,* **68**, 170–183.

Mylius, K. (1929) Spastische und tetanische Netzhautveranderungen bei der Eklampsie. *Bericht: Deutsche Ophthalmalogische Gesellschaft,* **47,** 379–386.

Skinner, H.A. (1970) *The Origin of Medical Terms,* 2nd ed., p. 149. New York: Hafner Publishing Co.

Stander, H.J. (1932) Haemorrhagic retinitis in vomiting of pregnancy. *Surgery, Obstetrics, and Gynecology,* **54**, 129–132.

Wagener, H.P. (1934) Lesions of the optic nerve and retina in pregnancy. *Journal of the American Medical Association,* **103**, 1910–1913.

Wagener, H.P. (1933) Arterioles of the retina in toxemia of pregnancy. *Journal of the American Medical Association,* **101**, 1380–1384.

Cerebrospinal Fluid

Fish, S.A., Morrison, J.C., Bucovaz, E.T., et al. (1972) Cerebral spinal fluid studies in eclampsia. *American Journal of Obstetrics and Gynecology,* **112**, 502–512.

Morrison, J.C., Whybrew, D.W., and Wiser, W.L. (1971) Enzyme levels in the serum and cerebrospinal fluid in eclampsia. *American Journal of Obstetrics and Gynecology,* **110,** 619–624.

Spillman, R. (1922) Lumbar puncture in the treatment of eclampsia. *American Journal of Obstetrics and Gynecology,* **4**, 568–571.

EEG in Eclampsia

Chiang, M., T'an, Y., and Feng, Y. (1964) Electroencephalographic study of toxemia of pregnancy. *China Medical Journal,* **83**, 227–240.

Gibbs, F.A., and Reid, D.E. (1942) The electroencephalogram in pregnancy. *American Journal of Obstetrics and Gynecology,* **44**, 672–675.

Jost, H. (1948) Electroencephalographic records in relation to blood pressure changes in eclampsia. *American Journal of Medical Science,* **216**, 57–63.

Kolstad, P. (1961) The practical value of electroencephalography in pre-eclampsia and eclampsia. *Acta Obstetrica et Gynecologica Scandinavica*, **40**, 127–138.

Rosenbaum, M., and Maltby, G.L. (1943) Cerebral dysrhythmia in relation to eclampsia. *Archives of Neurology and Psychiatry*. **49**, 204–213.

Rosenbaum, M., and Maltby, G.L. (1943) The relation of cerebral dysrhythmia to eclampsia. *American Journal of Obstetrics and Gynecology*, **45**, 992–1004.

Whitacre, F.E., Loeb, W.M., and Chin, H. (1947) A contribution to the study of eclampsia. *Journal of the American Medical Association*, **133**, 445–449.

Antihypertensive Treatment

Boulos, B.M., Davis, L.E., Almond, C.H., et al. (1971) Placental transfer of diazoxide and its hazardous effect on the newborn. *Journal Clinical Pharmacology*, **11**, 206–210.

British Medical Journal (1976) Management of eclampsia. *British Medical Journal*, **2**, 1485, 1486.

Cameron, D.I. (1976) Diazoxide in the treatment of hypertensive crisis: a series of 23 patients and a review of the literature. *East Africa Medical Journal*, **53**, 357–365.

Finnerty, F.A., Kakaviatos, N., Tuckman, J., et al. (1963) Clinical evaluation of diazoxide: A new treatment for acute hypertension. *Circulation*, **28**, 203–208.

Finnerty, F.A. (1974) Hypertensive emergencies. In *Hypertension Manual*, ed. Laragh, J.N., New York: Yorke Medical Books.

Harbert, G.M., Cornell, G.W., and Thornton, W.N. (1969) Effect of toxemia on uterine dynamics. *American Journal of Obstetrics and Gynecology*, **105**, 94–104.

Koch-Weser, J. (1976a) Drug therapy: Diazoxide. *New England Journal of Medicine*, **294**, 1271–1274.

Koch-Weser, J. (1976b) Drug therapy: Hydralazine. *New England Journal of Medicine*, **295**, 320–323.

Ladner, C., Brinkman, C.R., Weston, P., et al. (1970a) Dynamics of uterine circulation in pregnant and nonpregnant sheep. *American Journal of Physiology*, **218**, 257–263.

Ladner, C.N., Weston, P.V., Brinkman, C.R., et al. (1970b) Effects of hydralazine on uteroplacental and fetal circulations. *American Journal of Obstetrics and Gynecology*, **108**, 375–380.

Landesman, R., and Wilson, K.H., (1968) The relaxant effect of diazoxide on isolated gravid and nongravid human myometrium. *American Journal of Obstetrics and Gynecology*, **101**, 120–125.

Landesman, R., Coutinho, E.M., and Wilson, K.H., et al. (1968) The relaxant effect of diazoxide on nongravid human myometrium in vivo. *American Journal of Obstetrics and Gynecology*, **102**, 1080–1084.

McCall, M.L. (1954) Continuing vasodilator infusion therapy: Utilization of a blend of 1-hydrazinophthalazine and cryptenamine in toxemia of pregnancy. *Obstetrics and Gynecology*, **4**, 404–410.

Michael, C.A. (1972) The control of hypertension in labour. *Australian and New Zealand Journal of Obstetrics and Gynaecology*, **12**, 48–54.

Nuwayhid, B., Brinkman, C.R., Katchen, B., et al. (1975) Maternal and fetal hemodynamic effects of diazoxide. *Obstetrics and Gynecology*, **46**, 197–203.

Roe, T.F., Podosin, R.L., and Blaskovics, M.E. (1975) Drug interaction: Diazoxide and diphenylhydantoin. *Journal of Pediatrics*, **87**, 480–484.

Sullivan, J.M. (1974) Blood pressure elevation in pregnancy. *Progress in Cardiovascular Diseases*, **16**, 375–393.

Diazepam

Elliott, P.M. (1970) The management of eclampsia with intravenous diazepam and protoveratrine. *Australian and New Zealand Journal of Obstetrics and Gynaecology*, **10**, 99, 100.

Flowers, C.E., Rudolph, A.J., and Desmond, M.M. (1969) Diazepam (Valium) as an adjunct in obstetrics analgesia. *Obstetrics and Gynecology*, **34**, 68–81.

Joyce, D.N., and Kenyon, V.G. (1972) The use of diazepam and hydrallazine in the treatment of severe pre-eclampsia. *Journal of Obstetrics and Gynaecology of the British Commonwealth*, **79**, 250–254.

Kawathekar, P., Anusuya, S.R., Sriniwas, P., et al. (1973) Diazepam (calmpose) in eclampsia: A preliminary report of 16 cases. *Current Therapeutic Research,* **15**, 845–855.

McCarty, G.T., O'Connell, B., and Robinson, A.E. (1973) Blood levels of diazepam in infants of two mothers given large doses of diazepam during labour. *Journal of Obstetrics and Gynaecology of the British Commonwealth,* **80**, 349–352.

Niswander, K.R. (1969) Effect of diazepam on meperidine requirements of patients during labor. *Obstetrics and Gynecology,* **34**, 62–67.

Yeh, S.Y., Paul, R.H., Cordeno, L., et al. (1974) A study of diazepam during labor. *Obstetrics and Gynecology,* **43**, 363–373.

MAGNESIUM

del Castillo, J., and Engbaek, L. (1954) The nature of the neuromuscular block produced by magnesium. *Journal of Physiology,* **124**, 370–384.

del Castillo, J., and Stark, L. (1952) The effect of calcium ions on the motor end-plate potentials. *Journal of Physiology,* **116**, 507–515.

Fishman, R.A. (1965) Neurological aspects of magnesium metabolism. *Archives of Neurology,* **12**, 562–569.

Hoff, H.E., Smith, P.K., and Winkler, A.W. (1940) Effects of magnesium on the nervous system in relation to its concentration in serum. *American Journal of Physiology,* **130**, 292–297.

Randall, R.E., Cohen, M.D., Spray, C.C., et al. (1964) Hypermagnesemia in renal failure: Etiology and toxic manifestations. *Annuals of Internal Medicine,* **61**, 73–88.

Somjen, G., Hilmy, M., and Stephen, C.R. (1966) Failure to anesthetize human subjects by intravenous administration of magnesium sulfate. *Journal of Pharmacology and Experimental Therapeutics,* **154**, 652–658.

Wacker, W.E.C., and Parisi, A.F. (1968) Magnesium metabolism. *New England Journal of Medicine,* **278**, 658–663, 712–717.

CSF Magnesium

Bradbury, M.W.B. (1965) Magnesium and calcium in cerebrospinal fluid and in the extracellular fluid of brain. *Journal of Physiology,* **179**, 67P, 68P.

Greenberg, D.M., and Aird, R.B. (1937/8) Blood and spinal fluid magnesium and calcium levels in epilepsy and convulsive states. *Proceedings of the Society for Experimental Biology and Medicine,* **37,** 618–620.

Harris, W.H., and Sonnenblick, E.H. (1955) A study of calcium and magnesium in the cerebrospinal fluid. *Yale Journal of Biology and Medicine,* **27**, 297–303.

Hunter, G., and Smith, H.V. (1960) Calcium and magnesium in human cerebrospinal fluid. *Nature,* **186**, 161, 162.

Oppelt, W.W., MacIntyre, I., and Rall, D.P. (1963) Magnesium exchange between blood and cerebrospinal fluid. *American Journal of Physiology,* **205**, 959–962.

Magnesium and Eclampsia

Alton, B.H., and Lincoln, G.C. (1925) The control of eclampsia convulsions by intraspinal injections of magnesium sulfate. *American Journal of Obstetrics and Gynecology,* **9**, 167–177.

Chesley, L.C., and Tepper, I. (1957) Plasma levels of magnesium attained in magnesium sulfate therapy for preeclampsia and eclampsia. *Surgical Clinics of North America,* **37**, 353–367.

Flowers, C.E., Easterling, W.E., White, F.D., et al. (1962) Magnesium sulfate in toxemia of pregnancy. *Obstetrics and Gynecology,* **19**, 315–327.

Flowers, C.E. (1965) Magnesium sulfate in obstetrics: A study of magnesium in plasma, urine, and muscle. *American Journal of Obstetrics and Gynecology,* **91**, 763–776.

Lazard, E.M. (1925) A preliminary report on the intravenous use of magnesium sulfate in puerperal eclampsia. *American Journal of Obstetrics and Gynecology,* **9**, 178–188.

Pritchard, J.A. (1955) The use of the magnesium ion in the management of eclamptogenic toxemias. *Surgery, Gynecology, Obstetrics,* **100**, 131–140.

Pritchard, J.A., and Pritchard, S.A. (1975) Standardized treatment of 154 consecutive cases of eclampsia. *American Journal of Obstetrics and Gynecology,* **123**, 543–552.

Pritchard, J.A., and Stone, S.R. (1967) Clinical and laboratory observations on eclampsia. *American Journal of Obstetrics and Gynecology,* **99**, 754–765.

Winkler, A.W., Smith, P.K., and Hoff, H.E. (1942) Intravenous magnesium sulfate in the treatment of nephritic convulsions in adults. *Journal of Clinical Investigation,* **21**, 207–216.

Neonatal Hypermagnesemia

Aikawa, J.K., and Bruns, P.D. (1960) Placental transfer and fetal uptake of Mg^{28} in the rabbit. *Proceedings of the Society for Experimental Biology and Medicine,* **105,** 95–99.

Brady, J.P., and Williams, H.C. (1967) Magnesium intoxication in a premature infant. *Pediatrics,* **40**, 100–103.

Hutchinson, H.T., Nichols, M.M., Kuhn, C.R., et al. (1964) Effects of magnesium sulfate on uterine contractility, intrauterine fetus, and infant, *American Journal of Obstetrics and Gynecology,* **88**, 747–758.

Lipsitz, P.J. (1971) The clinical and biochemical effects of excess magnesium in the newborn. *Pediatrics,* **47**, 501–509.

Lipsitz, P.J., and English, I.C. (1967) Hypermagnesemia in the newborn infant. *Pediatrics,* **40**, 856–862.

Cerebral Edema Therapy

Fieschi, C. (1971) Regulation of cerebral vessels to CO_2 in acute brain disease and its importance to therapy. In *Cerebral Vascular Diseases, 7th Conference,* ed. Toole, J.F., Moosy, J., and Janeway, R., pp. 130–143. New York: Grune & Stratton.

Fishman, R.A. (1975) Brain edema. *New England Journal of Medicine,* **293**, 706–711.

Shenkin, H.A., and Bouzarth, W.F. (1970) Clinical methods of reducing intracranial pressure: Role of the cerebral circulation. *New England Journal of Medicine,* **282**, 1465–1470.

Pheochromocytoma

Awitti-Sunga, S.A., and Ursell, W. (1975) Phaeochromocytoma in pregnancy: Case report. *British Journal of Obstetrics and Gynaecology,* **82**, 426–428.

Brenner, W.E., Yen, S.S.C., Dingfelder, J.R., et al. (1972) Pheochromocytoma: Serial studies during pregnancy. *American Journal of Obstetrics and Gynecology,* **113**, 779–788.

Buzanowski, Z.Z., Jorgensen, E.O., and Rahimi, A. (1972) Pheochromocytoma in obstetric practice. *Obstetrics and Gynecology,* **39**, 120–124.

Cannon, J.F. (1958) Pregnancy and pheochromocytoma. *Obstetrics and Gynecology,* **11**, 43–48.

Davies, J.N.P., and Short, C.R. (1955) Phaeochromocytoma in a pregnant African Woman. *Journal of Obstetrics and Gynaecology of the British Empire,* **62**, 203, 204.

Dean, R.E. (1958) Pheochromocytoma and pregnancy. *Obstetrics and Gynecology,* **11**, 35–42.

El-Minawi, M.F., Paulino, E., Cuestra, M., et al. Pheochromocytoma masquerading as preeclamptic toxemia. *American Journal of Obstetrics and Gynecology,* **109**, 389–395.

Fox, L.P., Grandi, J., Johnson, A.H., et al. (1969) Pheochromocytoma associated with pregnancy. *American Journal of Obstetrics and Gynecology,* **104**, 288–295.

Geisler, H.E., and Lloyd, F.P. (1963) Pregnancy complicated by invasive pheochromocytoma and neurofibromatosis. *Obstetrics and Gynecology,* **21**, 614–617.

Gemmell, A.A. (1955) Phaeochromocytoma and the obstetrician. *Journal of Obstetrics and Gynaecology of the British Empire,* **62**, 195–202.

Gilstrap, L.C., Brekken, A.L., and Harris, R.E. (1976) Sipple syndrome and pregnancy. *Journal of the American Medical Association,* **235**, 1136, 1137.

Griffith, M.I., Felts, J.H., and James, F.M. (1974) Successful control of pheochromocytoma in pregnancy. *Journal of the American Medical Association,* **229**, 437–439.

Hendee, A.E., Martin, R.D., and Waters, W.C. (1969) Hypertension in pregnancy: Toxemia or pheochromocytoma? *American Journal of Obstetrics and Gynecology,* **105**, 64–72.

Pestelek, B., and Kapor, M. (1963) Pheochromocytoma and abruptio placentae. *American Journal of Obstetrics and Gynecology,* **85**, 538–540.

Roland, C.B. (1959) Pheochromocytoma in pregnancy: Report of a fatal reaction to phentolamine (regitine) methanesulfonate. *Journal of the American Medical Association,* **171**, 1806–1809.

Schenker, J.G., and Chowers, I. (1971) Pheochromocytoma and pregnancy: Review of 89 cases. *Obstetric and Gynecologic Survey,* **26**, 739–747.

Simanis, J., Amerson, J.R., and Hendee, A.E. (1972) Unresectable pheochromocytoma in pregnancy: Pharmacology and biochemistry. *American Journal of Medicine,* **53**, 381–385.

Smith, A.M. (1973) Phaeochromocytoma and pregnancy. *Journal of Obstetrics and Gynecology of the British Commonwealth,* **80**, 848–851.

Sprague, A.D., Thelin, T.J., and Dilts, P.V. (1972) Pheochromocytoma associated with pregnancy. *Obstetrics and Gynecology,* **39**, 887–891.

Thiery, M., Derom, R.M.J., Van Kets, H.E., et al. (1967) Pheochromocytoma in pregnancy. *American Journal of Obstetrics and Gynecology,* **97**, 21–29.

CATECHOLAMINE EXCRETION

Axelrod, J. (1962) Purification and properties of phenylethanolamine-N-methyl transferase. *Journal of Biological Chemistry,* **237**, 1657–1660.

Burn, G.P. (1953) Urinary excretion of the pressor amines in relation to phaeochromocytoma. *British Medical Journal,* **1**, 697–699.

Crout, J.R., Pisano, J.J., and Sjoerdsma, A. (1961) Urinary excretion of catecholamines and their metabolites in pheochromocytoma. *American Heart Journal,* **61**, 375–381.

Crout, J.R., and Sjoerdsma, A. (1964) Turnover and metabolism of catecholamines in patients with pheochromocytoma. *Journal of Clinical Investigation,* **43**, 94–102.

Hashimoto, Y., Kurobe, Y., and Hirota, K. (1974) Effect of delivery on serum dopamine-β-hydroxylase activity and urinary vanillyl mandelic acid excretion of normal pregnant subjects. *Biochemical Pharmacology,* **23**, 2185–2187.

Pekkarinen, A., and Castren, O. (1968) Excretion of vanilmandelic acid (VMA) in the third trimester of normal and toxaemic pregnancy and other clinical conditions. *Annales Chirurgiae et Gynaecologiae Fenniae,* **57**, 373–381.

Zuspan, F.P. (1970) Urinary excretion of epinephrine and norepinephrine, *Journal of Clinical Endocrinology,* **30**, 357–361.

Zuspan, F.P. (1972) Adrenal gland and sympathetic nervous system response in eclampsia. *American Journal of Obstetrics and Gynecology,* **114**, 304–313.

FETAL EFFECTS

Beard, R.W. (1962) Response of human foetal heart and maternal circulation of adrenaline and noradrenaline. *British Medical Journal,* **1**, 443–446.

Morgan, C.D., Sandler, M., and Panigel, M. (1972) Placental transfer of catecholamines in vitro and in vivo. *American Journal of Obstetrics and Gynecology,* **112**, 1068–1075.

Thiery, M., Derom, R.M.J., and Van Kets, H.E. (1967) Pheochromocytoma in pregnancy. *American Journal of Obstetrics and Gynecology,* **97**, 21–29.

Thrombotic Thrombocytopenic Purpura

Amorosi, E.L., and Ultmann, J.E. (1966) Thrombotic thrombocytopenic purpura: Report of 16 cases and review of the literature. *Medicine,* **45**, 139–159.

Barrett, C., and Marshall, J.R. (1975) Thrombotic thrombocytopenic purpura. *Obstetrics and Gynecology,* **46**, 231–235.

Case records of the Massachusetts General Hospital, case 74-1963 (1963) *New England Journal of Medicine,* **269**, 1195–1203.

Case records of the Massachusetts General Hospital, case 50-1966 (1966) *New England Journal ofMedicine,* **275**, 1125–1133.

Chung, E.B., and Gomez-Acebo, J. (1960) Thrombotic thrombocytopenic purpura. *Georgetown Medical Bulletin,* **14**, 137–143.

Harrison, H.N. (1958) Thrombotic thrombocytopenic purpura occurring in the puerperium. *Archives of Internal Medicine,* **102**, 124–130.

McElin, T.W., Mussey, R.D., and Watkins, C.H. (1950) Splenectomy during pregnancy with a report of 5 cases and review of the literature. *American Journal of Obstetrics and Gynecology,* **59**, 1036–1044.

Miner, P.F., Nutt, R.L., and Thomas, M.E. (1955) Thrombotic thrombocytopenic purpura occurring in pregnancy. *American Journal of Obstetrics and Gynecology,* **70**, 611–617.

Moon, E.C., and Kitay, D.Z. (1972) Hematologic problems in pregnancy: II. Thrombotic (thrombohemolytic) thrombocytopenic purpura. *Journal of Reproductive Medicine,* **9**, 212–221.

O'Brien, J.L., and Sibley, W.A. (1958) Neurologic manifestations of thrombotic thrombocytopenic purpura. *Neurology,* **8**, 55–64.

O'Leary, J.A., and Marchetti, A.A. (1962) Thrombotic thrombocytopenic purpura in pregnancy. *American Journal of Obstetrics and Gynecology,* **83**, 214–219.

Perel, I.D., and Forgan-Smith, W.R. (1972) Thrombotic thrombocytopenic purpura presenting as eclampsia. *Australian and New Zealand Journal of Obstetrics and Gynaecology,* **12**, 257–262.

Piver, M.S., Lisker, S.A., Rowan, N., et al. (1968) Thrombotic thrombocytopenic purpura during pregnancy. *American Journal of Obstetrics and Gynecology,* **100**, 302–304.

Pritchard, J.A., Cunningham, F.G., and Mason, R.A. (1976) Coagulation changes in eclampsia: Their frequency and pathogenesis. *American Journal of Obstetrics and Gynecology,* **124**, 885–864.

Reisfield, D.R. (1959) Thrombotic thrombocytopenic purpura and pregnancy. *Obstetric and Gynecologic Survey,* **14**, 303–321.

Reisfield, D.R. (1962) Death from thrombotic thrombocytopenic purpura during pregnancy. *Obstetrics and Gynecology,* **19**, 517–519.

Rodriguez, H.F., Babb, D.F., Santiago, E.P., et al. (1957) Thrombotic thrombocytopenic purpura: Remission after splenectomy. *New England Journal of Medicine,* **257**, 983–985.

Richardson, J.H., and Smith, B.T. (1968) Thrombotic thrombocytopenic purpura: Survival in pregnancy with heparin sodium therapy. *Journal of the American Medical Association,* **203**, 176, 177.

Solomon, W., Turner, D.S., Block, C., et al. (1963) Thrombotic thrombocytopenic purpura in pregnancy. *Journal of the American Medical Association,* **184**, 587–590.

Zilliacus, H. (1964) Thrombocytopenia in pregnancy. *Clinical Obstetrics and Gynecology,* **7**, 404–425.

Water Intoxication

Abdul-Karim, R., and Assali, N.S. (1961) Renal function in pregnancy: V. Effects of oxytocin on renal hemodynamics and water and electrolyte excretion, *Journal of Laboratory and Clinical Medicine,* **57**, 522–532.

Abdul-Karim, R.W., and Rixk, P.T. (1970) The effect of oxytocin on renal hemodynamics, water, and electrolyte excretion. *Obstetric and Gynecologic Survey,* **25**, 805–813.

Arieff, A.I., Llach, F., and Massry, S.G. (1976) Neurological manifestations and morbidity of hyponatremia: Correlation with brain water and electrolytes. *Medicine,* **55**, 121–129.

Burt, R.L., Oliver, K.L., and Whitener, D.L. (1969) Water intoxication complicating elective induction of labor at term. *Obstetrics and Gynecology,* **34**, 212–214.

Goodner, D.M., Arnas, G.M., Andros, G.J., et al. (1971) Psychogenic polydipsia causing acute water intoxication in pregnancy at term. *Obstetrics and Gynecology,* **37**, 873–876.

King, T.M., and Hall, D.G. (1966) Water intoxication in obstetrics, *Missouri Medicine,* **63**, 359–362.

Leventhal, J.M., and Reid, D.E. (1968) Oxytocin-induced water intoxication with grand mal convulsion. *American Journal of Obstetrics and Gynecology,* **102**, 310, 311.

Liggins, G.C. (1962) The treatment of missed abortion by high dosage syntocinon intravenous infusion. *Journal of Obstetrics and Gynaecology of the British Commonwealth,* **69**, 277–281.

Lilien, A.A. (1968) Oxytocin-induced water intoxication: A report of a maternal death. *Obstetrics and Gynecology,* **32**, 171–173.

Pittman, J.G. (1963) Water intoxication due to oxytocin. *New England Journal of Medicine,* **268**, 481, 482.

Potter, R.R. (1964) Water retention due to oxytocin. *Obstetrics and Gynecology,* **23**, 699–702.

Self, J. (1966) Water intoxication induced by oxytocin administration. *American Journal of the Medical Sciences,* **252,** 573, 574.

Silva, P., and Allan, M.S. (1966) Water intoxication due to high doses of synthetic oxytocin. *Obstetrics and Gynecology,* **27**, 517–520.

Whaley, P.J., and Pritchard, J.A. (1963) Oxytocin and water intoxication. *Journal of the American Medical Association,* **186**, 155–157.

Toxicity of Local Anesthetics

Alper, M.H. (1976) Toxicity of local anesthetics. *New England Journal of Medicine,* **295,** 1432, 1433.

Berger, G.S., Tyler, C.W., and Harrod, E.K. (1974) Maternal deaths associated with paracervical block anesthesia. *American Journal of Obstetrics and Gynecology,* **118**, 1142–1143.

deJong, R.H., and Heavner, J.E. (1972) Local anesthetic seizure prevention: Diazepam versus pentobarbital. *Anesthesiology,* **36**, 449–457.

Foldes, F.F., Davidson, G.M., Duncalf, D., et al. (1965) The intravenous toxicity of local anesthetic agents in man. *Clinical Pharmacology and Therapeutics,* **6**, 328–335.

Foldes, F.F., Molloy, R., McNally, P.G., et al. (1960) Comparison of toxicity of intravenously given local anesthetic agents in man. *Journal of the American Medical Association,* **172**, 1493–1498.

Grimes, D.A., and Cates, W. (1976) Deaths from paracervical anesthesia used for first-trimester abortion, 1972–1975. *New England Journal of Medicine,* **295**, 1397–1399.

Mark, L.C., Brand, L., and Goldensohn, E.S. (1964) Recovery after procaine-induced seizures in dogs. *Electroencephalography and Clinical Neurophysiology,* **16,** 280–284.

Smith, B. E., Hehre, F. W., and Hess, O. W. (1964) Convulsions associated with anesthetic agents during labor and delivery. *Anesthesia and Analgesia,* **43,** 476–482.

Usubiaga, J.E., Wikinski, J., Ferrero, R., et al. (1966) Local anesthesia-induced convulsions in man. *Anesthesia and Analgesia,* **45**, 611–620.

Wagman, I.H., deJong, R.H., and Prince, D.A. (1967) Effects of lidocaine on the central nervous system. *Anesthesiology,* **28**, 155–172.

CHAPTER TWELVE

Peripartum Psychiatric Disease

Childbirth is a psychological milestone. Mature parents grow emotionally during the process by adaptive mechanisms. A psychotic or potentially psychotic individual lacks the resilient psyche needed to handle either pregnancy or the subsequent presence of a child. Hormonal changes probably play a role which cannot at present be defined. Unresolved conflicts and other psychological factors have been identified in pregnant and puerperal women who develop mental illness. These factors are operable in situations where no hormonal changes can be implicated—after adoption (Tetlow, 1955) and in fathers (Zilboorg, 1931; Wainwright, 1966; Asch and Rubin, 1974).

PSYCHIATRIC DISEASE DURING PREGNANCY

The initial hospitalization for psychiatric illness infrequently occurs during pregnancy (Fig. 12.1). It is more common to see women with preexisting psychiatric disease become pregnant. Successful treatment may increase the pregnancy rate. In either case, any treatment beyond psychotherapy is complicated by concern for the fetus.

Phenothiazines

Phenothiazines have been a keystone of psychiatric treatment since the mid-1950's. In spite of their extensive use, critical observations of their effects during pregnancy are sparse. This may indicate either few complications in pregnancy or few critical observers or both.

Phenothiazines freely cross the placenta and are metabolized by the

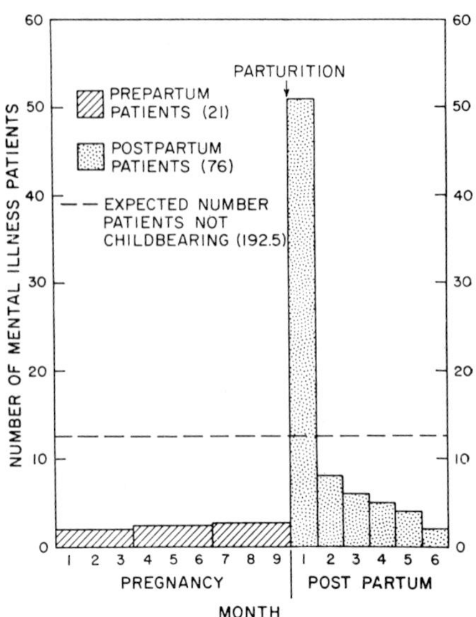

Figure 12.1. Incidence of peripartum psychiatric admissions, Hamilton County, Ohio, 1957–1958. From Paffenbarger, R. S., and McCabe, L. J. (1966) The effects of obstetric and perinatal events on risk of mental illness in women of childbearing age. *American Journal of Public Health,* **56**, 401.

fetus and neonate. Experiments with mice in late gestation found that ^{35}S-chlorpromazine crossed the placenta within 5 minutes. Within 1 hour, over half of the transferred drug had been metabolized (Mirkin, 1976). Phenothiazine given to humans shortly before delivery has been detected in cord blood (Potts and Ullery, 1961), amniotic fluid, and neonatal urine (O'Donoghue, 1971). Administration of 1 mg of chlorpromazine to infants of untreated mothers demonstrated that the neonate is able to metabolize the drug. Chlorpromazine and six of its metabolites were found in the infant's urine within 24 hours of birth (O'Donoghue, 1971). Chlorpromazine and other phenothiazines are excreted in breast milk (Knowles, 1965).

Maternal Complications. Relatively low doses of phenothiazines have been used during early gestation to lessen nausea and vomiting and during labor to potentiate analgesic drugs without increasing central nervous system depression. An acute dystonic reaction is an alarming neurologic complication which can occur after only one exposure to the drug. Contortions abate after administration of diphenhydramine, 50 mg IM, or benztropine, 1 or 2 mg IV. This syndrome is distinct from chorea gravidarum (see Chapter 4). Long-term administration of phenothiazine, often in high doses, can cause Parkinson's syndrome, akathisia, and tardive dyskinesia. A relatively benign cause of first trimester jaundice is phenothiazine-induced cholestasis.

Fetal Complications. Fetal and neonatal complications of phenothiazines are rare whether the drug is given acutely during labor (Carroll and Moir, 1958) or chronically throughout pregnancy to treat psychoses (Ayd, 1963; Sobel, 1960; Kris, 1962; Catz and Yaffee, 1976). Phenothiazines are not known to be human teratogens (Wilson, 1976; Sobel, 1960).

Neonatal movement disorders attributed to maternal phenothiazine ingestion are rare. Abnormal neonatal posturing accompanying acute maternal dystonia has not been reported. Transient neurologic abnormalities have been observed in four infants, including two siblings born of schizophrenic mothers who were receiving phenothiazine on a long-term basis (Hill et al., 1966; Tamer et al., 1969). However, no attempt was made to document the presence and persistence of phenothiazines in the urine of these infants. In one patient, signs including coarse flapping intention tremor, hypertonic arm muscles, abnormal hand posturing, and a very active Moro reflex followed by tremulousness lasted up to 10 months. Diphenhydramine was beneficial in this patient (Tamer et al., 1969).

There is concern that placentally transferred phenothiazines, probably those containing a piperidine side chain (e.g., thioridazine), could cause retinopathy by binding to melanin in the developing eye (Lancet, 1971). There have been no reports that chlorpromazine causes this problem (Catz and Yaffee, 1976).

Children exposed in utero to chronic phenothiazine therapy have developed normally both physically and intellectually with a 6-year follow-up period (Ayd, 1963; Kris, 1962).

No adverse neonatal effect has been attributed to phenothiazine excreted in breast milk.

MAO Inhibitors

Monoamine oxidase (MAO) inhibitors have a place in the treatment of depression but are a danger to any pregnant women because the need for narcotic analgesics or anesthesia can be expected during delivery. If toxemia develops, she will need antihypertensive and diuretic drugs. All these drugs are contraindicated if the patient is taking an MAO inhibitor. For this reason it is recommended that administration of MAO inhibitors be stopped should a patient become pregnant (Tylden, 1968). After waiting at least 1 week, a tricyclic antidepressant can be substituted if needed. MAO inhibitors have not prevented postpartum depression in a group of women considered at high risk of developing that condition (Tod, 1964). MAO inhibitors may interfere with placental implantation of a fertilized ovum (Robson et al., 1961).

Tricyclic Antidepressants

Tricyclic antidepressants (i.e., dibenzazepine derivatives) can be used during pregnancy with the safety of clinical experience, although manufacturers warn of potential fetal complications for legal reasons. These compounds can be teratogenic in rabbits (Robson and Sullivan, 1963). With the exception of three cases of limb deformities which were well publicized in the lay press (McBride, 1972; Barson, 1972), no adverse effects have been noted among children of women taking therapeutic doses of these drugs (Wilson, 1976). In a retrospective study of other children with similar limb deformities, maternal use of tricyclic depressants could not be identified as a cause (Wilson, 1976).

Lithium

Lithium, administered as lithium carbonate, effectively treats acute mania and prevents recurrent bipolar swings of depression and mania. Lithium can be used during pregnancy if proper precautions are taken.

Lithium is distributed throughout the body as a monovalent cation. Therapeutic effects are achieved with serum levels of 0.7 to 1.2 mEq/1, and toxicity occurs with serum concentrations of over 1.5 mEq/1. Manifestations of toxicity include sluggish behavior, anorexia, nausea, and a coarse tremor proceeding to chorea, ataxia, stupor, convulsions, and death as blood levels increase. Dialysis is indicated if the patient is severely toxic or if renal failure occurs.

Excretion of lithium is analogous to that of sodium (Thomsen and Schou, 1968). The clearance of lithium can increase 50 to 100 per cent during pregnancy and drop to prepregnancy levels about the time of delivery (Schou et al., 1973). On the other hand, restriction of salt and administration of diuretics can induce lithium retention and toxicity even though the oral intake is unchanged. Even if lithium levels have been tightly controlled during pregnancy, toxicity can develop during labor and can progress during the early puerperium (Woody et al., 1971). To prevent this, the lithium dose should be halved in the week before the expected date of confinement (Fig. 12.2). Lithium should not be ingested during labor. Biweekly or weekly lithium levels are warranted during pregnancy and in the early puerperium (Weinstein and Goldfield, 1975).

Fetal Effects. High concentrations of lithium are teratogenic in rodents. Lithium administered orally to rabbits and monkeys resulted in neither alterations in pregnancy nor malformations of the fetus (Gralla and McIlhenny, 1972). Human leukocyte chromosomes are undamaged by lithium concentrations in the therapeutic range (Friedrick and Nielsen, 1969; Timson and Price, 1971). There is conflicting evidence about whether high toxic doses can cause human chromosomal damage. As a theoretical consideration, pulses in the lithium level caused by administration of the drug once or twice a day should be prevented by spreading out the doses and by administering no more than 300 mg at any one time.

An international register of lithium babies suffered from reporting bias: unfortunately, not all babies exposed were reported. Although the incidence of lithium-induced fetal abnormalities can be calculated only from a large comprehensive prospective study, data from the registry shows that lithium does not add much, if at all, to the risk of human malformation (Schou et al., 1973; Weinstein and Goldfield, 1975).

Lithium concentrations in maternal and fetal blood are identical (Sykes et al., 1976) (Fig. 12.2). Maternal toxicity produces fetal or neonatal toxicity, but neonatal toxicity can develop without maternal intoxication (Weinstein and Goldfield, 1975) Excretion of lithium may be slower in the neonatal kidney than in the adult. Neonatal lithium toxicity is characterized by hypotonia, low Apgar scores, failure of temperature control, and an absent Moro reflex. Recovery requires 1 to 2 weeks of supportive care. No residual effects have been noted.

Human breast milk has a lithium concentration of between 30 and 100 per cent of maternal blood (Schou and Amdisen, 1973; Sykes et al., 1976). Serum levels of lithium in breast-fed infants can approximate therapeutic levels (Fig. 12.2). Toxicity from this source has not been reported. Breast feeding by lithium-treated mothers is to be discouraged (Weinstein and Goldfield, 1975), but it is not contraindicated (Sykes et al., 1976).

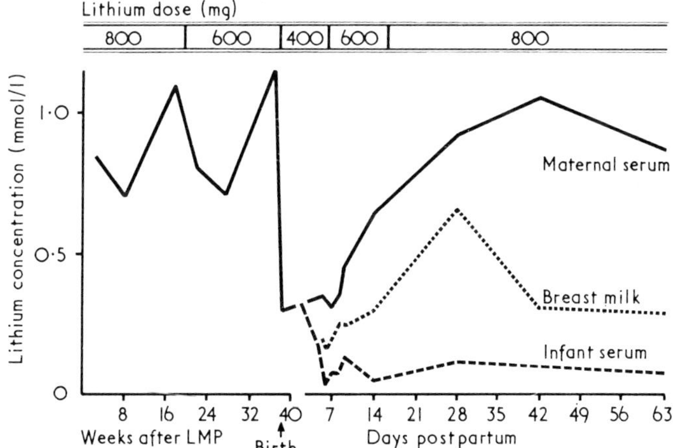

Figure 12.2. Concentration of lithium in maternal serum, breast milk, and infant serum. From Sykes, P. A., Quarries, J., and Alexander, F. W. (1976) Lithium carbonate and breast feeding. *British Medical Journal,* **4,** 1299.

Electroconvulsive Therapy

Uncontrollable psychotic violence and catatonic withdrawal combined with potential malnutrition and dehydration have been considered clinical justification for electroconvulsive therapy during pregnancy (Sobel, 1960). Electroconvulsive therapy has not been reported to provoke abortion or fetal damage (Sobel, 1960), although animal experiments indicate that in early gestation it is a risk to the fetus (Rosvold, 1949). Neither a review of reported cases nor a survey of the experience of eight New York State mental hospitals which used 202 pregnant psychotic patients not treated with electroconvulsive therapy as a control group showed an increased incidence of fetal death or abnormality (Sobel, 1960). Uncontrolled clinical experience supports this conclusion.

Insulin Coma Therapy

Pregnancy is a contraindication to insulin coma therapy (ICT). Over one-third of pregnant women so treated expelled a macerated fetus or a malformed infant. A follow-up study has never been conducted of the development and intelligence of infants at risk who were declared normal at birth. Insulin injected into chick embryos resulted in major defects of whatever organs were actively developing at the time of administration (Duraiswami, 1950).

PUERPERAL PSYCHOSIS

Ancient physicians believed puerperal psychosis to be a specific disease. Hippocrates considered it to be caused by cerebral engorgement from misdirected milk ("per lactis migrationem ad cerebrum") (Zilboorg, 1929). A scanty lochia, failure of lactation, and expression of blood from the nipple were ominous signs. This view persisted, although milk could not be found within the brain. Marcé (1858) broke with tradition when he declared that all types of psychoses occurred during the puerperium and that no type was unique to that period. It took a generation for this concept to be accepted on both sides of the Atlantic (Lloyd, 1889).

Epidemiology

The incidence of postpartum psychoses is one to two cases per 1000 live births (Esquirol, 1845; Paffenbarger and McCabe, 1966). This rate increases with age but not necessarily with parity (Pugh et al.,

1963; Paffenbarger and McCabe, 1966). Although this rate is low enough that the problem is seen infrequently by any one obstetrician, it is high enough and the population is large enough for postpartum psychoses to be a familiar problem to psychiatrists. One-sixth of the women who become psychotic after one pregnancy will become psychotic again from a future pregnancy, but not necessarily the next one (Martin, 1958; Paffenbarger and McCabe, 1966).

Women who develop postpartum psychoses tend to be older than control groups of puerperal women. On an age-adjusted basis, women in the psychotic group bear fewer children and wait longer between pregnancies (Paffenbarger and McCabe, 1966). Age of menarche and age at marriage are irrelevant. As a group, social factors (i.e., race, religion, occupation of the father, sex of the child, and illegitimacy) are irrelevant but may have a role in an individual case (Fondeur et al., 1957; Thomas and Gordon, 1959; Paffenbarger and McCabe, 1966).

The mix of postpartum psychoses varies little if at all from that of a general psychiatric population. The relative proportion of the types of psychoses diagnosed varies among psychiatrists and with the era in which they practice. The distribution of postpartum psychoses among the major categories of mental disease was almost identical to the distribution in a control group in which disease had not been precipitated by childbirth; the groups were matched for age, sex, hospital, and year of admission (Fondeur et al., 1957). Another study found the incidence of manic-depressive illness to be increased (Pugh et al., 1963). Recurrences after another pregnancy mimic the initial episode in quality.

The time limit following childbirth for the definition of a puerperal psychosis is arbitrary. If a 6 month period is surveyed, half of the psychotic reactions occur within a fortnight, two-thirds within a month (Martin, 1958; Paffenbarger and McCabe, 1966). Six weeks is a commonly accepted limit (Herzog and Detre, 1976).

Clinical Presentation

The "baby blues" not infrequently experienced by mature women are distinct from psychotic postpartum reactions, but both share some psychodynamic elements (Markham, 1961).

A transient postpartum depression or regression typically occurs 3 to 5 days after delivery; it is somewhat similar to that observed during serious illness or after an operation. The initial elation has passed, and the new mother becomes irritable, withdrawn, and tearful. Although ambivalence toward the infant exists, she is preoccupied by concerns for the baby and herself. A mature woman has the ego strength to grow emotionally and be strengthened by this ultimate feminine role.

The women who develop postpartum psychoses do not grow from the experience. Basic elements in their psyche have not withstood the challenge. In retrospect, it is evident that these women complained of more headaches and backaches or exhibited pathologic anxiety in other ways while bearing the child (Paffenbarger and McCabe, 1966). Dystocia is more common. After childbirth, insomnia and agitation often precede psychotic behavior. These women do not "take to the baby," have difficulty nursing, ignore the infant, or, in extreme cases, commit infanticide (Tetlow, 1955; McIlroy, 1928).

The psychodynamics of any individual's reaction do not fit a mold, but several factors have been identified in the group as a whole. A weak ego is basic. Often this results from a symbiotic parent-dominated relationship which makes it difficult for the child to assume the adult role of a parent. In other cases the infant may be identified with a hated person. For some masculine-aggressive women, childbirth painfully resurrects the castration complex. The instinctive desire to become pregnant clashes with the commitment to rear a child. Parenthood is not necessarily a solution for a neurotic woman's problems.

Differential Diagnosis

A young woman with postpartum mental illness deserves to have organic diseases firmly excluded. Psychotic behavior beginning immediately after childbirth should be suspect. The most important step is a thorough neurologic history and examination. A few simple tests can eliminate other possibilities. The list of possible diagnoses is endless, but a few deserve special mention.

A "toxic exhaustive psychosis" can occur during or immediately after sleepless, hard labor lasting over 36 hours (Strecker and Ebough, 1926). Intensive-care-unit psychosis is its modern counterpart. Modern obstetricians rarely allow labor to last that long, especially if the membranes have ruptured.

Scopolamine, once commonly used during labor, can cause frightful hallucinations and wild behavior. Dilated pupils and a dry fever support the diagnosis. Physostigmine, 1 mg intravenously and repeated every 2 to 4 hours as needed, is effective treatment which should be used after delivery.

Barbiturates unwittingly administered to a woman with latent acute intermittent porphyria will precipitate a crisis. Neuropathy, tachycardia, and other features previously reviewed may suggest the diagnosis on clinical grounds. A Watson-Schwarz test is diagnostic (see p. 39).

In countries where beriberi is prevalent, the increased metabolic demands of labor and lactation are known to precipitate Wernicke's encephalopathy (see p. 36).

A lumbar puncture may reveal either blood or infection. Intrapartum subarachnoid hemorrhage can mimic postpartum catatonic schizophrenia (Hanson and Brown, 1973). Personality change may be an early sign of tuberculous meningitis (see p. 92).

Cerebral vasculitis or treatment of it with steroids can cause psychoses. Systemic lupus erythematosus is exacerbated by pregnancy. An electroencephalogram and an erythrocyte sedimentation rate are helpful.

The torpor of Sheehan's postpartum pituitary necrosis develops in the months and years after delivery, but not in the immediate puerperium.

Treatment

Treatment varies with the individual situation but does not differ basically from the treatment of patients whose illness was not precipitated by childbirth. Sex hormones have proved to be ineffective (Normand, 1967).

Prognosis

The prognosis is at least as good as nonpuerperal psychoses in both schizophrenic and manic-depressive patients (Fonduer et al., 1957). Future pregnancies in 15 to 20 per cent of these women will be followed by another postpartum psychosis similar to the first.

REFERENCES

Asch, S. S., and Rubin, L. J. (1974) Postpartum reactions: Some unrecognized variations. *American Journal of Psychiatry,* **131**, 870–873.

Brown, W. A., and Shereshefsky, P. (1972) Seven women: A prospective study of postpartum psychiatric disorders. *Psychiatry,* **35,** 139–159.

Douglas, G. (1968) Some emotional disorders of the puerperium. *Journal of Psychosomatic Research,* **12,** 101–106.

Esquirol, E. (1845) *Mental Maladies: A Treatise on Insanity,* transl. Hunt, E. K. Philadelphia: Lea & Blanchard.

Fondeur, M., Fixsen, C., Triebel, W. A., et al. (1957) Postpartum mental illness: A controlled study. *Archives of Neurology and Psychiatry,* **77**, 503–512.

Hanson, G. D., and Brown, M. J. (1973) Waxy flexibility in a postpartum woman—A case report and review of the catatonic syndrome. *Psychiatric Quarterly,* **47**, 95–103.

Herzog, A., and Detre, T. (1976) Psychotic reactions associated with childbirth. *Diseases of the Nervous System,* **37,** 229–235.

Lloyd, J. H. (1889) Puerperal insanity and the insanity of pregnancy and lactation. In *A System of Obstetrics,* Vol. 2. Philadelphia: Lea Brothers.

Marcé, L. V. (1858) *Traité de la Folie des Femmes Encientes, des Nouvelles Accouchées et des Nourices.* Paris: Baillière et Fils.

Markham, S. (1961) A comparative evaluation of psychotic and nonpsychotic reactions to childbirth. *American Journal of Orthopsychiatry,* **31,** 565–578.

Martin, M. E. (1958) Puerperal mental illness: A follow-up study of 75 cases. *British Medical Journal,* **2,** 773–777.

McIlroy, A. L. (1928) The influence of parturition upon insanity and crime. *British Medical Journal,* **1,** 303, 304.

Normand, W. C. (1967) Postpartum disorders. In *Comprehensive Textbook of Psychiatry,* ed. Freedman, A. M. and Kaplan, H. I. Baltimore: The Williams & Wilkins Co.

Paffenbarger, R. S., and McCabe, L. J. (1966) The effect of obstetric and perinatal events on risk of mental illness in women of childbearing age. *American Journal of Public Health,* **56,** 400–407.

Pugh, T. F., Jerath, B. K., Schmidt, W. M., et al. (1963) Rates of mental disease related to childbearing. *New England Journal of Medicine,* **268,** 1224–1228.

Sim, M. (1968) Psychiatric disorders of pregnancy. *Journal of Psychosomatic Research,* **12,** 95–100.

Strecher, E. A., and Ebaugh, F. G. (1926) Psychoses occurring during the puerperium. *Archives of Neurology and Psychiatry,* **15,** 239–252.

Tetlow, C. (1955) Psychoses of childbearing. *Journal of Mental Science,* **101,** 629–639.

Thomas, C. L., and Gordon, J. E. (1959) Psychosis after childbirth: Ecological aspects of a single impact stress. *American Journal of the Medical Sciences,* **238,** 363–388.

Tod, E. D. M. (1964) Puerperal depression: A prospective epidemiological study. *Lancet,* **2,** 1264–1266.

Trethowan, W. H. (1968) The Couvade syndrome—Some further observations. *Journal of Psychosomatic Research,* **12,** 107–115.

Wainwright, W. H. (1966) Fatherhood as a precipitant of mental illness. *American Journal of Psychiatry,* **123,** 40–44.

Zilboorg, G. (1929) The dynamics of schizophrenic reactions related to pregnancy and childbirth. *American Journal of Psychiatry,* **8,** 733–767.

Zilboorg, G., (1931) Depressive reactions related to parenthood. *American Journal of Psychiatry,* **10,** 927–962.

Phenothiazines

American College of Neuropsychopharmacology–Food and Drug Administration Task Force (1973) Neurologic syndromes associated with antipsychotic drug use. *New England Journal of Medicine,* **289,** 20–23.

Ayd, F. J. (1963) Chlorpromazine: Ten years' experience. *Journal of the American Medical Association,* **184,** 51–54.

Carroll, J. J., and Moir, R. S. (1958) Use of promethazine (phenergan) hydrochloride in obstetrics. *Journal of the American Medical Association,* **169,** 2218–2224.

Catz, C. S., and Yaffee, S. J. (1976) Environmental factors: Pharmacology. In *Prevention of Embryonic, Fetal, and Perinatal Disease,* Ch. 6. Washington: U. S. Govt. Printing Office.

Flanagan, T. L., Lin, T. H., Novick, W. J., et al. (1959) Spectrophotometric method for the determination of chlorpromazine and chlorpromazine sulphoxide in biological fluids. *Journal of Medicinal and Pharmaceutical Chemistry,* **1,** 263–273.

Hill, R. M., Desmond, M. M., and Kay, J. L. (1966) Extrapyramidal dysfunction in an infant of a schizophrenic mother. *Journal of Pediatrics,* **69,** 589–595.

Knowles, J. A. (1965) Excretion of drugs in milk: A review. *Journal of Pediatrics,* **66,** 1068–1082.

Kris, E. B. (1962) Children born to mothers maintained on pharmacotherapy during pregnancy and postpartum. In *Recent Advances in Biological Psychiatry,* ed. J. Wortis, Vol. 4, Ch. 18. New York: Plenum Press.

Kris, E. B., and Carmichael, D. M. (1957) Chlorpromazine maintenance therapy during pregnancy and confinement. *Psychiatric Quarterly,* **31,** 690–695.

Lancet, (1971) Drugs and the foetal eye. *Lancet,* **1,** 122.

Mirkin, B. L. (1976) *Perinatal Pharmacology and Therapeutics.* New York: Academic Press.

O'Donoghue, S. E. F. (1971) Distribution of pethidine and chlorpromazine in maternal, foetal, and neonatal biological fluids. *Nature,* **229,** 124, 125.

Potts, C. R., and Ullery, J. C. (1961) Maternal and fetal effects of obstetric analgesia: Intravenous use of promethazine and meperidine. *American Journal of Obstetrics and Gynecology,* **81,** 1253–1259.

Sobel, D. E. (1960) Fetal damage due to ECT, insulin coma, chlorpromazine or reserpine. *Archives of General Psychiatry,* **2,** 606–611.

Tamer, A., McKey, R., Arias, D., et al. (1969) Phenothiazine-induced extrapyramidal dysfunction in the neonate. *Journal of Pediatrics,* **75,** 479, 480.

Wilson, J. G. (1976) Environmental factors: Teratogenic drugs. In *Prevention of Embryonic, Fetal, and Perinatal Disease,* Ch. 7. Washington: U.S. Govt. Printing Office.

Monoamine Oxidase (MAO) Inhibitors

Robson, J. M., Poulson, E., and Lindsay, D. (1961) Mechanism of action of some amines and amine oxidase inhibitors on pregnancy. *Journal of Reproductive Fertility,* **2,** 530, 531.

Tod, E. D. M. (1964) Puerperal depression: A prospective study, *Lancet,* **2,** 1264–1266.

Tylden, E. (1968) Pregnancy and monoamine oxidase inhibitors. *British Medical Journal,* **2,** 698.

Tricyclic Antidepressants

Barson, A. J. (1972) Malformed infant. *British Medical Journal,* **2,** 45.

Cassano, G. B., and Hansson, E. (1966) Autoradiographic distribution studies in mice with C^{14}-imipramine. *International Journal of Neuropsychiatry,* **2,** 269–278.

Cassano, G. B., Sjöstrand, S. E., and Hansson, E. (1965) Distribution and fate of C^{14}-amitriptyline in mice and rats. *Psychopharmacologica,* **8,** 1–11.

Crombie, D. L., Pinsent, R. J. F. H., and Fleming, D. (1972) Imipramine in pregnancy. *British Medical Journal,* **1,** 745.

Kuenssberg, E. V., and Knox, J. D. E. (1972) Imipramine in pregnancy. *British Medical Journal,* **2** 292.

McBride, W. G. (1972) The teratogenic effects of imipramine. *Teratology,* **5,** 262A.

Robson, J. M., and Sullivan, F. M. (1963) The production of foetal abnormalities in rabbits by imipramine. *Lancet,* **1,** 638–639.

Scanlon, F. J. (1969) Use of antidepressant drugs during the first trimester. *Medical Journal of Australia,* **2,** 1077.

Sim, M. (1972) Imipramine and pregnancy. *British Medical Journal,* **2,** 45.

Wilson, J. G. (1976) Environmental Factors: Teratogenic drugs. In *Prevention of Embryonic, Fetal, and Perinatal Disease,* Ch. 7. Washington: U.S. Govt. Printing Office.

Lithium

Aoki, F. Y., and Ruedy, J. (1971) Severe lithium intoxication: Management without dialysis and report of a possible teratogenic effect of lithium. *Canadian Medical Association Journal,* **105,** 847, 848.

Friedrich, U., and Nielsen, J. (1969) Lithium and chromosome abnormalities. *Lancet,* **2,** 435, 436.

Fries, H. (1970) Lithium in pregnancy. *Lancet,* **1,** 1233.

Gralla, E. J., and McIlhenny, H. M. (1972) Studies in pregnant rats, rabbits, and monkeys with lithium carbonate. *Toxicology and Applied Pharmacology,* **21,** 428–433.

Schou, M. (1973) Lithium and pregnancy: III. Lithium ingestion by children breast-fed by women on lithium treatment. *British Medical Journal,* **2,** 138.

Schou, M., and Amdisen, A. (1970) Lithium in pregnancy. *Lancet,* **1,** 1391.

Schou, M., Amdisen, A., and Steenstrup, O. R. (1973) Lithium and pregnancy: II. Hazards to women given lithium during pregnancy and delivery. *British Medical Journal,* **2,** 137–138.

Schou, M., Goldfield, M. D., Weinstein, M. R., et al. (1973) Lithium and pregnancy: I. Report from the Register of Lithium babies. *British Medical Journal,* **2,** 135, 136.

Silverman, J. A., Winters, R. W., and Strande, C. (1971) Lithium carbonate therapy during pregnancy: Apparent lack of effect upon the fetus. *American Journal of Obstetrics and Gynecology,* **109,** 934–936.

Sykes, P. A., Quarries, J., and Alexander, F. W. (1976) Lithium carbonate and breast feeding. *British Medical Journal,* **4**, 1299.

Thomsen, K., and Schou, M. (1968) Renal lithium excretion in man. *American Journal of Physiology,* **215,** 823–827.

Timson, J., and Price, D. J. (1971) Lithium and mitosis. *Lancet,* **2,** 93.

Weinstein, M. R., and Goldfield, M. D. (1975) Administration of lithium during pregnancy. In *Lithium Research and Therapy,* ed. Johnson, F. N., Ch. 15. London: Academic Press.

Woody, J. N., London, W. L., and Wilbanks, G. D. (1971) Lithium toxicity in a newborn. *Pediatrics,* **47,** 94–96.

Electroconvulsive Therapy and Insulin Coma

Charatan, F. B., and Oldham, A. J. (1954) Electroconvulsive treatment in pregnancy. *Journal of Obstetrics and Gynaecology of the British Empire,* **61,** 665–667.

Duraiswami, P. K. (1950) Insulin-induced skeletal abnormalities in developing chickens. *British Medical Journal,* **2,** 384–390.

Gralnick, A. (1946) Shock therapy in psychoses complicated by pregnancy. *American Journal of Psychiatry,* **102,** 780–782.

Laird, D. M. (1955) Convulsive therapy in psychoses accompanying pregnancy. *New England Journal of Medicine,* **252,** 934–936.

Rosvold, H. E. (1949) The effects of electroconvulsive shocks on gestation and maternal behavior. *Journal of Comparative and Physiological Psychology,* **42,** 207–219.

Sobel, D. E. (1960) Fetal damage due to ECT, insulin coma, chlorpromazine, or reserpine. *Archives of General Psychiatry,* **2**, 606–611.

Index

Note: Numbers in italics indicate illustrations.

A

Abortion, criminal, 134
  habitual, 66, 99
  saline, 137
Abruptio placentae, 118
Acetazolamide, 193
Acoustic neuroma, 157, 158, *159*
Acroparesthesias, 27, 33
Acute intermittent porphyria, 37–42
Addison's disease, 171
ADH. See *Antidiuretic hormone.*
After-pains, 5, 7
Air embolus, 133–135
Amenorrhea
  after cord transection, 12
  with galactorrhea, 163
  in myotonic dystrophy, 66
  in Sheehan's syndrome, 144
  in Wilson's disease, 81
Amitriptyline, 15, 182, 254
Amniotic fluid
  catecholamines, 238
  embolus, 118, 132, *133*, 222, 223
  after mannitol, 128
  phenothiazine concentration, 252
  polyhydramnios, 67
  porphyrins, 42
Anemia
  folate deficiency, 201, 202
  sickle cell, 133, 135, 137
  in TTP, 238, 239
Anesthesia
  general, in myasthenia, 58, 61
    in myotonia, 66
  regional, 8, 10, 11
    in myasthenia, 58, 61
    in poliomyelitis, 91
    toxicity, 241, 242
    and Valsalva's maneuver, 123, 164
Aneurysms, 115–128
  aortic, 125
  arterial, 125
  cerebral, 124–127
  mycotic, 119
  splenic artery, 125
Angiomas
  cerebral, 117–127, *122*
  cutaneous, 79, 121, *122*, *169*
  retinal, 121
  spinal, 118, 120, 167–170, *169*
Anticholinesterases, 57, 63. See also individual drugs.
Anticoagulants
  in cerebral phlebitis, 143, 144
  subarachnoid hemorrhage, 118
  teratogenicity, 118
Anticonvulsants. See also individual agents.
  in eclampsia, 225, 229, 232–234
  in epilepsy, 201–206
  hematologic effects, 201, 202
  teratogenicity, 199–201
Antidepressants, 253–255
  antepartum use, 253–255
  dibenzazepine, 15, 182, 254
  for headache, 182
  teratogenicity, 254, 255
Antidiuretic hormone
  in diabetes insipidus, 16
  and oxytocin, 16, 240, 241
  in porphyria, 39
Antihypertensive treatment, 225, 226
  diazoxide, 226–229
  hydralazine, 225, 226
Arteriography
  in arteritis, 130
  in brain tumor, *160*
  in cerebral aneurysms, 120
  in cerebral phlebitis, 143

Arteriography (*Continued*)
during pregnancy, 120
in stroke, 130
Arteriovenous malformations, cerebral, 117–127, *122*
spinal, 118, 120, 167–170, *169*
Arteritis, 118, 119, 130, 131
Arthrogryposis multiplex congenita, 67, 103
Astrocytoma, 158, *160*
Atropine, 58, 62
Autonomic hyperreflexia
in Guillain-Barré syndrome, 31
in paraplegia, 12
in porphyria, 38, 39
in tetanus, 102
Autoregulation, 216–219, *216*

B

Baby blues, 257
Baby, floppy, 63, 64, 202, 232, 233, 255
Backache, 43
Barbiturates. See *Phenobarbital.*
Bell's palsy, 24–27
Benign intracranial hypertension, 171–175
Benzodiazepenes. See *Diazepam.*
Beri beri, 36, 258
Blindness
in carotid-cavernous fistulae, 148
in eclampsia, 219–221
in parasellar tumors, 159–163
Brachial neuritis, 30
Brain tumor, 157–167. See also names of specific tumors, *e.g., Meningioma, Pinealoma.*
Breast, innervation, 14
stimulation, 15, 16. See also *Galactorrhea, Milk.*
Bromide, 196, 202

C

Carbamazepine, 200, 206
Cardiomyopathy, peripartum, *131*, 132
Carotid-cavernous fistula, *136,* 147–148
Carpal tunnel syndrome, 27, 28
Catamenial epilepsy, 191, *192,* 193
Catamenial migraine, 184
Catamenial sciatica, 23, *24*
Catecholamines
in paraplegia, 13
in pheochromocytoma, 236–238
placental transfer, 238
in porphyria, 39
in tetanus, 102
Cauda equina
anesthesia, 10, 11, 91

Cauda equina (*Continued*)
choriocarcinoma, 165, 166
cyst, 168
disc, 43
endometriosis, 23
paraplegia, 12
Cavernous sinus thrombosis, 136
Centrencephalic epilepsy, 197
Cerebellar hemangioblastoma, 158
Cerebral edema
in eclampsia, 214, 216, 218
treatment, 127, 128
in tumors, 164
Cerebrospinal fluid
antibiotic concentrations. See names of individual drugs.
in benign intracranial hypertension, 171, 173
calcium, 230
cerebral phlebitis, 142
chorionic gonadotropin, 166
in eclampsia, 224
in Guillain-Barré syndrome, 31
in listerial meningitis, 99, 100
magnesium, 230, *231*
in multiple sclerosis, 111
in poliomyelitis, 88
pressure, 123, *124*. See also *Valsalva's maneuver, Papilledema.*
in subarachnoid hemorrhage, 116, 117
in tuberculous meningitis, 93
Cerebrovascular disease
aneurysm, 115–128
arterial occlusions, 128–135
in arteritis, 130, 131
with choriocarcinoma, 131, 165, 166
embolic, 130–135
with the Pill, 128–130
arteriovenous malformations, 117–124, 167–170
carotid-cavernous fistula, *136,* 147, 148
with rheumatic fever, 78
venous thrombosis, 119, 135–144
cavernous sinus thrombosis, 136
cortical vein thrombosis, 137, *138, 139*
lateral sinus thrombosis, 136, 137
with the Pill, 135, 137, *138, 139,* 141, 142
during pregnancy, 142
prognosis, 143
sagittal sinus thrombosis, 137, 171
treatment, 143, 144
Ceruloplasmin, 80, 82
Chastek's paralysis, 35
Chiari-Frommel syndrome, 16
Cholinesterase deficiency, 242
Cholinesterase inhibitors, 57, 63, 242. See also names of individual drugs.

Chorea
with encephalitis lethargica, 83
gravidarum, 74–80
Huntington's, 79
lithium-induced, 254
Pill-induced, 79
Sydenham's, 77–80
treatment, 77
Choriocarcinoma, 119, 131, 143, 164–167
infantile, 167
neurologic presentations, 165, 166
testicular, 16
Chorionic gonadotropin, 166
Clefts, orofacial, 199, 200
Coagulopathy
with abruptio placentae, 118
with amniotic fluid embolus, 132
with anticonvulsants, 201, 202
with purpura, 238–240
Coitus
and epilepsy, 190, 191
and narcolepsy, 191
and paraplegia, 12
and subarachnoid hemorrhage, 123
Coma, in eclampsia, 213
in subarachnoid hemorrhage, 116
Congenital defects. See *Teratogenicity* and names of individual drugs.
Congenital listeriosis, 98
Congenital myasthenia gravis, 62, 63
Congenital poliomyelitis, 92
Congenital syphilis, 103, 104
Congenital tuberculosis, 97
Contraceptives, oral. See *Pill, the.*
Cortical blindness, 219
Cortical vein thrombosis, 137, *138*, *139*
Corticosteroids
antenatal effects, 128
in Bell's palsy, 26, 27
in benign intracranial hypertension, 171, 173
in carpal tunnel syndrome, 28
in cerebral edema, 128
in chorea gravidarum, 77
in Guillain-Barré syndrome, 31
in lupus erythematosus, 259
in multiple sclerosis, 111
in myasthenia gravis, 58
and peripartum psychosis, 259
in polymyositis, 69
in TTP, 240
in tuberculous meningitis, 94
CSF. See *Cerebrospinal fluid.*
Curare
and arthrogryposis, 103
in myasthenia, 58
in myotonia, 66
in tetanus, 102, 103

D

Dexamethasone. See *Corticosteroids.*
Diabetes insipidus, 16, 17, 144
Diazepam
in eclampsia, 225, 233
in epilepsy, 206, 225, 233
in headache, 182, 183
in lumbar disc disease, 43
neonatal metabolism, 183
placental transfer, 183
in status epilepticus, 225, 233
in tetanus, 102
Diazoxide
and neonatal hyperglycemia, 229
and uterine inertia, *228*
for hypertensive encephalopathy, 225–229
Dibenzazepine antidepressants, 15, 182, 254
Diet
in benign intracranial hypertension, 173, 175
in epilepsy, 194, 201
in gestational neuropathy, 33
in migraine, 184, 187
Diphenylhydantoin. See *Phenytoin.*
Diphtheria, 31
Disc disease, 23, 43
Disproportion, cephalopelvic, 45
Disseminated intravascular coagulopathy, 118, 132
Disseminated sclerosis, 111–114, 170
Dysmenorrhea, 4

E

Eclampsia, 211–234
atypical, 116, 141, 211, 213
cerebral blood flow, 216, 219
cerebrospinal fluid, 118, 119, 224, 225
differential diagnosis, 222–224
amniotic fluid embolus, 132
anesthetic toxicity, 241, 242
beri beri, 36, 258
epilepsy, 197
paraplegia, 12, 13
pheochromocytoma, 235
porphyria, 41
subarachnoid hemorrhage, 116
TTP, 239
water intoxication, 240, *241*
early, 211, 222
EEG in, 224
late, 213
vs. cerebral phlebitis, 141, 211
treatment, 225–229, 232–234
anticonvulsants, 225, 232–234
antihypertensive drugs, 225–229
cerebral edema, 234

Eclampsia (*Continued*)
treatment, magnesium sulfate, 229–232
visual changes, 234
Ectopic pregnancy, 37
Edrophonium, 57, 63
Electroconvulsive therapy, 256
Electroencephalogram
in cerebral phlebitis, 142
in chorea, 78
in coitus, 191
in eclampsia, 224
in hypermagnesemia, 232
in hyponatremia, 240
during menses, 192, *193*
in petit mal, 197
with the Pill, 193, *193*
in TTP, 239
Embolism
air, 133–135
amniotic fluid, 132, *133*
fat, 132, 133, *134*
paradoxical, 132
Empty sella syndrome, 173
Encephalitis lethargica, 82–84
Encephalopathy
hypertensive, 171, 213–219
rheumatic, 78
Wernicke's, 23–37, 258
Endocarditis, 118, 119, 131
Endometriosis, sciatica, 23, *24*
subarachnoid hemorrhage, 23, 120
Endometritis, listerial, 98, 99
tuberculous, 97
Ependymoma, 167
Epidural anesthesia, *10,* 11
Epidural hematoma, spinal, 168
Epilepsy, 190–206
catamenial, 191–193
counselling, 197–201
genetics, 197, 198
gestational, 196
lactation, 196
sexual, 190, 191
teratogenicity, 199–201
treatment during pregnancy, 194, 201–206
Ergonovine, 186
Ergotamine, 186
Erythema, palmar, 121
Estrogens
and arteriovenous shunting, 121, 170
in benign intracranial hypertension, 174, 175
extra-ovarian production, 174, 175
in migraine, 184
in myasthenia gravis, 59
in obesity, *175*
Estrogens (*Continued*)
in porphyria, 40, 41
in Wilson's disease, 82
Ethambutol, 94, 96
Ethionamide, 98
Ethosuximide, 197, 200, 206

F

Facial paralysis, 24–27
Fallopian tube, innervation, 23, 67
Fat embolus, 132, 133, *134*
Femoral neuropathy, 44, 47, *47,* 48
Floppy baby, 63, 64, 202, 232, 233, 255
Folate deficiency, 201, 202
Foot drop, 43–47, *45*
Frankenhauser's plexus, 7, 8
Furosemide, 225–227

G

Galactorrhea
amenorrhea, 163
drug-induced, 15
nonpuerperal, 15, 16, 172
Gestational seizure, 196, 197
Gliomas, of brain, 158, *160,* 164
of spinal cord, 167
Gonadotropin, chorionic, 166
Guillain-Barré syndrome, 30–32, 171, 173

H

Haloperidol, 77
Headache, 182–187
in benign intracranial hypertension, 171
in cerebral phlebitis, 137, 142
in eclampsia, 214
menstrual, 184, *185*
migraine, 183–187
muscle contraction, 182, 183
in pheochromocytoma, 235
with the Pill, 184, 185
tension, 182, 183
toxic, 183
treatment during pregnancy, 182, 186, 187
in tuberculous meningitis, 92
Hematin, 42
Hemoglobinopathy, S–C disease, 133
sickle cell disease, 133, 135, 137
Hepatolenticular degeneration, 79–82
Herpes zoster, 15, 25
Huntington's chorea, 79
Hydatidiform mole, 165, 166, 222
Hydralazine, 225, 226
Hyperemesis gravidarum, 33
in porphyria, 41

Hypermagnesemia, in eclampsia, 229–232
in myasthenia gravis, 58, 61
Hypernatremia, 137
Hyperosmolar therapy, 128, 164, 234
Hypertension
benign intracranial, 171–175
differential diagnosis, 222, *223*, 224
in paraplegia, 12, 13
in porphyria, *38*, 41
in pheochromocytoma, 235
in subarachnoid hemorrhage, 116
in TTP, 239
encephalopathy, 171, 213–219
hematoma, intracerebral, 213, *213*
treatment in eclampsia, 225–229
Hyperthyroidism, 79, 80
Hyperventilation, 123, 127, 164, 222, 225, 234
Hypogastric plexus, *2*, *3*, 6, 7
Hyponatremia, 146, 223, 240, 241
Hypoparathyroidism, 79, 80, 171
Hypophysis. See *Pituitary*.
Hypopituitarism, 144–146
Hypothalamus, 16, 17
Hypothermia, 126–128, 164, 225, 234
Hypothyroidism, 146
Hypotonia, in chorea, 74. See also *Floppy baby*.

I

Idiopathic thrombocytopenic purpura, 239, 240
Innervation. See *Nerve(s)* or specific organ.
Insufflation, tubal, 5
vaginal, 135
Insulin coma therapy, 256
Intervertebral disc, 23, 43
Isoniazid
and phenytoin, 95, 205
placental transfer, 95
pyridoxine deficiency, 95
in tuberculosis, 94, 95

K

Knee-chest exercises, 135
Korsakoff's psychosis, 33–37, 258
Kuru, 104

L

Labor
CSF pressures, 123, *124*
intrauterine pressures, 4
pain, 4
after subarachnoid hemorrhage, 126, 127
Lactation. See also *Galactorrhea*, *Milk*.
in diabetes insipidus, 16, 17
Lactation (*Continued*)
in epilepsy, 196
failure of, 16, 144
in myasthenia gravis, 60
neurohormonal control, 14
in postpartum psychosis, 256
in quadriplegia, 13
in Sheehan's syndrome, 144
in syringomyelia, 15
Wernicke's encephalopathy, 258
Lateral femoral cutaneous nerve, 28–30, *29*
Lateral sinus thrombosis, 136, 137
Let-down reflex, 14–16. See also *Milk-ejection reflex*.
Lidocaine, in myasthenia gravis, 61, 242
toxicity, 241, 242
Listeriosis, 98–100
Lithium, 254, 255
Local anesthesia. See *Anesthesia, regional*.
Lumbar disc disease, 43
vs. endometriosis, 23
Lumbosacral plexus
in choriocarcinoma, 166
endometriosis, 23, 24
intrapartum injury, 30, 43–47
Lupus erythematosus 69, 77, 79, 80, 119, 131, 259

M

Magnesium, 229–232
in myasthenia gravis, 58–61
Mannitol, 128, 164, 234
MAO inhibitors, 253
Marfan's syndrome, 125
McArdle's disease, 69
Menarche, 172, 190
Meningioma, 121, 157, 158, *162*, 167
parasellar, 159–161
Meningitis, listerial, 98–100
tuberculous, 92–98
vs. subarachnoid hemorrhage, 116
Meningocele, 168
Menopause, 190
Menses
Bell's palsy, 25, *26*
benign intracranial hypertension, 172
brain tumor and, 162
EEG changes, 192, *193*
epilepsy, 191, *192*, 193
myasthenia gravis, 59
poliomyelitis, *89*
porphyria, 40, 41
sciatica, 23, *24*
spinal arteriovenous malformations, 168
Meralgia paresthetica, 28–30, *29*

Merkel's discs, 8, 9
Microangiopathy, thrombotic, 238–240
Migraine, 130, 183–187
Milk
  bromide, 196, 202
  chlorpromazine, 253
  diazepam, 183
  ergot, 186
  isoniazid, 95
  lithium, *255*
  phenobarbital, *203*
  phenytoin, 205, 206
Milk-ejection reflex, 14–16
  in paraplegia, 13, 15
Monoamine oxidase inhibitors, 253
Mononeuritis multiplex, familial, 30
Multiple sclerosis, 111–114, 170
Myasthenia gravis, 56–65
  congenital, 62, 63
  management of delivery, 61, 62
  neonatal, 56, 62–65
Myelography
  antenatal risk, 13, 14, 170
  in catamenial sciatica, 23
  in disc disease, 43
  in spinal arteriovenous malformation, 168, 170
Myelomalacia, 170
Myophosphorylase deficiency, 69
Myotonia congenita, 68, 69
Myotonic muscular dystrophy, 65–68
  counselling, 67, *68*
  neonatal, 67
Myxoma, atrial, 131

N

Narcolepsy, 191
Neonatal bromism, 202
Neonatal choriocarcinoma, 167
Neonatal coagulopathy, 202
Neonatal hypermagnesemia, 232
Neonatal listeriosis, 98, 99
Neonatal lithium toxicity, 255
Neonatal myasthenia gravis, 56, 62–65
Neonatal myotonic dystrophy, 67
Neonatal phenobarbital withdrawal, 203, 204
Neonatal poliomyelitis, 92
Neonatal seizures, 95
Neonatal tetanus, 100, 103
Neostigmine, 57, 63, 64
Nerve(s)
  anterior crural, 47, 48
  to breast, 15
  to cervix, *2, 3,* 6–8
  facial, 24–27
  femoral, *3, 44, 47,* 48
  lateral femoral cutaneous, 28–30, *29*
Nerve(s) (*Continued*)
  obturator, *48,* 49
  to ovaries, *2, 3,* 6
  to oviduct, *2, 3,* 6–8
  peroneal, 43–47
  to perineum, 8
  presacral, 7, 10, 11
  pudendal, *2, 3,* 8
  to uterus, *2, 3,* 6–8
  to vagina, 8, *9*
Neuralgic amotrophy, 30
Neurectomy, presacral, 10
Neuritis. See *Neuropathy.*
Neurofibromatosis, 167, 168, 236
Neuroma, acoustic, 157, 158, *159*
Neuropathy. See also *Polyneuropathy.*
  beri beri, 36
  brachial, 30
  catamenial, 23, *24*
  facial, 24–27
  femoral, *44,* 47, *48*
  gestational, 33–37
  median, 27, 28
  meralgia paresthetica, 28, *29,* 30
  obturator, *44, 48,* 49
  optic. See *Optic neuritis.*
  peroneal, 43–47
  with the Pill, 32, 33
  porphyric, 37–42
Neuropraxis, 46
Neurotemesis, 46
Nevus, spider, 79, 121, 170

O

Obesity, 29, 172, 173, 175
Obstetric palsy, 43–49, 101
Obturator neuropathy, *44, 48,* 49
Oligodendroglioma, 158, 167
Optic neuritis
  in multiple sclerosis, 111
  in Sheehan's syndrome, 144, *146*
  in Wernicke's encephalopathy, 34
Oral contraceptives. See *Pill, the.*
Otitic hydrocephalus, 136, 137, 171
Ovary, innervation, *2, 3,* 6, *10*
  in myotonic dystrophy, 66
Oviduct, innervation, *2, 3,* 6–8
Oxytocin
  ADH effect, 240, *241*
  and diazoxide, *228*
  response to suckling, 14
  uterine effect, 5, 186, *228*

P

Pain
  after-pain, 5, 7
  dysmenorrhea, 4

Pain (*Continued*)
  labor, 4
  pathways, 10
  referred, 5, 7, 8, *10,* 11
  visceral, 1
Pantothenic acid, 36
Papilledema, 31, 78, 138, 171, 174, 221
Paracervical anesthesia, 8, 10
Paracervical ganglia, *2, 3,* 7, 8
Paradoxical embolus, 132
Paraplegia, 12–14, 167–170
Paravertebral anesthesia, 10, 11
Parkinson's syndrome, 82–84, 252
Penicillamine, 81
Petit mal, 197
Phenobarbital, 202–204, 234
  clearance, 203, *204*
  in eclampsia, 225, 234
  in milk, 203
  neonatal withdrawal, 203, 204
  in porphyria, 37, 41, 42
  teratogenicity, 200, 201
Phenothiazine
  antepartum use, 251–253
  in chorea, 77
  galactorrhea, 15
  in milk, 253
  movement disorders, 79, 252
  neonatal effects, 253
  in porphyria, 42
Phenytoin, 204–206, 233
  clearance, *204, 205*
  in eclampsia, *225,* 233
  and isoniazid, 95, *205*
  in milk, 205, 206
  in myotonia, 65
  neonatal metabolism, 205
  in porphyria, 40
Pheochromocytoma, 234–238
  vs. autonomic stress syndrome, 13
  vs. eclampsia, 222, 223, 235
Physostigmine, 258
Pill, the
  aortic strength, 125, *126*
  benign intracranial hypertension, 172
  cerebral venous thrombosis, 135, 137, *138, 139,* 141, 142
  ceruloplasmin, 82
  chorea, 79
  EEG changes, *193*
  epilepsy, 193
  green plasma, 82
  headache, 172
  myasthenia gravis, 59
  polyneuropathy, 32, 33
  porphyria, 40, 41
  rifampin, 97
  stroke, 128–130
  Wilson's disease, 82
Pinealoma, 16
Pituitary
  in amenorrhea-galactorrhea, 163
  blood supply, *146*
  diabetes insipidus, 16, 144
  postpartum necrosis, 144, *145,* 146
  tumors, 16, 157, 158, 161, *162,* 163
Placenta
  abruptio, 118
  in listeriosis, 98
  in TTP, 239
  in tuberculosis, 97
Plexus
  brachial, 30
  Frankenhauser's, 7, 8
  hypogastric, *2, 3,* 6, 7
  lumbosacral, *44,* 166
  paracervical, *2, 3,* 7, 8, 10
Poliomyelitis, 88–92, 171
Polycythemia, 79, 80, 131, 135, 171
Polyhydramnios, 67
Polymyositis, 69
Polyneuropathy
  gestational distal, 33–37
  Guillain-Barré syndrome, 30–32
  pyridoxine deficiency, 36, 95
  recurrent with pregnancy or the Pill, 32, 33
  thiamine deficiency, 33–37
  porphyric, 37–42
Porphyria, 37–42
  genetic defects, *39,* 40
  hormonal effects, 40
  vs. eclampsia, 41
  vs. Guillain-Barré syndrome, 31
  vs. postpartum psychosis, 37, *38,* 258
Prednisone. See *Corticosteroids.*
Presacral neurectomy, 10
Primidone, *203,* 206
Procaine. See also *Anesthesia.*
  in myasthenia gravis, 58, 61, 242
  toxicity, 241, 242
Progesterone
  in endometriosis, 24
  in migraine, 184
  in myasthenia gravis, 60
  in porphyria, 40, 41
Prolactin, milk-ejection reflex, 14
  pituitary tumors, 163
Propranolol
  in autonomic stress syndrome, 13
  fetal effects, 187
  in migraine, 186
  in pheochromocytoma, 237
  in porphyria, 39, 42
  in tetanus, 102
Pseudotumor cerebri, 171–175
Psychosis
  antepartum, 251–256

Psychosis (*Continued*)
porphyric, 37, *38,* 258
postpartum, *252,* 256–259
in Sheehan's syndrome, 144–147, 259
Pudendal anesthesia, 8, 10
Pudendal nerve, 8
Puerperium
after-pains, 5, 7
cardiomyopathy, *131,* 132
cerebral phlebitis, 135–144
psychosis, *252,* 256–259
tetanus, 100, 101
Pyridostigmine, 57, 62, 64
Pyridoxine
with isoniazid, 95
neonatal seizures, 95
and penicillamine, 81
and polyneuropathy, 36

Q

Quadriplegia, 12, 13, 15
Queen Anne, 99
Quinine, 58, 65, 66

R

Referred pain, 5, 7, 8, *10,* 11
Regional anesthesia. See *Anesthesia regional.*
Retinal detachment, 219, *220*
Retinal edema, 219
Retinal venous occlusion, 135
Retinopathy, thioridazine, 253
Rheumatic fever, 77, 78
chorea, 77–80
Rifampin, 94, 97

S

Sagittal sinus thrombosis, 137, 171
Salpingitis, 5
Scopolamine, 61, 258
Seizure disorder, 190–206, 222–224. See also *Epilepsy, Eclampsia.*
Sexual seizure, 190, 191
Sheehan's syndrome, 144–147, 259
Sickle cell anemia, 133, 135, 137
Sinus, cavernous, *136*
lateral, *136*
sagittal, *136,* 137
Spider nevus, 79, 121, 170
Spinal tumors, 167, 168, 171, 173
Status epilepticus, 164, 171, 225, 232, 233
Streptomycin, 58, 94–96
Stroke. See *Cerebrovascular disease.*
Subarachnoid hemorrhage, 115–128
aneurysm, 117–128
arteriovenous malformation, 117–128
cerebral venous thrombosis, 119, 142
Subarachnoid hemorrhage (*Continued*)
choriocarcinoma, 119
eclampsia, 116, 119, 224
endometriosis, 23
treatment, 126–128
Suckling. See *Lactation, Galactorrhea.*
Sydenham's chorea, 77–80
Syphilis, 11, 12, 16, 103, 104
Syringomyelia, 75
Systemic lupus erythematosus, 69, 77, 79, 80, 119, 131

T

Tabes dorsalis, 11, 12, 15, 16
Teratogenicity
anticoagulants, 118
anticonvulsants, 199–201
antituberculous drugs, 95, 97, 98
fetal hypoglycemia, 256
fetal irradiation, 13
imipramine, 254
lithium, 254, 255
phenobarbital, 200, *201*
phenothiazines, 253
phenytoin, 199–201, *201*
Tetanus, 100–103
Thiamine, 36, 37
Thioridazine, 253
Thomsen's disease, 253
Thrombocytopenia
ITP, 239, 240
TTP, 131, 222, *223,* 238–240
Thymectomy, 58, 59, 62
Thymoma, in myasthenia, 58–60, 62
during pregnancy, 60, 61
Tricyclic antidepressants, 15, 182, 254
Tridione, 200
Toxemia. See *Eclampsia.*
Tuberculosis, 92–98, 259
meningitis, 92, 93
during pregnancy, 93, 94
treatment, 94–97
Tumor(s)
brain, 157–167
pituitary, 16, 157, 158, 161, *162,* 163
spinal cord, 167–168

U

Uterus, nerve supply, *2, 3,* 5–8, *10*
perfusion, 225, 229

V

Vagina
insufflation, 135
nerve supply, *2, 3, 9, 10*
Valsalva's maneuver, 121, 123, *124,* 126, 148, 164, 168, 213

Vanillylmandelic acid, 236, 237
Vasculitis. See *Arteritis.*
Vasopressin. See *Antidiuretic hormone.*
Visual symptoms. See also *optic neuritis.*
  carotid-cavernous fistula, 147, 148
  eclampsia, 219–221
  parasellar tumors, 159–163
Vitamin A, 171
Vitamin B_1, 36, 37
Vitamin B_6, 36, 81, 95
Vitamin K, 202
VMA, 236, 237
Von Recklinghausen's neurofibromatosis, 167, 168, 236

W

Water intoxication, 146, *223*, 240, *241*
Wernicke's encephalopathy, 33–37, 258
Wilson's disease, 79–82